Occupational Disorders of the Upper Extremity

Occupational Disorders of the Upper Extremity

Edited by

Lewis H. Millender, M.D.

Clinical Professor, Department of Orthopedic Surgery
Tufts University School of Medicine
Lecturer, Department of Orthopedic Surgery
Harvard Medical School
Surgeon, Department of Orthopedic Surgery
New England Baptist Hospital and
Brigham and Women's Hospital
Boston, Massachusetts

Dean S. Louis, M.D.

Professor, Department of Surgery
University of Michigan Medical School
Chief, Division of Orthopedic Hand Surgery
Department of Orthopedics
University of Michigan Hospitals
Ann Arbor, Michigan

Barry P. Simmons, M.D.

Associate Professor, Department of Orthopedic Surgery
Harvard Medical School
Chief, Hand Surgery Service
Department of Orthopedics
Brigham and Women's Hospital
Boston, Massachusetts

Churchill Livingstone
New York, Edinburgh, London, Melbourne, Tokyo

Library of Congress Cataloging-in-Publication Data

Occupational disorders of the upper extremity / edited by Lewis H.
  Millender, Dean S. Louis, Barry P. Simmons.
        p. cm.
    Includes bibliographical references and index.
    ISBN 0-443-08797-0
    1. Extremities, Upper—Wounds and injuries. 2. Occupational
diseases. 3. Overuse injuries. 4. Disability evaluation.
I. Millender, Lewis H., date –. II. Louis, Dean S., date –.
III. Simmons, Barry P.
    [DNLM: 1. Arm. 2. Arm Injuries. 3. Occupational Diseases.
4. Workman's Compensation. WE 805 0145]
RD557.027 1992
617.5'7044—dc20
DNLM/DLC
for Library of Congress   91-34012
                                                                               CIP

Distributed in the United Kingdom by Churchill Livingstone, Robert Stevenson House, 1–3
Baxter's Place, Leith Walk, Edinburgh EH1 3AF, and by associated companies, branches,
and representatives throughout the world.

Accurate indications, adverse reactions, and dosage schedules for drugs are provided in this
book, but it is possible that they may change. The reader is urged to review the package
information data of the manufacturers of the medications mentioned.

The Publishers have made every effort to trace the copyright holders for borrowed material.
If they have inadvertently overlooked any, they will be pleased to make the necessary
arrangements at the first opportunity.

Acquisitions Editor: *Leslie Burgess*
Copy Editor: *David Terry*
Production Designer: *Jill Little*
Production Supervisor: *Sharon Tuder*
Production services provided by Bermedica Productions, Ltd.

Printed in the United States of America

First published in 1992   7 6 5 4 3 2 1

To my wife, Bonnie, for her support and encouragement in this and all my projects
L.H.M.

To my children, Brett, Stacy, Todd, and Amy
D.S.L.

To my father, Arthur M. Simmons, M.D.
By his example as a loving, caring father and physician
he molded my career as a parent and as a doctor.
B.P.S.

Contributors

Thomas J. Armstrong, Ph.D.
Associate Professor, Department of Industrial Health, University of Michigan School of Public Health, Ann Arbor, Michigan

William H. Bowers, M.S., M.D.
Associate Professor, Divisions of Orthopedic Surgery and Plastic and Reconstructive Surgery, Department of Surgery, Virginia Commonwealth University Medical College of Virginia School of Medicine; Chief, Upper Extremity Service, Children's Medical Center, Richmond, Virginia

Gail F. Brain, R.N., B.S., CRRN, CIRS
Independent consultant (workers' compensation issues), Boston, Massachusetts

Michael E. Charness, M.D.
Associate Professor, Department of Neurology, Harvard Medical School; Director, Performing Arts Clinic, Division of Neurology, Department of Medicine, Brigham and Women's Hospital, Boston, Massachusetts; Staff Physician, Section of Neurology, West Roxbury Veterans Administration Medical Center, West Roxbury, Massachusetts

Evelyn R. Davis, M.S., CRC, CIRS
Corporate Director of Staff Development, Comprehensive Rehabilitation Associates, Inc., Boston, Massachusetts

Susan A. Emerson, M.Ed., OTR/L, CHT
Director, Seacoast Hand Rehabilitation Center, Dover, New Hampshire

William W. Eversmann, Jr., M.D.
Hand Surgeon, Iowa Medical Clinic, Cedar Rapids, Iowa

Don L. Goldenberg, M.D.
Professor, Department of Medicine, Tufts University School of Medicine; Chief, Department of Rheumatology, Newton-Wellesley Hospital, Newton, Massachusetts

Damian C.R. Ireland, M.D.
Clinical Assistant Orthopaedic Surgeon, Department of Surgery, Alfred Hospital; Consultant Orthopaedic Surgeon, Royal Australian Navy; Director, Melbourne Hand Surgery and Rehabilitation Centre, Melbourne, Australia

Mark J. Koris, M.D.
Instructor, Department of Orthopedic Surgery, Harvard Medical School; Associate Surgeon, Hand Surgery Service, Brigham and Women's Hospital and Children's Hospital Medical Center, Boston, Massachusetts

Elaine LaCroix, MHSM, OTR/L, CHT
Director, Hand Rehabilitation Associates, Brookline, Massachusetts, and Nashua, New Hampshire

Robert D. Leffert, M.D.
Professor, Department of Orthopedic Surgery, Harvard Medical School; Chief, Surgical Upper Extremity Rehabilitation Unit, Massachusetts General Hospital, Boston, Massachusetts

Dean S. Louis, M.D.
Professor, Department of Surgery, University of Michigan Medical School; Chief, Division of Orthopedic Hand Surgery, Department of Orthopedics, University of Michigan Hospitals, Ann Arbor, Michigan

Lewis H. Millender, M.D.
Clinical Professor, Department of Orthopedic Surgery, Tufts University School of Medicine; Lecturer, Department of Orthopedic Surgery, Harvard Medical School; Surgeon, Department of Orthopedic Surgery, New England Baptist Hospital and Brigham and Women's Hospital, Boston, Massachusetts

Theodore Nadelson, M.D.
Clinical Professor, Department of Psychiatry, Tufts University School of Medicine; Chief, Department of Psychiatry, Department of Veterans Affairs Medical Center, Boston, Massachusettes

Barry P. Simmons, M.D.
Associate Professor, Department of Orthopedic Surgery, Harvard Medical School; Chief, Hand Surgery Service, Department of Orthopedics, Brigham and Women's Hospital, Boston, Massachusetts

Andrew L. Terrono, M.D.
Instructor, Department of Orthopedic Surgery, Tufts University School of Medicine; Staff Member, Department of Orthopedic Surgery, New England Baptist Hospital, Boston, Massachusetts

Edward M. Welch, J.D.
Lecturer, Department of Labor and Industrial Relations, Michigan State University College of Social Science, East Lansing, Michigan

Edwin T. Wyman, Jr., M.D.
Assistant Clinical Professor, Department of Orthopedic Surgery, Harvard Medical School; Visiting Orthopedic Surgeon, Department of Orthopedic Surgery, Massachusetts General Hospital, Boston, Massachusetts

Preface

The incidence of work-related disorders in the upper extremity has dramatically increased over the past decade, and there is no indication that this will change. The causes are myriad and complicated, and there is no clear consensus why significant increases in these problems have occurred. Numerous studies have related these injuries—defined as cumulative trauma disorders—to repetitive motions, excessive force, and/or abnormal positioning of the joints in an increasingly mechanized and stressful industrial setting. Other studies attribute these chronic painful syndromes to sociopolitical and economic forces that are associated with a changing work ethic and outdated, unworkable workers' compensation laws that encourage workers to remain sick rather than motivate them to return to work.

Whatever the cause, physicians are called upon to examine, diagnose, and treat these patients. The physician confronted with the injured worker must have a clear understanding of the many factors that can affect the outcome of any treatment program. The traditional methods we use to treat most musculoskeletal conditions are often ineffective in these situations, and surgery is often counterproductive, resulting in prolonged and even permanent disability. Indications for operative treatment must be carefully evaluated; they are different in the injured worker.

Our purpose in writing this book is to present a guide for the physician managing these problems. To achieve this, the book is divided into four sections.

Section I presents a historical perspective of work-related injuries and then discusses the epidemiology of and biomechanical studies on cumulative trauma disorders.

Section II is a description of the workers' compensation system. It includes a general overview of the program, presenting the perspectives of the insurance company, the plaintiff, and the employer. The chapters discuss how the system's adversarial approach often leads to patient frustration, anger, and resentment, which is manifested as chronic pain resulting in long-standing disability.

Section III provides an overall approach to evaluation and management of the injured worker. This approach is based on our understanding of (1) the diagnosis and prognosis for recovery; (2) the patient's job and industry characteristics; (3) pertinent additional medical information; and (4) nonmedical factors, including legal, socioeconomic, and psychological issues. Chapter 9 presents a stepwise approach based on the four factors listed above. The remaining chapters in Section III review disorders of the upper extremity in detail. Two important chapters on medical problems and psychological problems that affect the worker are presented.

Section IV discusses rehabilitation of these complicated problems. The role for therapy and work hardening is covered. The rehabilitation specialist is a new player in this expanding field. The responsibility of the rehabilitation specialist and how such a specialist interacts with the physician, patient, employer, and insurer is discussed in detail. When the patient is unable to return to work, vocational rehabilitation is necessary; this is discussed in Chapter 19. Finally, the physician must evaluate impairment; the latest methods of impairment evaluation based on American Medical Association guidelines are presented in Chapter 20.

As a group, we would like to thank our contributors. We hope their work will help to improve patient care.

I would like to thank our publisher, Churchill Livingstone, whose staff helped to make the work go smoothly; in particular, the professionalism, concern, and care of our Editor, Leslie Burgess, made this project an enjoyable one. I also want to thank my office staff, Christine Woodruff and Deborah Cram, for their efforts and hard work (L.H.M.).

I would like to thank my secretary, Gwendolyn Stewart, for her tireless assistance (D.S.L.).

My thanks go to Stacy Lewis for her help in preparing the manuscripts and organizing the chapters (B.P.S.).

Lewis H. Millender, M.D.
Dean S. Louis, M.D.
Barry P. Simmons, M.D.

Contents

IV. REHABILITATION

Occupational Disorders of the Upper Extremity: Orthopaedic, Psychosocial, and Legal Implications

Lewis H. Millender, M.D.

Physicians who evaluate and treat patients with occupational disorders of the upper extremity must use more than traditional medical methods. They must strive to understand the myriad of physical, psychological, and social problems that affect patients and impede their ability to manage a work-related disorder. The purpose of this book is to present physicians and surgeons with an overview of the medical and nonmedical issues that have an impact upon work-related disorders of the upper extremity and to provide a treatment strategy for the successful management of these problems.

Successful treatment depends upon a multidisciplinary team that includes the physician, therapists, rehabilitation counselors, attorneys, and insurance claims personnel—even industry representatives. Today a team approach is manda-tory in patient care because nonmedical issues often play a significant role in the lives of patients and in their attitude toward a work-related disorder (Fig. 1-1). How nonmedical issues are handled can determine the success or failure of treatment, sometimes even more than can the prescribed medical treatment. Therefore, in addition to addressing specific musculoskeletal disorders that affect workers, the chapters in this book include such topics as insurance, union policy, workers' compensation law, and employment. With this perspective, physicians can discern the interrelated elements that can affect patients and then assess how a team approach might possibly work for their patients.

The incidence of occupational disorders has steadily increased over the past decade, and evidence indicates that this

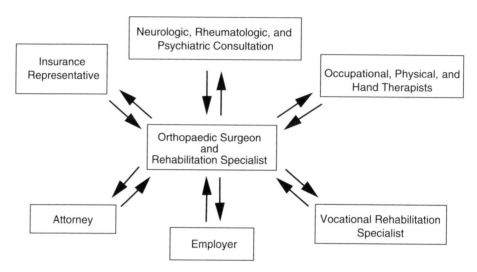

Fig. 1-1. Chronic work-related disorders require a multidisciplinary approach. Because of the nature of the condition, the orthopaedic surgeon usually manages the case along with a rehabilitation specialist. Close cooperation with various professionals is necessary for successful management.

trend will continue.[1-3] As an epidemic of cumulative trauma disorders has hit many industries, the cost of disability insurance and workers' compensation benefits has skyrocketed. These problems have become a national concern and are the topic for television discussion and articles in newspapers and national magazines.[4] Employers know that these problems have a direct effect on profitability and their ability to compete with foreign competitors. Today industry has mounted a national campaign to try to determine the cause of these problems and methods to decrease the cost of occupational disorders.[5,6]

The causes of occupational disorders are complex, diverse, and incompletely understood. Many well designed and carefully conducted studies have shown that the incidence of cumulative trauma disorders is increasing in direct relationship to a changing work environment. As automation has developed and production requirements changed, employees are required to carry out more repetitive jobs at a faster pace. Studies have shown that repetition, forcefulness, and awkward positions have a direct effect on the development of cumulative trauma disorders.[7-9] Assembly lines, job pacing, and job incentives have been associated with an increased incidence of cumulative trauma disorders. Recent reports have shown that poultry workers, butchers, electronic assembly personnel, packaging and grocery checkout workers, and stitchers have an increased incidence of these disorders.[7,10-13] More recently there have been reports of increased cumulative trauma among computer operators and journalists.[4]

Others have questioned whether the increased incidence of cumulative trauma disorder is entirely the result of changes in industrial production. Some researchers feel that these ailments are related to a changing work ethic, a more informed public, and liberalized workers' compensation laws that reward sickness instead of wellness.[4–17] Additionally, a more adversarial public and our litigious society are blamed for many of these problems. Others question whether the health care industry has fueled the fire with the development of a multitude of clinics, an increased number of therapists, and the dissemination of massive amounts of educational information about cumulative trauma disorders.[14] All of these factors, plus employees who are unhappy with their jobs, boredom in the work place, and a level of generalized stress in society, tend to foster more occupational disorders.

APPROACH TO THE INJURED WORKER

When dealing with a disabled worker the physician must consider four general areas. Because each patient is different, different areas will be more important in each case. However, in most chronic situations each of these areas must be resolved successfully in order to return the patient to the job.

> - Establish specific musculoskeletal diagnosis. Determine appropriate methods for treatment. Determine prognosis for returning to work.
> - Evaluate general medical and psychiatric issues that influence the treatment.
> - Understand job, company, industry, and union factors that influence the treatment.
> - Evaluate legal issues that influence return to work.

ESTABLISH SPECIFIC MUSCULOSKELETAL DIAGNOSIS, DETERMINE APPROPRIATE METHODS FOR TREATMENT, DETERMINE PROGNOSIS FOR RETURNING TO WORK

Establishing the correct diagnosis is the key to proper management. In most acute injuries the diagnosis is easily established by a simple history and physical examination and is confirmed with routine radiographs or additional laboratory tests. The treatment is usually straightforward, and prognosis is related to the severity of the problem.

In contrast, the work disorders that are the focus of this book are chronic or recurrent; for example, patients with a longstanding musculoskeletal condition or who have had recurrent episodes of disability preventing them from returning to work. The diagnosis, treatment, and prognosis of these problems are more difficult than for an acute disorder.

To establish a treatment plan and prognosis for return to work it is helpful to place patients into one of four categories.

- CATEGORY 1: Diagnosis is easily established, good methods are available for treating the condition, and the prognosis for returning to work is good.
- CATEGORY 2: Diagnosis is established, but neither nonsurgical nor surgical treatment is always successful in returning the patient to the original job.
- CATEGORY 3: The condition combines definite physical problems and additional nonmedical issues.
- CATEGORY 4: Diagnosis is unclear.

Category 1

> The diagnosis is easily established, good methods are available for treating the condition, and the prognosis for returning to work is good.
> **FACTORS**
> 1. The patient has a correctable musculoskeletal disorder.
> 2. The patient is highly motivated, often skilled, and highly paid.
> 3. There are no adverse legal, emotional, or company conflicts.

This group comprises patients who present with well-defined musculoskeletal disorders in which the diagnosis is clear and defined methods of nonsurgical and surgical treatment have been established. The results of treatment are good, and studies report a large percentage of patients returning to work following treatment. There are many examples of patients who fit this group. Dental hygienists or typists who fail conservative treatment for carpal tunnel syndrome can be treated with surgery and generally return to work. Dentists, electricians, and carpenters who develop trigger fingers and de Quervain's tenosynovitis can be successfully treated with injections or surgery and are able to return to their work. In many cases tenolysis, joint releases, and bone grafting for non-union of fractures restore adequate function to allow patients to return to work.

The common denominator in this group is that the patients are highly motivated, often skilled, highly paid employees who have a correctable medical problem. There are no adverse company, legal, or emotional conflicts that have a negative impact upon their musculoskeletal injury.

The physician's role in these cases is to provide appropriate nonsurgical or surgical treatment and appropriate therapy. Today, highly trained occupational, physical, and hand therapists can rehabilitate patients to their maximum degree of recovery. Work-hardening programs are effective, and physical capacity evaluations are available when needed.[18] Close cooperation between the physician and therapist is the prescription for the successful return to work.[20]

Category 2

> The diagnosis has been established, but neither surgical nor nonsurgical treatment is always successful, and the patient may not be able to return to the original job.
> **FACTORS**
> Group 1. Patients with serious musculoskeletal injuries that prevent them from returning to the original job. Vocational rehabilitation is necessary.
> Group 2. Patients for whom a return to the original job is questionable. Careful evaluation of the job and job alternatives is important before making final recommendations.
> Group 3. Patients with cumulative trauma disorders who require careful evaluation before recommending surgery. Attempts at job modification or retraining are often preferable to surgery.

This is an important and difficult group of patients whose treatment recommendations require considerable judgment by the physician. These patients fall into three categories.

Certain patients have serious injuries that preclude them from returning to their previous occupation. Machinists, carpenters, and technicians who have thumb or multiple digital amputations or serious tendon, joint, or nerve injuries obviously will need job rehabilitation. When such patients are motivated, and adverse industry, insurance, emotional, and legal issues do not impede rehabilitation, they can be retrained and become productive employees. In these situations highly skilled rehabilitation specialists are invaluable in guiding the patient through the complicated legal and administrative processes toward successful employment.[18,19] In other cases because of age, additional medical problems, or the magnitude of the injury, total disability or retirement is the appropriate way to resolve the problem.

In addition to the above type of patient for whom job rehabilitation or retirement is obvious, there are two additional groups for whom surgical considerations are more complicated and difficult. Group two comprises patients for whom the prognosis for returning to work after surgery is unclear, and in the third group is a special category of patients who suffer from cumulative trauma disorders. In both of these groups unwise operations can result in prolonged and permanent disability.

Group 2 patients have well-defined injuries that may prevent them from returning to work. Some of these patients, regardless of the type of surgical or nonsurgical treatment, will not be able to carry out their previous job; for example, a laborer with a painful wrist following an intra-articular radius fracture, a carpenter with a distal radioulnar joint injury, or an electrician with a stiff proximal interphalangeal joint from a fracture. In these cases, before recommending surgery a careful evaluation by a therapist and careful evaluation of the job requirements are necessary. Is rehabilitation preferable to surgery? What is the likelihood that surgery will restore the patient to the original job? In the example cited above, a laborer who has a painful distal radioulnar joint problem will not return to work after a distal ulnar excision, so it should not be done for this reason alone. Alternatively, an electrician might return to work after tenolysis, and so surgery could be recommended.

The final group of patients comprises those with cumulative trauma problems. Experience has shown that unskilled workers with carpal tunnel syndrome, de Quervain's tenosynovitis disease, trigger fingers, or certain proximal nerve entrapments usually do not return to work after surgery. These patients frequently have complicated painful postoperative courses and often become chronically disabled. Adverse psychosocial issues are often responsible. Job modification is preferable to surgery, and one should be very careful before recommending surgery to this group of patients.[3] Studies have shown that motivated workers suffering from cumulative trauma disorders can return to the same job after work hardening, job modification, and education in joint and tendon protection.[20]

Management of these last two groups of patients requires close cooperation with allied health professionals. The hand therapist and physical therapist are skilled in evaluating workers and their jobs. In many cases after maximum recovery has been obtained, a physical capacity evaluation can be carried out to determine if the patient can return to the previous job. The therapist can help the physician make the difficult decisions regarding surgical reconstruction in some of these patients.

Vocational specialists and case managers are important when alternate work or rehabilitation is needed. They work with companies and insurers and provide the patient guidance and advice. In some cases the nonmedical issues are clear cut and easily resolved. When the company has alternate work and is responsive, the transition to a new job is easy. When no alternative work is available, the nonmedical issues are more difficult to resolve.[6,19] Formal rehabilitation, which includes testing and schooling, require skilled vocational counselors.

Category 3

> The condition combines definite physical problems and additional nonmedical issues.
> **FACTORS**
> 1. Patient presents with chronic pain out of proportion to the work-related musculoskeletal disorder.
> 2. Chronic pain is a manifestation of the patient's anger, frustration, and depression associated with the injury, as well as psychosocial or economic issues.

This group includes patients with musculoskeletal problems who also have major nonmedical issues that must be resolved. They are frequently angry and frustrated because the system has not responded to their perceived needs. Some may have a difficult musculoskeletal problem that has been difficult to resolve and are frustrated with their physician. Inappropriate surgical procedures that fail engender anger and resentment. Frustration with the legal system and anger and resentment with employers or insurance companies are also seen. Litigation and adversarial attitudes that are fostered by attorneys are additional causes of patient frustration.[21]

Patients in this group demonstrate pain out of proportion to the musculoskeletal condition. The pain is a manifestation of anger, frustration, and often depression that is associated with the failure to resolve the medical and nonmedical issues.[17,22]

These are the most difficult patients to cure, and there is a high percentage of failure among this population. Such patients often are on the disability rolls for years, cost society enormous amounts of money, and clog the legal system. They usually end up in pain clinics and many become totally and permanently disabled.[23]

In cases in which there is a degree of motivation and the patient has some emotional stability, the cycle can be broken before the orthopaedic surgeon makes the referral to a pain clinic. Together the physician and the rehabilitation counselor can try to break the cycle of anger and depression. The basic ingredients of success are the concern and care for the patient shown by the physician and rehabilitation counselor and the patient developing complete trust in this team. When this trust develops, patients will express their feelings about previous treatments, company conflicts, home problem, and fears of returning to work. Sometimes then the pain and hand function begin to improve, and a move toward rehabilitation is possible. This process requires considerable time, and the surgeon must be interested and skilled in dealing with this type of problem. The rehabilitation counselor must also have special skills in understanding this group of patients.

Category 4

An increasingly larger number of cumulative trauma patients being seen today fall into this category. The basic

Diagnosis is unclear.
FACTORS
1. Patient presents with generalized, vague aching discomfort in the hands or arms and no specific musculoskeletal diagnosis can be established.
2. Symptoms can represent chronic fibromyalgia or other rheumatologic abnormalities.
3. Symptoms often represent RSI or "repetitive strain injury," a psychosomatic disorder associated with psychological, social, or economic issues.

issue is pain that is difficult to diagnose as a specific musculoskeletal condition. The classic presentation is a patient with diffuse, generalized vague aching or discomfort that may extend from the wrists to the forearm. The pain may be localized over the lateral or medial epicondyle or around the wrist area, or there may be a shoulder or neck component. The only physical findings are tenderness and weakness. No anatomic distribution or evidence of inflammation is apparent.

Some of these patients have chronic tendinitis or fibromyalgia, a condition that is becoming more defined.[24,25] Some may have early nerve entrapments. Thoracic outlet syndrome can produce very obscure symptoms. Careful rheumatologic and neurologic consultation may be needed to rule out a definite physiologic cause for the pain. Some recent research attributes some of these obscure conditions to an inflammatory process in the muscle; however, it is difficult to confirm this in most cases.

A condition that has been called repetitive strain injury or RSI is being reported more frequently.[26,27] This condition was studied extensively in Australia in the mid-1980s. Many feel that RSI, which became of epidemic proportions in Australia, is a psychosomatic disorder associated with job stress, secondary gain issues and liberalized compensation laws (see Chapter 7). The condition has been diagnosed in most industrialized countries. When confronted with this diagnosis one must understand that the underlying cause is psychological and not primarily a musculoskeletal problem, and it must be treated from this approach.

After one is certain that there is no organic etiology for the problem, psychological evaluation is indicated. The use of rehabilitation specialists is very helpful in these difficult long-standing cases. The patients are generally emotionally fragile, usually have employment, legal, and other mitigating concerns that need to be addressed. Rehabilitation counselors have a clear understanding of all the issues, are able to support and advise the patient, and can interact with the multiple parties that are involved in the problem.

EVALUATE GENERAL MEDICAL AND PSYCHIATRIC ISSUES THAT INFLUENCE THE TREATMENT

Other medical issues affect work-related disorders. The general health of the worker, especially pre-existing medical illnesses, such as cardiovascular conditions, diabetes, or respiratory conditions, must be considered. More specifically, such conditions as osteoarthritis, rheumatoid arthritis, fibromyalgia, or remote traumatic musculoskeletal conditions may affect the present disorder (Fig. 1-2). These pre-existing conditions are partic-

```
MEDICAL
ISSUES
```

● General medical
  health

● Age

● Osteoarthritis

● Rheumatoid
  arthritis

● Fibromyalgia

● Diabetes

● Previous
  injury

● Traumatic
  arthritis

Fig. 1-2. Workers' hand disorders: medical issues.

ularly important in the older worker and must influence one's decision regarding treatment. It would probably be inappropriate to carry out a trapezium arthroplasty in a 63-year-old woman with arthritis in the thumb carpometacarpal joint if the sole reason was attempting to enable her to work as a stitcher for another 2 years. Patients with generalized arthritis or chronic recurrent tendinitis are difficult to rehabilitate to assembly-line jobs.

Most chronic work-related injuries eventually come under the care of the orthopaedic or hand surgeon. However, consultation with a rheumatologist is often very helpful. Consultation and management of these patients with the rheumatologist can make the difference in enabling some of these patients with combined disorders to return to work. The rheumatologist's knowledge of drug man-

agement, in combination with the orthopaedic surgeon's knowledge of the specific injury, is necessary to treat such patients.

Psychiatric factors always play a major role in patients with chronic work-related disorders and can be the major stumbling block to rehabilitation. These problems are difficult to recognize and are even more difficult for the surgeon, who is usually the attending physician, to treat. The emotional issues are complicated, and the physician must be aware of them and make efforts to recognize and treat them.

Patients may be distressed for several reasons. They have a chronic musculoskeletal problem that has not been resolved. This problem affects their work and deprives them of a livelihood, which alone can cause significant emotional distress. Another factor that engenders distress is the workers' compensation system. This system, which was established to care for and compensate injured workers and eliminate the adversarial climate that develops after work injuries, in fact often fosters mistrust, confusion, anger, and depression. Employees fear the loss of job, loss of wages, and an inability to care for their family. The system engenders a litigious atmosphere which further confuses the worker and they do not know whom to trust. This distress may be manifested as chronic pain, and the physician is presented with a patient who has chronic pain that is unexplainable and resistant to all forms of treatment.

The third cause of patient distress is that the treating physician is not trained and often not interested in this type of problem. Often, patients with chronic disorders are seen and treated by orthopaedic surgeons who have not been trained in understanding and dealing with chronic pain that is associated with emotional problems. When medical or surgical treatment is unsuccessful and physicians cannot explain the reason for the failure, blame is sometimes placed upon the patient. This aggravates an already explosive situation. The result is the total failure of treatment, chronic disability, and prolonged litigation. The orthopaedic surgeon who is not interested in this patient population or who feels unqualified to manage the complicated issues often associated with work-related disorders should refer the patient to physicians who are interested in these problems.

UNDERSTAND JOB, COMPANY, INDUSTRY, AND UNION FACTORS THAT INFLUENCE THE TREATMENT

An understanding of the patient's job requirements, company policy, industry, and union issues is necessary for the phy-

sician attempting to decide about treatment and return to work issues after occupational disorders (Fig. 1-3).[6]

Employee's Job

An understanding of the specific requirements of the patient's job helps the physician diagnose the problem, evaluate the prognosis for return to work, and respond to legal issues regarding etiology or causation (Fig. 1-4). The mechanism of injury is important in acute situations. If the injury was an acute torque, the radioulnar joint might be injured. Acute extension or flexion forces could injure the wrist. In chronic conditions the amount of repetition and force becomes important. Is there repetitive elbow flexion or long periods of overhead work? Does the job require awkward positions?

When return to work issues arise, physicians must have a very clear understanding of the job requirements. They may be asked to evaluate a job specification and state if the worker is able to carry out this job. The therapist is more often equipped to make this evaluation than the physician. Physical capacity evaluations can be ordered, as can specific on-site job evaluations. After physical capacity and job evaluation, a good hand therapist can recommend if the patient can return to the specific job.[28,29]

In addition to studying the specific job requirements, the physician and therapist should evaluate what opportunities exist to lessen the risks for reinjury. Is the job machine paced, and is the pace too rapid? Is this job an incentive job, and can the job be modified for this employee? Many times we find that the employee enjoys the work, and with small adjustments, such as job rotation, job enlargement, or eliminating incentive pay, the problem can be solved.

Another issue is the employee's skill.

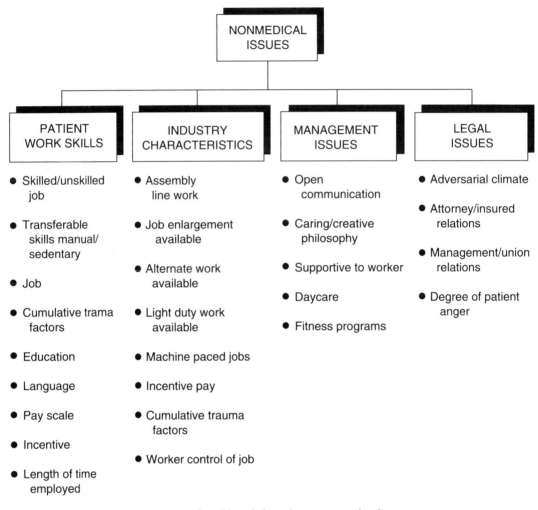

Fig. 1-3. Workers' hand disorders: nonmedical issues.

Is the patient a highly skilled, highly paid employee or an unskilled worker? Highly skilled workers generally have more transferable skills and can find alternate work more easily than can workers with fewer skills. The carpenter, electrician, or heavy duty machine operator may find it easier to obtain alternate work than the unskilled or uneducated worker who does not speak English. Some of the most difficult employment situations are found in this latter group.

Industry and Company Issues

One must understand the industry and company policy regarding injured workers. Some industries have a high percentage of strenuous manual jobs, and little alternative work is available. In these situations job rotation or alternate or light work is limited. This becomes a problem when trying to return a patient to work.

Company attitudes and policy influ-

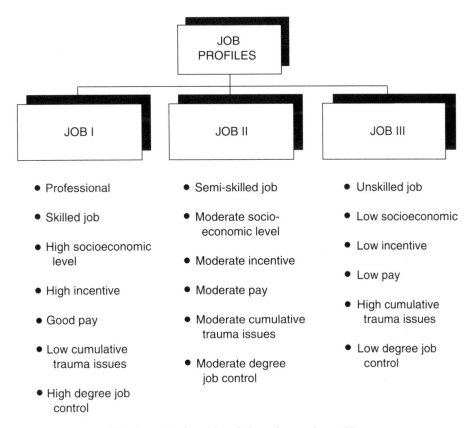

Fig. 1-4. Workers' hand disorders: job profiles.

ence whether an employee can be returned to work successfully.[5,7,30,31] Today progressive companies have developed work policies that have had a significant effect in decreasing the number of workers' compensation claims, shortening the disability time, and cutting disability costs after injury. Many companies have established safety committees to monitor safety and investigate jobs that have high rates of injury. After the cause is established, steps are taken to correct the problem or modify the jobs. Employees are educated in safety issues and are instructed to report early symptoms before serious problems develop.[6]

Another area that industry is focusing on is fitness. Many companies now have on-site fitness centers and athletic trainers available to instruct employees in fitness programs. Studies have shown that fitness programs, including stretching and strengthening programs, can decrease cumulative trauma injuries. Fitness and recreational programs also increase employee morale and job satisfaction. A positive work environment has been shown to decrease work-related disorders.[6]

Another issue is a willingness of the company to accommodate the injured worker.[6] Today, more companies are offering light or alternate work for the injured employee. Attempts are made to return the worker either to adjusted work or to part-time work as soon as possible.

Progressive companies have human resource and health facilities that are proactive and establish early contact with the physician and patient and attempt to facilitate a quick return to work. Many studies have shown that, if workers can be returned to their company in a modified job soon after injury, long-standing chronic disability can be eliminated.

Probably the most important factor in cutting disability costs is an enlightened management that cares about its employees, listens to their concerns, and responds to their needs. Many studies have demonstrated that companies that have sensitive, open, concerned management and develop programs such as those discussed above will significantly decrease disability costs.

EVALUATE LEGAL ISSUES THAT INFLUENCE RETURN TO WORK

Physicians who treat workers injuries must have a general understanding of the laws in their state that pertain to work-related injuries. Our ability to return the worker to the workforce is affected by these laws. In chronic long-standing cases, the legal system can become cumbersome and the stumbling block preventing successful treatment of the patient.

Ideally when patients are injured they are treated for the injury, rehabilitated, and return to the same or to another job depending upon the results of treatment. All medical bills are paid by the insurer, the workers are paid a portion of their weekly wage, and depending upon the loss of function as determined by the physician based upon certain published guidelines, they receive a lump sum settlement. However, in reality, this often does not happen. Injured workers usually obtain attorneys whose purpose is to represent their best interest and ensure that they will be protected from termination by their employer, not be required to return to work prematurely, and will receive proper compensation when the case is settled.

When the patient obtains counsel an adversarial climate may result between the attorney, the insurer, and the employer. This adversarial and litigious climate is detrimental to the patient's medical recovery because it causes confusion, and uncertainty. The patient often does not know whom to believe and is fearful of losing his or her job. The process is slow, causing frustration. Anger ensues, depression is frequently the next element in the equation, and the physician is presented with a patient demonstrating chronic pain. Orthopaedic surgeons must realize that many of the patients with chronic pain are suffering from chronic depression often associated with a flawed workers' compensations system.

MANAGED CARE PLANS

A new approach to dealing with work-related disorders is through managed care plans. As the costs to industry have skyrocketed, attempts have been made to control both the incidence and costs of work-related disorders. Managed care plan organizations contract with companies to manage all aspects of work-related injuries. Depending on the needs of the specific company, various types of programs are available.

These programs all revolve around a case manager who is trained to respond to the needs of the injured worker at any point of the disability process following the injury. Acute injuries are given prompt medical care by the physician trained in industrial medicine. When specialized care is needed it is arranged promptly. Prognosis for return to work is established early and adjusted work or job change arranged. When therapy or work hardening is needed it is also available. Each step is carefully orchestrated by the case manager, and conflicts and misunderstandings are minimized. The employee is supported at each step.

Most managed care facilities are staffed by trained industrial physicians, industrial therapists, and psychologists. Sometimes, vocational rehabilitation specialists are also on staff. Psychiatrists, neurologists, and rheumatologists who are interested in these types of problems are available for consultation. In chronic cases of either serious injury of overuse disorders the employee is evaluated, and the appropriate steps are taken to restore the worker to health. These steps range from physical means of rehabilitating the worker to vocational rehabilitation or psychological counseling. Sometimes it is preferable to recommend settlement of the case.

This new approach to managing these complicated problems has proven successful. By understanding the various issues that have impeded the worker from returning to work and attempting to eliminate some of the correctable industrial and legal issues, we can prevent long-standing hard-core disability.

REFERENCES

1. Blair SJ, McCormick E: Prevention of trauma: cooperation toward a better working environment. J Hand Surg 10A:953, 1985
2. Blair SJ, Bear-Lehman J: Editorial comment: prevention of upper extremity oc-

cupational disorders. J Hand Surg 12A:821, 1987
3. Louis DS: Cumulative trauma disorders. J Hand Surg 12A:823, 1987
4. Kilborn PT: Automation: pain replaces the old drudgery. New York Times, Sunday, June 24:1, 1990
5. Lutz G, Hansford T: Cumulative trauma disorder controls: the ergonomics program at Ethicon, Inc. J Hand Surg 12A:863, 1987
6. Welch EM: Workers' Compensation: Strategies for Lowering Costs and Reducing Workers' Suffering. LRP Publications, Fort Washington, PA, 1989
7. Feldman RG, Travers PH, Chirico-Post J et al: Risk assessment in electronic assembly workers: carpal tunnel syndrome. J Hand Surg 12A:849, 1987
8. Armstrong TJ, Fine LJ, Goldstein SA et al: Ergonomics considerations in hand and wrist tendinitis. J Hand Surg 12A:830,1 987
9. Arndt R: Work pace, stress, and cumulative trauma disorders. J Hand Surg 12A:866, 1987
10. Masear VR, Hayes JM, Hyde AG: An industrial cause of carpal tunnel syndrome. J Hand Surg 11A:222, 1986
11. Silverstein B, Fine L, Stetson D: Hand-wrist disorders among investment casting plant workers. J Hand Surg 12A:838, 1987
12. Howard FM, Eversman WW, Light TR et al: Cumulative trauma disorders in the home and in the work place. Cont Orthopaed 21:489, 1990
13. Tanaka S, Seligman P, Halperin W et al: Use of workers' compensation claims data for surveillance of cumulative trauma disorders. J Occup Med 30:488, 1988
14. Hadler NM: Illness in the workplace: the challenge of musculoskeletal symptoms. J Hand Surg 10A:451, 1985
15. Talso S, Hendler N, Brodie J: Effects of active and completed litigation on treatment results: workers' compensation patients compared with other litigation patients. J Occup Med 31:265, 1989
16. Melzack R, Katz J, Jeans ME: The role of compensation in chronic pain: analysis using a new method of scoring the McGill Pain Questionnaire. Pain 23:101, 1985

17. Brena SF, Chapman SL: Pain and litigation. p. 832. In Wall PD, Melzak R (eds): Textbook of Pain, Churchill Livingstone, Edinburgh, 1984

18. Herbin ML: Work capacity evaluation for occupational hand injuries. J Hand Surg 12A:958, 1987

19. Berryhill BH: Returning the worker with an upper extremity injury to industry: a model for the physician and therapist. J Hand Ther 3:56, 1990

20. Flinn-Wagner S, Mladonicky A, Goodman G: Characteristics of workers with upper extremity injuries who make a successful transition to work. J Hand Ther 3:51, 1990

21. Block AR, Kremer E, Gaylor M: Behavioral treatment of chronic pain: variables affecting treatment efficacy. Pain 8:367, 1980

22. Swanson DW: Less obvious aspects of chronic pain. Postgrad Med 60:130, 1976

23. Painter JR, Seres JL, Newman RI: Assessing benefits of the pain center: why some patients regress. Pain 8:101, 1980

24. Goldenberg DL: Diagnostic and therapeutic challenges of fibromyalgia. Hosp Pract 30:39, 1989

25. Goldenberg DL: Fibromyalgia syndrome: an emerging but controversial condition. JAMA 257:2782, 1987

26. Hopkins A: The social recognition of repetition strain injuries: an Australian/American comparison. Soc Sci Med 30:365, 1990

27. Ireland CR: Psychological and physical aspects of occupational arm pain. J Hand Surg 13B:5, 1988

28. Benner CL, Schilling AD, Klein L: Coordinated teamwork in California industrial rehabilitation. J Hand Surg 12A:936, 1987

29. Schultz-Johnson K: Assessment of upper extremity-injured persons' return to work potential. J Hand Surg 12A:950, 1987

30. Smith BL: An inside look: hand injury-prevention program. J Hand Surg 12A:940, 1987

31. Muffly-Elsey D, Flinn-Wagner S: Proposed screening tool for the detection of cumulative trauma disorders of the upper extremity. J Hand Surg 12A:931, 1987

2

A Historical Perspective of Workers and the Work Place

Dean S. Louis, M.D.

Although recently we have become increasingly aware of the problems of workers and the difficulties that they experience, these problems are not of recent origin. Ramazzini's work in 1700 and 1713[1,2] presented the first comprehensive treatise on the subject, long before the Industrial Revolution and long before the intense mechanization that now exists. Rosen[3] cited even earlier works by Ellenbog in 1473 devoted to goldsmiths and by Paracelsus in 1567 relating to diseases of miners. No doubt, others whose works have yet to receive credit made observations relating to workers and problems they confronted in the workplace, but Ramazzini stands alone as the first to present a comprehensive overview of the general problem.

His observations, now almost 300 years old, are still at the heart of the problem:

> Various and manifold is the harvest of diseases reaped by certain workers from the crafts and trades that they pursue. All the profit that they get is fatal injury to their health, mostly from two causes.

> The first and most potent is the harmful character of the materials they handle. The second I ascribe to certain violent and irregular motions and unnatural postures of the body, by reason of which, the natural structure of the vital machine is so impaired that serious disease gradually develops therefrom.[1,2]

Ramazzini was aware of the health problems caused by toxic exposure, poor ventilation, awkward posture, and repetitive actions in the work place, especially as they related to the hand and upper extremity. Regarding potters, who used heavy metals, he observed, "First their *hands become palised*, and then they become paralytic, splenic, lethargic, cachectic, and toothless, so that one rarely sees a patient whose face is not cadaverous, and the color of lead." He noted that these workers failed to seek treatment until they were so terribly crippled that they were beyond help, and yet when told that they must refrain from their trades, they would refuse to do so because it was their only means of sustenance. Obviously, the workers' compensation system was not yet in existence.

Compensation for injury has a long and complicated history. The roots of the concept—that a worker should be compensated for loss—date to about 2050 B.C. As detailed in the Nippur Tablet No. 3191[4] dealing with the law of Ur-Nammu, King of Ur in Samaria, compensation was given for the injury of body parts, such as fractures of the hand, foot, and nose. Monetary relief for the loss was given, but at times there were also rewards for lost wages and doctors' fees.

The direct recompense for loss was later replaced by the law of Moses—"an eye for an eye, a tooth for a tooth"—which provided direct recourse for the loss. The early laws of the Greeks, Romans, Arabs, and Chinese provided for recompense for bodily harm, including a life for a life. Under early Arab law, for example, the loss of a portion of a thumb or a great toe was considered to be equivalent to the loss of one half of a finger. Compensation for the loss of a penis was based upon its length, and for an ear, its surface area was considered. Injuries to the head were compensated in camels. Thus, we have the camel-brain equivalent: a simple scratch was equivalent to one camel; if the injury involved the dura mater, it was recompensed by 33 camels; if there was brain damage then the recompense was 100 camels. Brain damage was considered to be fatal in those days, so that one life was considered to be worth 100 camels. Sand[5] reported that the Lombards (circa 600 A.D.) had a system of compensation in which injured workers did not have to prove blame.

As society became more complex and industrialized, so did the laws regarding workers' compensation. Germany developed the first comprehensive workers' compensation system in the late 1880s. This replaced the earlier system in which an injured worker had to prove that the employer was at fault. Most workers were not financially able to pursue such a path through the legal system. The advent of the workers' compensation laws and reforms changed this situation.

Coincident with the development of laws regarding workers' compensation was an observed change in the attitude of workers. This was noted specifically by McKendrick[6] after the Workman's Compensation Act of 1906 in Great Britain. He noted, that workers applied for benefits for even the most trivial problems that would have been tolerated without medical attention before the enactment of the legislation. Sir John Collie[7] was so upset with this alteration in behavior that he wrote a book about it in 1913: *Malingering and Feigned Sickness*. McKendrick also devoted a book to the subject in which he classified malingerers as real, partial, or unconscious according to his appreciation of intent.

In 1934, Hammer[8] described a condition in workers that was characterized by pain and swelling and was accompanied by burning and numbness in the fingers. He was aware of de Quervain's earlier work and recognized part of the symptom complex for what it was. However, he did not further pursue the symptoms, which were no doubt the carpal tunnel syndrome. He observed,

> The advent of the Workmen's Compensation Act has placed upon the surgeon the added responsibility of making careful inquiry into the subject of tenosynovitis in so far as that condition relates to the continued use of certain sets of muscles in daily occupation.... It should not then be surprising to find that certain industrial pursuits require the continuous use of special groups of muscles, constituting "high speed hand operations" and that such oft-repeated manipulations predispose to the development of tenosynovitis.

In 1931 Conn[9] commented on the Ohio

State Workers' Compensation Act of 1929. Primary tenosynovitis, characterized by a passive effusion or crepitus into the tendon sheath of the flexor or extensor muscles of the hand due to frequently repetitive motions or vibration, was then considered compensable. The new code abandoned the need for an etiologic diagnosis and recognized repetitive motion and vibration by themselves as causative factors.

Arthur,[10] in discussing Conn's paper, noted the high incidence of tenosynovitis in newly hired employees and those who had returned from vacation. In 1947 in an extensive review of the problems of median nerve compression, Brain et al.[11] concluded that occupation was a causal factor. Each of his six patients had a history of recent or chronic repetitive hand use.

In recent decades the concept that work could be the cause of disease has been the subject of heated debates in the literature relating to two basic issues: (1) whether an activity can cause "disease" and (2) the extent that emotional or psychological problems may amplify and prolong physical symptoms.

The literature about "epidemic" of repetitive strain injury (RSI) that plagued Australia in the late 1970s and early 1980s illustrates this polarization of thought (see Chapter 8). Hocking[12] reviewed this problem in 1987, citing the increased incidence of RSI in Telecom, a governmental authority that at that time employed over 90,000 telecommunications workers in Australia. He reported rates of 343 cases of RSI per 1000 keyboard staff members during a 50-year period. Other employees, including clerical workers, telegraphists, and process workers, were also involved. Sixteen percent of the affected group experienced symptoms for over 26 weeks. The overall costs were in excess of $15 million. He suggested that psychosocial stress and neurosis were a

basis upon which physical stress precipitated symptoms. He was unable to account for the reasons why this epidemic peaked in 1984 and then dramatically declined in 1986, although he did observe that job satisfaction appeared to be a key factor in the genesis of the problem. The dramatic fall in the incidence of this problem in Australia remains a matter of speculation. The resulting literature placed a great emphasis upon the psychological aspects of the problem.[13–17] The issues of causality and the extent of the emotional components of the situation are still unresolved.

Hershenson[18] perhaps summarized the problems of work-related disorders in the United States best when he observed their total effect upon the entire U.S. economy.

> There is little doubt that the growing incidence of cumulative injuries is placing serious strain on employers and insurers who finance the workers' compensation system. There are tremendous cost problems facing the industry today. A basic principle of insurance is the ability to predict costs of future losses and to set aside adequate reserves to pay them. This has become very difficult in cumulative injury cases because of the long tail, and because of different and new benefits that are granted each year by the legislators as well as through judicial decision. Thus we are paying out dollars on an increasing number of different kinds of occurrences which yesterday were not considered to have been covered by compensation, or were compensated on a much lower benefit schedule. Expenses of administration, and of litigating cumulative injury cases are extremely high. The inflationary impact of cumulative injury on consumers, resulting in higher prices for goods and services, cannot be ignored any longer.

Cumulative trauma[19] is now a major problem in the United States. The issues of compensation and impairment as they relate to the work place and cumulative trauma are covered elsewhere in the book, as are details of specific cumulative trauma disorders. It is clear that we are in a time of transition in our understanding and management of musculoskeletal problems in the work place. One newly initiated to these problems might feel an overwhelming frustration with the situation. This historical review is intended to give a proper perspective to that emotion, which is not new to this situation, having been recognized for over 500 years.

REFERENCES

1. Ramazzini B: DeMorbis artificum diatriba. Diseases of Workers. Translated by Wilmer Cave Wright. University of Chicago Press, Chicago, 1940
2. Ramazzini B: Diseases of Workers. Translated by Wilmer Cave Wright. Hafner Publishing Co, New York, 1964
3. Rosen G: The Worker's Hand. CIBA Symposium, 1942
4. Geerts A, Kornblith B, Urmson J: Compensation for Bodily Harm. Fernand Nathan, Editions Labor, Brussels, 1977
5. Sand R: Vers La Medecine Sociale. Paris, 1948 p 344
6. McKendrick A: Malingering and Its Detection. E & S. Livingstone, Edinburgh, 1912
7. Collie, Sir John: Malingering and Feigned Sickness. Edward Arnold, London, 1913
8. Hammer AW: Tenosynovitis. Med Rec 140:353, 1934
9. Conn HR: Tenosynovitis. Ohio State Med J 9:713, 1931
10. Arthur WC: Discussion of paper by Conn. Ohio State Med J 9:715, 1931
11. Brain WR, Wright AD, Wilkinson M: Spontaneous compression of both median nerves in the carpal tunnel. Lancet 1:277, 1947
12. Hocking B: Epidemiologic aspects of "repetitive strain injury" in Telecom, Australia. Med J Aust 147:218, 1987
13. Ferguson DA: RSI: putting the epidemic to rest. Med J Aust 147:213, 1987
14. Wright GD: The failure of the RSI concept. Med J Aust 147:233, 1987
15. Cleland LG: RSI: a model of social iatrogenesis. Med J Aust 147:236, 1987
16. Ireland DCR: Psychological and physical aspects of occupational arm. J Hand Surg 13B:5, 1988
17. Hadler N: Illness in the work place: the challenge of musculoskeletal symptoms. J Hand Surg 10A:451, 1985
18. Hershenson A: Cumulative injury: a national problem. J Occup Med 21:674, 1979
19. Putz-Anderson V (ed): Cumulative Trauma Disorders: A Manual For Musculoskeletal Diseases of the Upper Limbs. Taylor and Francis, New York, 1988

3

Cumulative Trauma Disorders of the Upper Limb and Identification of Work-Related Factors

Thomas J. Armstrong, Ph.D.

Ergonomics is concerned with the design of work equipment, procedures, and environments so that people can achieve maximum performance without an undue risk of injury or disease. The literature contains many studies of work design, productivity, and quality control. It also contains studies that demonstrate some of the adverse effects of excessive work demands, ranging from fatigue to chronic muscle, tendon, and nerve disorders. One of the earliest references to to these problems is from Bernard Ramazzini, who in 1713 wrote,

> Various and manifold is the harvest of diseases reaped by workers from the crafts and trades they pursue. The first cause I ascribe to the nature of the materials they handle. The second to certain violent and irregular motions and unnatural postures by which the natural structure of the vital machine is so impaired that serious diseases develop therefrom.[1]

The terms "various and manifold" and "harvest of diseases" suggest that multiple effects and disorders may result when work requirements exceed an individual's capacity. The current literature has succeeded in naming some of these disorders. In some cases these conditions are named for their affected tissues or symptoms; for example, myalgia, tendinitis, epicondylitis, carpal tunnel syndrome, and cubital tunnel syndrome. In other cases these conditions are named for the activities that are associated with their development; examples include washer woman's sprain, gamekeeper's thumb, drummer's palsy, flute player's hand, pizza cutter's palsy, pipetter's thumb, reedmaker's elbow, tobacco-primer's wrist, and wall washer's thumb.[2–15] Because the development and manifestation of these disorders share common elements, they are treated as a group and referred to as "cumulative trauma disorders." Cumulative trauma disorders are

19

defined as those disorders that are caused, precipitated, or aggravated by repeated or sustained exertions of the body.[16-18] Although these disorders can occur in many locations in the body, this chapter is concerned with the hand, wrist, and forearm.

In addition to "cumulative trauma disorder," other terms widely used to refer to disorders with these characteristics include repetitive trauma disorder,[19,20] repetitive strain injury,[21-24] overuse syndrome,[25] work-related disorder,[26] and regional musculoskeletal disorders.[27] Although differences among these terms and concepts can be debated, the similarities outweigh the differences.

CHARACTERISTICS OF CUMULATIVE TRAUMA DISORDERS

Their pathogenesis involves both mechanical and physiologic processes. The mechanical processes result from the exertion of force and the development of tissue stresses and strains. The tissues of the body, as do materials, deform when subjected to forces or mechanical stresses. These deformations may interfere with basic physiologic processes and result in mechanical failure.[28-32] Unlike nonliving materials, several factors help prevent the body from reaching the breaking point. One is the stimulation of nerves that produce pain or discomfort. These can be thought of as the body's way of telling us to slow down or stop so that it can recover.[33-35] The second is the repair mechanism, which immediately begins repairing the damaged tissues and adapting them to those work stresses.[36,37] Cumulative trauma disorders can be thought of as a condition in which activity produces a mechanical or physiologic disturbance that results in persistent symptoms or signs. When these activities are a result of work, the resulting disorders are work related.[26]

Cumulative trauma disorders are multifactorial. Multifactorial implies that there may be more than one factor that causes aggravates, precipitates a cumulative trauma disorders.[26] These factors may pertain to personal conditions or activities, as well as work activities. As a practical matter, work activities appear to account for the greatest proportion of cases.[38-41]

These disorders generally develop over periods of weeks, months, and years. There are not yet rigorous data on how much time is required for cumulative trauma disorders to develop. It suffices to say that they usually are not the result of a single exertion or a sudden event. Usually, workers have been experiencing symptoms or episodes of symptoms for some time before they seek medical attention.

These disorders often are unreported. Although they may result in considerable discomfort and may affect performance of work and daily living tasks, only in extreme cases are they completely disabling. Workers may be very resourceful in finding ways of coping with the effects of cumulative trauma disorders. These include modification of the work equipment and procedures and of their lifestyle. Even when conditions do result in disability, they may be handled as a personal problem rather than as work-related problems.

These common characteristics must be considered in developing an ergonomics prevention program for cumulative trauma disorders.

FATIGUE

Symptoms and signs of fatigue include discomfort, loss of strength, reduced motor control, and electrical

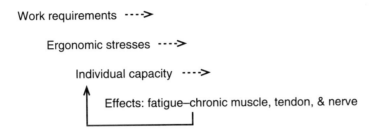

Fig. 3-1. Simplification of the progression of work activities to fatigue and cumulative trauma disorders.

changes.[34,35,42–47] The symptoms of fatigue may be confused with those of cumulative trauma disorders because they occur under similar circumstances; that is, work that entails repetitive, sustained, or forceful exertions. Fatigue is similar to cumulative trauma disorders in that it also involves mechanical and physiologic processes. However, in contrast to those disorders, the symptoms of fatigue develop and recover in periods of seconds, minutes, or hours. If symptoms persist from one shift to the next, then that person should be evaluated by a physician to determine the presence of a condition more serious than fatigue.

It can be argued that cumulative trauma disorders develop when the time between successive exertions or work periods is insufficient for recovery or adaptation and the affected tissues remain irritated or inflamed.[47,48] A simplified process is shown in Figure 3-1. It also can be argued that prevention of fatigue will result in prevention of cumulative trauma disorders. This may be a reasonable assumption in the absence of definitive data; however, it is yet to be proven.

RISK FACTORS

Risk factors of cumulative trauma disorders can be classified as work related or personal, depending on whether they occur as a result of the job or other activities. The considerable clinical, biomechanical, and epidemiologic data supporting the relationship between work factors and cumulative trauma disorders have been reviewed elsewhere.[16,40,41,49–52] This chapter focuses on the analysis of work factors in selected occupations. The most important work-related risk factor of upper limb cumulative trauma disorders is the use of the hands. Use of the hands can be characterized in terms of exertion frequency, and duration. The effect of the exertions may be enhanced by

- force
- localized mechanical stresses
- certain postures
- low temperatures
- vibration

For the purposes of this discussion, these work-related factors are referred to as "ergonomic factors." There is an abundance of clinical, biomechanical, and epidemiologic evidence supporting the relationship between ergonomic factors and cumulative trauma disorders; however, most of it is qualitative, and it is not yet possible to predict acceptable levels for these factors either alone or in combination with one another. As a result, problems often are not identified until after the fact when workers complain of pain or other problems with their hands. Even when a good faith effort is made to eliminate all possible stresses from the job, some workers may still be affected. Therefore, it is advisable to establish a control program that includes a sensitive surveillance program for identification of affected workers and jobs so that interventions can be devised before impairments develop into disabilities.

THE PROGRAM

The overall organization of the control program is shown in Figure 3-2. It includes surveillance, evaluation, and interventions for affected workers; evaluations and interventions for affected jobs; and evaluation of all interventions, and it is run by a team.

Surveillance is the cornerstone of the control program.[20,53–56] It should be designed to identify problems while they are in their earliest stages. This aim may be achieved through either passive or active surveillance. Passive surveillance relies on voluntary reporting of problems by workers. OSHA records, first aid reports, medical visits, and insurance claims generally require the worker to take the initiative to seek help. Passive surveillance data may be highly variable depending on the source of the information. Fine et al.[55] compared the incidence rates of cumulative trauma disorders for two automobile assembly plants located next to one another based on OSHA records, workers' compensation reports, personal medical absences, and plant medical visits. The rates on OSHA records were from three to ten times greater than those for workers' compensation. Rates based on personal medical absences were four to ten times greater than for workers' compensation reports. Worker visit rates to the plant medical department were sevenfold greater at one plant. These differences reflect differences in the way that worker health problems were managed at the two plants and in worker attitudes about the plant medical program. This variability makes it difficult to identify affected jobs and to evaluate interventions.

In the past, employers were afforded a great deal of latitude in how they classified chronic musculoskeletal disorders. In the late 1980s OSHA began the practice of citing employers for not classifying such disorders as work related.[57] In 1990 they published guidelines for what they considered work related as part of an *Er-*

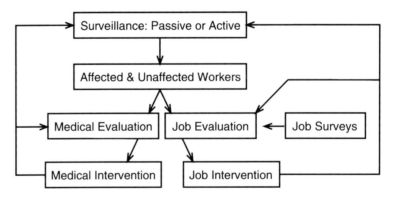

Fig. 3-2. An ergonomics control program for cumulative trauma disorders. Key features are the use of surveillance for identification of affected workers and evaluation of all medical and work interventions.

gonomics Guidelines for Meat Packing Plants.[54] These criteria included

- At least one physical finding (e.g., positive Tinel's, Phalen's, or Finkelstein's test; or swelling, redness, or deformity; or loss of motion; or
- At least one subjective symptom (e.g., pain, numbness, tingling, aching, stiffness, or burning), and at least one of the following:
  - • medical treatment (including self-administered treatment when made available to employees by their employer)
  - • lost work days (includes restricted work activity); or
  - • transfer/rotation to another job

OSHA guidelines should help eliminate inconsistencies between classification of cases and make the resulting data more useful.

Differences from one plant to another depend on the awareness and attitudes about work related health issues of workers, managers, and local medical personnel from plant to plant and area to area. Sometimes workers are afraid to accept the possibility that there is something wrong with them. They may also be afraid to report problems that jeopardize their employment, bonuses, or advancement. They can be very resourceful in finding ways of coping with the pain and impairment of upper limb disorders, such as modification of work activities, tools, and activities of daily living and leisure. Such behavior may be reinforced by a negative attitude by their employer or physician toward workers' compensation patients. Increased education of workers, managers, and medical personnel should result in improved reporting and more useful passive surveillance data.

Active surveillance entails the use of questionnaires, interviews, and physical examinations to survey the health status of the work force. Such surveys may be administered to the entire work force or to a representative sample of workers. Important qualities of active surveillance are that it should be sensitive and unbiased. Sensitive means that it should capture all possible cases even at the expense of a few false positive results.[58,59] These can be sorted out later with a medical examination. Unbiased means that the same protocol is used on all workers and that it does not suggest to workers that they should or should not be experiencing symptoms. One way of doing this is to ask workers to identify areas of discomfort. Workers can be asked to verbalize, point, or mark areas of discomfort on a drawing of the body. The surveyor then examines the data for similarities and differences. This approach was first described by Corlett and Bishop[60] and later by other investigators to look at comfort patterns.[18,40,61,62]

Analysis of surveillance data in most situations is qualitative. The number of workers usually is too small and unstable to establish statistically significant differences. For example, for an 80 percent chance of detecting the difference between one population with a prevalence of 10 percent and another with a prevalence of 20 percent with 95 percent certainty, over 200 workers would be required in each group.[59] About all that can be done in most cases is to calculate incidences rates by department. An incidence rate is the number of new cases per 200,000 workers. Cases of cumulative trauma disorders for a 6-month period at an instrument manufacturer are tabulated in Table 3-1. It was assumed that each person worked 1,000 hours during this 6-month period. Two departments, II and V, each had four cases; however, only 12 people were employed in Department II, resulting in an incidence rate of 66.7, whereas 39 people were employed in Department V, resulting in an incidence rate

Table 3-1.   Upper Limb Medical Complaints for 6 Months at an Electronics Engineering and Manufacturing Firm Grouped by Assembly Area and Hours Keying

	Assembly Area							Keying (Hours)			
	1	2	3	4	5	6	Total	<4	4–6	>6	Total
Number of workers	13	12	23	23	39	4	114	133	253	195	581
Cases	0	4	0	1	4	1	0	1	2	5	8
Incidence (%)[a]	0.0	66.7	0.0	8.7	20.5	50	17.5	1.5	1.6	5.1	2.8

[a] Cases per 100 workers per year
(From Armstrong,[51] with permission.)

of 20.5. Clearly the risk is much greater in Department II than Department V. All cases of cumulative trauma disorders should be investigated to ascertain their causes; however, departments with very high incidence rates should receive special attention and may receive special consideration for process changes and renovation.

Worker evaluations must be conducted by a licensed medical professional; however, ergonomists, safety professionals, supervisors, or engineers may assist by analyzing the job, providing information about the work exposure, and helping modify work procedures and equipment. Doing so will not only facilitate the return to work of the affected worker but also help prevent future occurrences.

A control program for cumulative trauma disorders draws on many resources: medical, supervision, management, safety, health, engineering, and labor. It therefore is recommended that a team of people from each of these areas be assembled to run the program.[63] The team should be provided with training so that they can interpret worker and job evaluation data to identify problems, set goals and priorities, and allocate or recommend resources. Specific activities may be delegated to team members or to persons from a team member's department or area. One person may be designated as team coordinator or leader to arrange and conduct meetings and to doc-

ument the progress of the program. Such documentation is important for identifying what works and what does not. Also, it provides evidence of an active program should the company come under investigation by OSHA. The frequency of formal team meetings will vary depending on the level of program activity.

JOB ANALYSIS

Job analysis is a systematic way of identifying and expressing in qualitative or quantitative terms what a worker does and, in this case, the stresses to which the employee is exposed.[64] This section describes procedures for assessing ergonomic stresses that result from hand work.[16,50,51] Three jobs are used to illustrate these procedures: an auto worker, a poultry processor, and a computer analyst. These jobs are described in Tables 3-2 to 3-4.

The analysis can be divided into two parts: documentation and the ergonomic assessment. The documentation is the identification and recording of the job-specific attributes that in turn determine the ergonomic stresses. It includes the following information:

• Objective: Why the job is performed
• Work standard: How much work the worker is expected to perform in a

Table 3-2. Documentation of Automobile Worker's Job

Title:	Auto worker—Headlight assembly
Objective:	Put headlight assembly together for installation in cars.
Standard:	Line speed 60 vehicles/hour; two headlights per vehicle
Work station:	Workbench; rack
Equipment:	Screwdriver; right angle powered screwdriver
Materials:	Headlights; headlight holders; headlight rims
Method:	1. Get holder and place in fixture on bench.
	2. Place headlight and place in holder.
	3. Get rim and place on bulb
	4a. Get screw and place in bit with one hand (four per headlight).
	4b. Drive screw with other hand (four per headlight).
	6. Get and place headlight assembly in rack.
Environment:	Inside—70–85°F

given amount of time, e.g., number of parts, number of transactions, detection of defects or problems
- Tasks: Activities that must be performed to accomplish the work objective; tasks need not be performed in the same sequence or for the same time; may be further divided into steps, which are usually performed in the same sequence
- Work objects: Objects on which work is performed; may be physical (e.g., subassemblies, assemblies, and carcasses) or nonphysical, e.g., inquiries, software, information, music, etc.
- Tools and equipment: Objects or devices held or manipulated with the hands that do something to the work object, e.g., screwdrivers, wrenches or knives, computers, instruments
- Work station: Physical surroundings that are used to hold or support work objects, tools, equipment, or the worker, e.g., the tables, chairs, conveyors, and assembly lines
- Environment: Where the work is performed and its physical characteristics, e.g., inside an air conditioned room with a constant temperature of 72°F with indirect fluorescent lighting
- Methods: A step-by step description of the exertions, motions, or acts required

Table 3-3. Documentation of Poultry Processor's Job

Title:	Turkey processing—Thigh boning
Objective:	Remove thigh bones from turkey carcasses.
Standard:	1,080 turkeys per hour line speed; 8-hour shift, 15 minute AM break, 30 minute lunch break and 15 minute PM break; four thigh boners each bone one thigh of every other turkey
Work station:	Overhead conveyor; shackles 112 cm above floor level; turkey thighs, 57 cm above floor level
Equipment:	Thigh boning knife; wire mesh glove for nonknife hand; optional rubber gloves for both hands; hard hat; smock; boots
Materials:	Turkeys
Method:	1. Grasp and position thigh with nonknife hand.
	2. Cut along thigh bone to separate meat from bone × 2–3 cuts.
	3. Cut remaining tendinous attachments (bone drops into conveyor as worker releases meat and bone).
Environment:	Air-conditioned turkey plant; turkeys 38°F; ambient air 45°F

Table 3-4. Documentation of Computer Analyst's Job

Title:	Computer analyst
Objective:	Assist computer network users with computer problems.
Standard:	Keep system operational and users happy.
Work station:	Modular work station; work surface 75 cm above floor
Equipment:	Personal computer connected to server via network; keyboard; monochrome monitor; work processing and electronic message system used to compose reports, letters, and messages; chair
Materials:	Inquiries from visitors, computer, and telephone; paper documents; manuals
Methods: (tasks)	Telephone conversations; meetings; interaction with computer to write letters, memos, and messages; create and de-bug software; and use reference documents
Environment:	Office with indirect lighting

to perform the job (e.g., get part, inspect part, insert part, drive screw, etc.); steps should be listed for the right and left hand, but one list is sufficient if both hands do the same actions

The documentation is used to assess each of the generic ergonomic factors. Persons learning to perform job analysis or who are not familiar with the jobs will find it is desirable to perform the documentation before performing the ergonomic assessment. However, with experience and familiarity, the two steps may be performed at the same time so that only the required documentation is recorded.

Repeated and Sustained Exertions

The frequency of exertions is related to the work rate and method. The steps in determining repetitiveness are as follows:

1. From the work standard, determine the number of work objects or tasks to be performed per hour.
2. Determine the work objects.
3. From the methods analysis, determine the number of steps required per work object.
4. Calculate repetitiveness as the number of exertions per hour.
5. Estimate the duration of exertion.
6. Classify rate repetition as follows:
   - High: the hands in constant rapid motion; wasted motions or difficulty with equipment would result in worker immediately falling behind
   - Medium: the hands in steady motion, but no difficulty keeping up; worker may pause or rest as necessary
   - Low: conspicuous pauses in each work cycle; worker may wait for equipment to cycle, the hands used only to remove an occasional defective part

Examples
Auto worker (Table 3-2)

1. Assemble two headlights per car while assembly line is moving at 40 cars per hour.
2. Headlight parts and assembly
3. Eight exertions per part
4. 60 cars/h × 2 bulbs per car × 8 exertions/assembly = 920 exertions/h
5a. Tool hand: continuous exertion
5b. Nontool hand: 50 percent of cycle time
6. Medium to high repetition: worker

works rapidly, but gets ahead of operation and can then rest

Poultry worker (Table 3-3)

1. Bone one thigh of 540 turkeys per hour
2. Turkeys
3a. Knife hand—three to four cuts per thigh
3b. Nonknife hand—one exertion per thigh
4a. Knife hand—540 birds/h × four cuts/bird
4b. Nonknife hand—540 birds/h × one exertion/bird
5a. Knife hand—continuous exertion
5b. Nonknife hand—50 percent of cycle time
6a. Knife hand—highly repetitive; hand is in near constant motion with no rest between cycles
6b. Nonknife hand: medium repetitiveness; the hand rests between turkeys as long as it holds thighs while cutting

Computer Analyst: (Table 3-4)

1. On demand
2. Inquiries
3. Variable depending on required resources, e.g., knowledge, manuals, or other people
4. Frequency of exertion is highly variable and related to use of keyboard, note taking, and handling of reference documents
5a. Shoulder, neck and elbows may involve prolonged static exertions while using keyboard
5b. Hand and fingers vary from high repetitive use of keyboard to idle while conducting telephone conversation

The computer analyst's routine and number of exertions are highly variable from day to day and from hour to hour. However, it may be possible to characterize in qualitative terms a typical day and an exceptional day from interviews with workers or supervisors. For example, a typical shift for a computer analyst is 50 percent keyboard work, 15 percent phone work, 20 percent using documents, and 30 percent meetings (note: the total may exceed 100 percent because more than one task may be performed at a time, e.g., using the phone and keyboard). On average of once per month, the computer analyst may work on the keyboard for 12 hours of continuous work.

Another way of determining work patterns is to do work sampling. Work sampling is a procedure in which the worker is observed at random or regular intervals throughout the work shift. It is then possible to calculate the percent of time that the worker performs each task or is exposed to given stresses. By taking at least 30 observations per shift, it can be assumed that the observed data follow a normal distribution. It can then be determined how many observations are required for a given level of statistical certainty.[65] An example of work sampling data for a programmer/analysis is shown in Table 3-5. In this example it was found that the worker spent 56 percent of his time keying, 11 percent writing, 7 percent on the phone, 7 percent in meetings, 32 percent reading, 25 percent handling papers, and 18 percent absent. The overall work pace was rated for each observation:

- Low: Intermittent keying, writing, handling; rest as desired
- Medium: Steady, but leisurely pace; rest as desired.

Therefore, the overall rating for this job is in the low to medium range.

Force

The force exerted by the hand is determined by load and friction. Friction is related to the material from

Table 3-5. Work Sampling Data for Computer Analyst

Time	Task 1	Task 2	Task 3	Overall Work Pace
9:40	reading			low
9:55	keying			medium
10:10	keying	writing		medium
10:25	reading	handling papers	medium	
10:40	keying	phone		medium
10:55	keying	reading		low
11:10	keying			medium
11:25	keying	medium		medium
11:40	absent			low
11:55	keying			medium
12:10	absent			low
12:25	absent			low
12:40	absent			low
12:55	absent			low
13:10	meeting			low
13:25	keying			low
13:40	reading			low
13:55	read	handling papers	low	
14:10	writing	phone		low
14:20	keying	reading	handling papers	low
14:35	keying			low
14:50	keying			medium
15:05	reading	handling papers	low	
15:20	keying			medium
15:50	keying			low
16:05	keying	reading	handling papers	medium
15:15	keying	docs		medium
15:30	keying	writing		medium

	TOTALS:	
	Keying	56%
	Writing	11%
	Phone	7%
	Absent	18%

which the work object is made and the moistness of the skin. Load forces are caused by gravity on work objects, tools, or the body; by friction; and by reaction forces. In addition, forces may be increased by bulky, poor fitting, or stiff gloves and by certain postures, e.g., more effort is required to hold something by pinching than by a power grip.

The steps for analyzing the force requirements are as follows.

1. Inspect the work method for all exertions of the hand. For example,
   - lifting or holding work objects
   - applying force to overcome resistance
   - resisting reaction forces
2. Identify and rate these factors affecting force.
   - weight
   - friction
   - gloves
   - hand posture
   - fit of parts
   - maintenance of blades/bits/gloves, etc.
3. Determine the duration of the force.
4. Estimate or rate force using
   - perceived exertion
   - electromyography
   - biomechanical analyses

Examples
Auto worker (see Table 3-2)

1. The forceful elements of the auto worker's job can be identified from inspection of the work elements in Table 3-2. They include transfer of parts and driving screws.
2a. Transfer of parts weighing less than 2 pounds. Requirements may be qualified further by reporting additional factors that affect force, e.g., parts are handled using a pinch grip and while wearing bulky gloves. In addition, parts occasionally stick together, and extra effort is required to pull them apart.
2b. Use of pistol screwdriver that produces 10 foot-pounds of torque
   - Holes occasionally do not line up, and extra effort is required to drive screws.
   - Worn Phillips screwdriver bits that require extra effort to engage in the screw are often used.
   - Screws are sometimes poorly formed and require extra effort.

3a. Force to transfer of parts occurs 960 times/h.
3b. Force to hold powered screwdriver occurs continuously.
3c. Force to drive screws occurs 480 times/h.
4. The force requirements often can be qualified or quantified further by using psychophysical methods. This entails asking workers to rate the force requirements of various aspects of the job. Care must be exercised to ask questions in a way that does not suggest how the worker should respond. One way of doing this is with a visual analogue scale. A visual analogue scale is a line with two or more verbal anchor points on which workers indicate the magnitude of their perceptions with check marks. An example of a survey of hand tool weight for an automobile trim department is shown in Figure 3-3.[66] This analysis shows that tools with a mass less than 1.5 kg usually are rated as "just right," whereas heavier tools are usually rated as "too heavy." It has yet to be shown that selection of tools in the "just right" range will reduce the risk of cumulative trauma disorder; however, analogous findings have been reported for lifting and overexertion disorders.[67,68]

Poultry Processor (see Table 3-3)

1. Forceful elements include
   - knife hand—holding knife, cutting thighs
   - nonknife hand—holding thighs for cutting
2a. Knife hand force factors: user technique, sharpness of blade
2b. Nonknife hand force factors—force depends on position of worker with respect to moving turkey
3a. Knife hand force frequency—continuous knife holding, 4,320 cuts/h

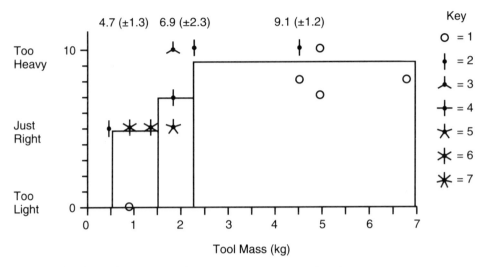

Fig. 3-3. Psychophysical ratings used to assess the weights of tools and to determine preferred weight ranges. (From Armstrong et al.,[66] with permission.)

3b. Nonknife hand force frequency—hold turkeys 1,080 times/h

4. The forces to hold the turkey and to hold and use the knife were quantified by using surface electromyography (emg). Figure 3-4 shows recordings of the forearm flexor muscle emgs for both the knife and nonknife hand.[69] The electromyograms were calibrated by having the subjects exert known forces with the same positions used to hold the knife and the thigh. It can be seen that the forces required for cutting are greater than those for holding the thighs. In addition, the hand holding the thighs rests between cuts, whereas the knife hand must maintain its grip on the knife.

Computer analyst (see Table 3-4)

1. Forceful elements include using the keyboard, handling documents, and pulling chair around work station
2. Force factors
   • force required to press keys is less than 100 g; however, workers usually exert more than the minimum required force—some exert considerably more
   • weight of documents
   • condition of chair casters, shape and slipperiness of work surface
3. The frequency of forceful exertions varies with the use of the keyboard.
4a. Key forces can be measured by using surface electromyograph or by placing the keyboard on a force platform.[65,70] A recording of average force exerted on the "e" key while typing text is shown in Figure 3-5.
4b. The force required to handle documents and move the chair around probably is greater than the keying force. These forces can be estimated from Amoton's law, which says that the friction force is equal to the contact force times the coefficient of friction. Figure 3-6 illustrates the forces required to move the chair, which can be estimated as the weight of the worker plus the chair times its rolling coefficient of friction. The weight of the worker and chair can be determined by weighing them; the coefficient of friction can be found in an

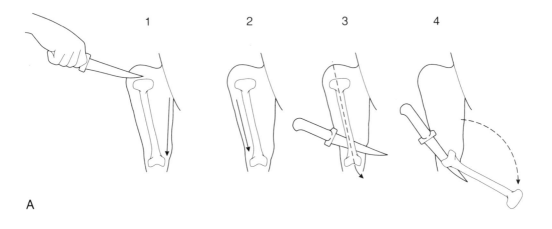

A

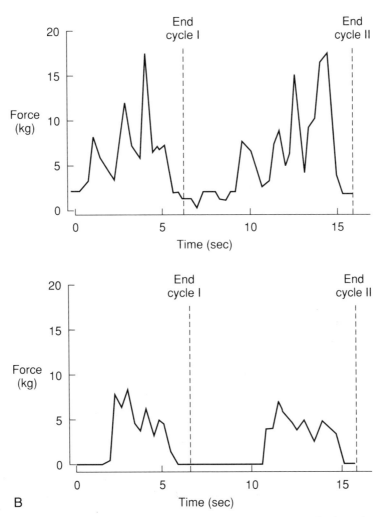

B

Fig. 3-4. Surface EMG recordings show that the force for trimming thighs (**A**) are greater and held longer than those for holding thighs (**B**). (From Armstrong et al.,[69] with permission.)

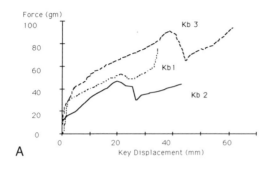

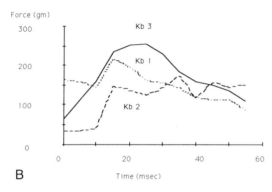

Fig. 3-5. Average key force displacement curves for computer keyboard. Average force exerted by ten subjects on "e" key while typing text is least for the light touch keyboard (**B**). (From Armstrong et al.,[65] with permission.)

engineering handbook. For this example with a worker-chair weight of 600 N (120 lb) and a coefficient of friction of 0.25, the required pull force will be 150 N (30 lb). The pull force, Fpull, is exerted by pinching, F_{pinch}, the edges of the work surface between the fingers and thumb. Friction is exerted on both sides of the work surface. The pinch force will be equal to

F_{pinch}
    $= F_{pull}/2 \times$ coefficient of friction

The coefficient of friction for the skin in contact with the vinyl lami-nate work surface is estimated from Table 3-6 as .0.50.[71] Therefore, the pinch force is equal to 75 N (15 lb.). Because this is more than most people can exert with one hand, two hands as well as the feet may be required in this case

A similar analysis can be applied to the handling of bundles of documents and manuals. The force requirements are likely to increase with handling of paper documents due to drying of the fingers.

Localized Mechanical Stresses

A mechanical stress is produced any time that a force is exerted on a material or a tissue. It is calculated as the force divided by the area. For example, Figure 3-7A shows the area of contact made by someone's forearm and hand as it rests on a flat surface; it can be calculated as 174 square centimeters. If it is assumed that the weight of the forearm and hand is 25 N and that the work surface is compliant so that the force is distributed uniformly over the surface, the contact stress between the work surface and the body is 1,435 N per square meter. Figure 3-7B shows the weight of the forearms and hand supported by the arm rests of a chair. In this case the surface area is found to be 25 square centimeters, and the average contact stress in this case is calculated as 9,687 N per square meter. The level of insult and discomfort increases with the magnitude contact stress.[72] Some parts of the body are more tolerant than others. For example, 1,435 N per square meter contact force may be tolerated longer if it is distributed in the fleshy areas of the forearm than over the ulnar nerve at the elbow or the finger flexor tendons and median nerve at the

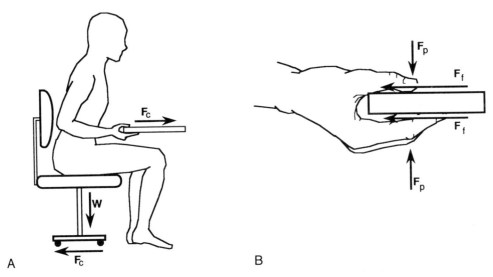

Fig. 3-6. (**A**) Workers pull on the work surface to overcome friction between chair and floor. (**B**) Workers must pinch work surface to produce enough friction force to move their seat.

wrist.[29] It is possible to apply sufficient pressure on the volar surface of the wrist to interfere with median nerve function.

The steps for analyzing contact force are as follows:

1. Identify all contact points between the body, work objects, and work surfaces from the methods analysis.
2. Determine the force of contact, e.g., weight of body segment, weight of work object, reaction force, etc. and the area and location of contact. Areas of contact may be expressed qualitatively (e.g., sharp edge or rounded edge) or quantitatively in centimeters square.
3. Determine the frequency and duration of contact.

Examples

Automobile worker (see Table 3-2)

Table 3-6. Coefficients of Friction for Skin and Various Materials As Used to Estimate Hand Force Requirements*

Material	Dry (n = 42)	Moist (n = 42)	Combined (n = 84)
Sand paper (#320)	—	—	0.61 + 0.10
Smooth vinyl	—	—	0.53 + 0.18
Textured vinyl	—	—	0.50 + 0.11
Adhesive tape	0.41 + 0.10	0.66 + 0.14	—
Suede	0.39 + 0.06	0.66 + 0.11	—
Aluminum	—	—	0.38 + 0.13
Paper	0.27 + 0.09	0.42 + 0.07	—

* (From Buchholz et al.,[71] with permission.)

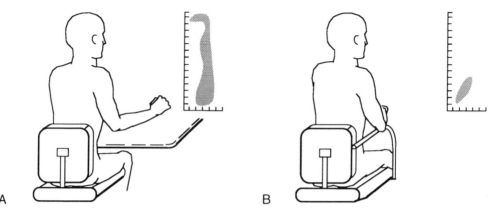

A   B

Fig. 3-7. Localized mechanical stresses are estimated by dividing the weight of the forearm and hand by the area of contact. The area of contact is approximately 175 square centimeters when the forearm and hand are lying on a flat work surface (**A**) and 25 cm when they are supported by a tubular arm rest (**B**).

1. Localized contact stresses between fingers and edges of parts (Fig. 3-8A) and between tool and fingers-palm and handle (Fig. 3-8B)
2. Localized contact stress factors
   • Parts weigh less than 10 N, but have sharp edges.
   • Tool weighs less than 15 N but produces 1.5 N-meter torque; edges of handle are well rounded, but there are sharp edges around the trigger.

3. Frequency of mechanical stresses— same as forceful exertions

Poultry worker (see Table 3-3)

1. Localized contact stresses between knife, finger, and palm (Fig. 3-9)
2. Localized contact stress factors:
   • position of finger on blade (Fig. 3-10)
   • shape of handle
   • use of gloves

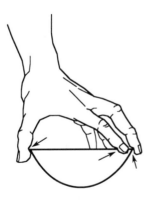

Fig. 3-8. Localized contact stresses occur between fingers and edges of parts while transferring the headlight assembly.

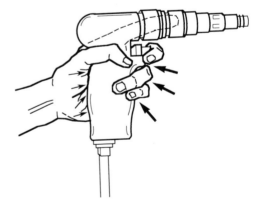

Fig. 3-9. Localized contact stresses occur between the palm, fingers, handle, and trigger of powered screwdriver.

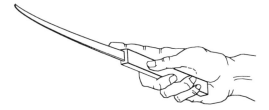

Fig. 3-10. Localized contact stresses occur between the palm and handle and finger and blade of the boning knife.

3. Frequency of mechanical stresses— same as knife force

Computer analyst (see Table 3-4)

1. Localized contact stresses between
   • keying—wrist and edge of work surface (Fig. 3-11) and between forearm and armrest (Fig. 3-7B).
   • moving chair—fingers, palm, and edge of work surface (Fig. 3-4)
2. Localized contact stress factors
   • keying—weight of forearms wrist, curvature of corners of work surface; forearm and armrest
   • moving chair—condition of casters, floor covering, shape and friction of work surface
3. Frequency of mechanical stresses— same as force

Posture Stresses

All postures are stressful if they are maintained long enough. Probably everyone is familiar with the discomfort associated with spending several days in bed convalescing from an illness. Similarly, even the most stressful postures may feel good for a brief period. For example, the seventh inning stretch feels good for a minute or two, but would not be tolerable for the entire ballgame. One posture may be more stressful than another for two reasons. First, some postures require more effort than others. For example, the body must work harder to produce the same force in a pinch position than a grip position. That is why there are handles on luggage and many other objects. Second, some postures produce pressure in certain parts of the body. For example, exertion of the fingers with a flexed wrist position results in pressure on the median nerve. This maneuver forms the basis of the wrist flexion or Phalen's test for carpal tunnel syndrome.[73,74] Similarly, extreme extension of the wrist causes increased pressure inside the carpal tunnel and tension on the median nerve.[75,76] It also can be shown that deviation of the wrist causes tension on the extrinsic abductor and extensor tendons of the thumb. Forced deviation of the wrist with the fingers wrapped around the thumb is used as a diagnostic test of de Quervain's disease.

Stressful upper limb postures for repeated or prolonged work are shown in Figure 3-12.[77] They include elevation of the elbows, reaching behind the torso, extreme elbow flexion, extreme forearm rotation, wrist deviation, flexion or hyperextension, and pinching. As a general rule, it is desirable to design work so that the wrist and forearm are in the same position as when they hang relaxed at the side of the body.

The steps for assessing postural stresses are as follows.

1. Observe the worker on a videotape; identify stressful postures and corresponding work elements.
2. Identify factors affecting posture, e.g., work location, orientation, tool shape, etc.
3. Determine the frequency and duration of stressful postures.
4. Quantify postures using psychophysical methods or gonimeters.

Examples
Automobile worker (see Table 3-2)

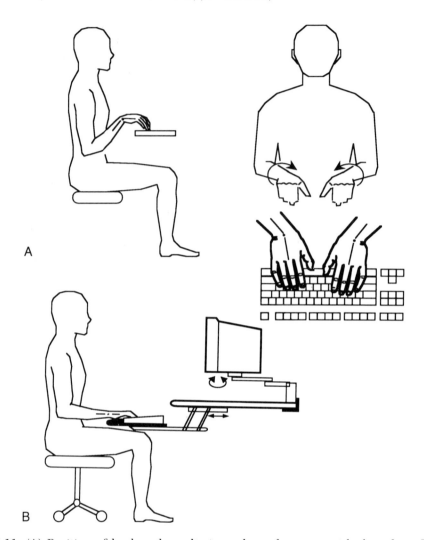

Fig. 3-11. (A) Position of keyboard results in prolonged contact with the edge of the work surface and wrist flexion, ulnar deviation, and inward forearm rotation. **(B)** Contact stresses and wrist posture may be controlled by placing the keyboard on an adjustable keyboard tray. (From Armstrong,[51] with permission.)

1. Stressful postures and work elements—elevation of the elbow, inward rotation of the forearm, and wrist flexion to drive screws (Fig. 3-13)
2. Posture factors—pistol-shaped tool, used on horizontal bench surface 100 cm above the floor
3. Posture frequency—driving 480 screws per hour
4. Postures were quantified in an automobile trim operation by having workers rate posture on a scale of zero (very comfortable) to ten (very uncomfortable).[66] The ratings for 33 workers using 23 tools are plotted as a function of vertical and horizontal location in Figure 3-14. These results show that preferred vertical work

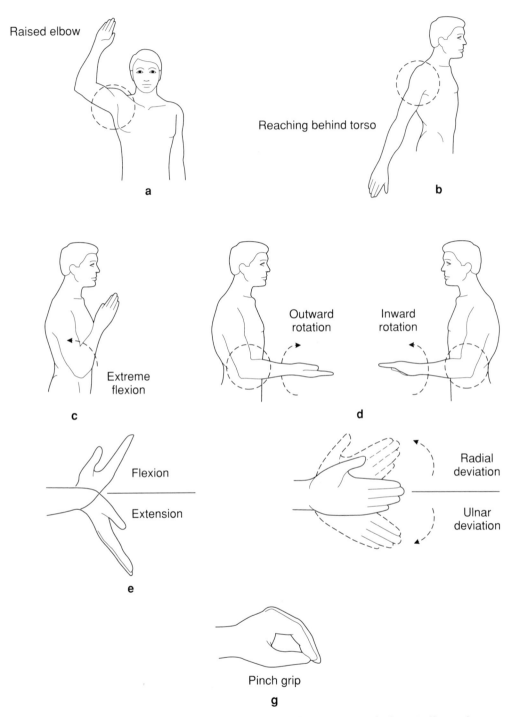

Fig. 3-12. Stressful postures for prolonged or repeated exertions include (**A**) elbow elevation, (**B**) reaching behind the torso, (**C**) extreme elbow flexion, (**D**) extreme forearm rotation, (**E**) wrist flexion or extreme wrist extension, (**F**) wrist deviation, and (**G**) pinching. (From Armstrong,[77] with permission.)

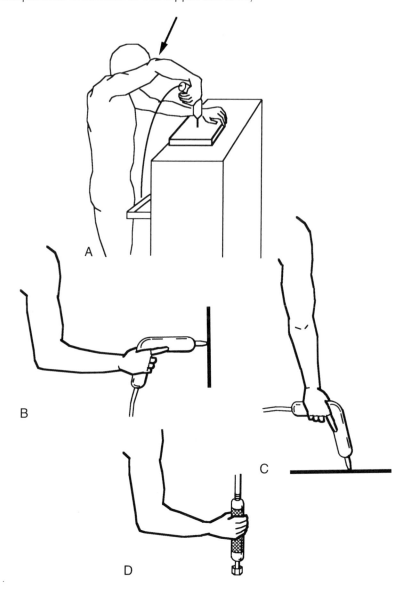

Fig. 3-13. (**A**) Driving screws into headlights requires workers to flex their wrist. This posture can be controlled by reorientation of the work object, (**B**) relocation of the work object, (**C**) or by using a different tool (**D**). From Armstrong,[50,51] with permission.)

locations were between 100 and 150 cm and horizontal locations within 40 cm.

Poultry worker (see Table 3-3)

1. Stressful postures and work elements—radial and ulnar deviation of the wrist inward rotation of the forearm while cutting thighs
2. Posture factors—straight knife, type of cut, and turkey location and orientation

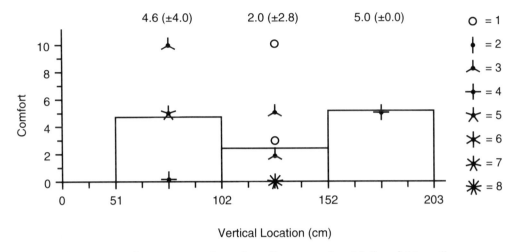

Fig. 3-14. Posture comfort ratings, where 0 = "very comfortable" and 10 = "very uncomfortable," plotted as a function of vertical (**A**) and horizontal (**B**) work location for 23 workers using 33 tools in automobile trim operation. Workers are most comfortable when work is located between 100 and 150 cm. (From Armstrong et al.,[66] with permission.)

3. Posture frequency—4,320 cuts per hour
4. Postures were quantified by observing films taken at three frames per second.[69] Films were replayed using a stop action camera, and observers classified flexion-extension into one of five posture ranges and radial-ulnar deviation into one of three ranges. The results show that poultry workers flex and deviate their wrist with each cut (Fig. 3-15).

Computer analyst (see Table 3-4)

1. Stressful postures and work elements—inward rotation of forearms, ulnar deviation and flexion of wrists while keying (Fig. 3-11)
2. Posture factors—sitting height of worker, elevation and orientation of keyboard and keys
3. Posture frequency—none to continuous
4. No further analysis was performed.

Low Temperature

Cooling of the highly innervated skin of the fingers to 0 to 20°C has been shown to profoundly affect strength, dexterity, and sensitivity.[78] When working in a cold environment, people with normal finger sensory function usually exert slightly more force than is required to keep objects from slipping out of the hand. For example, Flatt[79] estimated that normal subjects exert approximately 4 pounds per square inch on the handle of a hammer; however, when the hand is anesthetized they responded by exerting as much as 16 pounds per square inch. Most people have experienced this effect when working outside on a cold day. Increased force due to low temperatures will make the job more stressful. Cases of tenosynovitis due to frostbite have been reported even when there is no dermal necrosis.[80] Sources of cold exposure include ambient

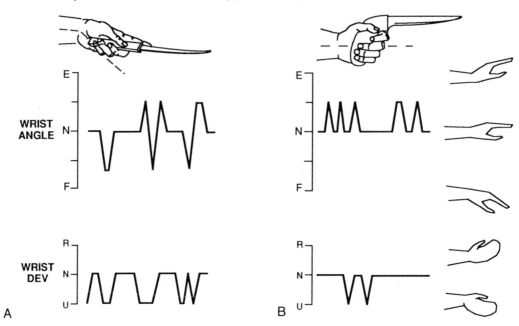

Fig. 3-15. (A) Trimming turkey thighs requires repeated deviation and flexion of the wrist. (B) This posture can be controlled by using a pistol-shaped handle. (From Armstrong et al.,[69] with permission.)

air, work materials, and the exhaust from air tools.

The steps for identification of cold exposure include the following:

1. Identify cold objects or materials that contact the body, particularly the hands, e.g., work objects, materials, air, etc.
2. Assess factors that affect cooling of the hand, e.g., temperature, thermal conductivity, gloves, clothing, etc.
3. Determine duration of exposure.

Examples
Automobile worker (see Table 3-2)

1. Cold exposure—exhaust air leaking around trigger cooling handle and fingers
2. Cooling factors:
   • temperature of exhaust air

• high thermal conductivity of metal handle
• absence of gloves
• exhaust air leaks around the trigger, continuous exposure
3. Frequency of cold exposure—continuous

Poultry worker (see Table 3-3)

1. Cold exposure
   • ambient air 5°C
   • turkeys—2°C
2. Cooling factors—clothing and gloves
3. Frequency of cold exposure
   • continuous exposure to ambient air
   • holding turkey thighs approximately 50 percent of time—air exposure 50 percent

Computer analyst (see Table 3-4)—no significant cold exposure

Vibration

Vibration is a frequently reported caus-ative factor of upper limb cumulative trauma disorders, particularly peripheral nerve disorders. Vibration exposure may result from using some power tools, hold-ing the controls of a powered machine, or using percussion tools, such as hammers and chisels. Exposure to vibration can be identified from the methods analysis; however, measurement of vibration re-quires special equipment and training. A discussion of vibration measurement is beyond the scope of this chapter, and the reader is referred to one of the many ex-cellent works on this subject.[81]

The steps for determining vibration ex-posure are as follows.

1. Identify vibration exposure from in-spection of work elements or obser-vation of worker.
2. Identify factors affecting vibration ex-posure.
3. Determine frequency of exertion.

Auto worker (see Table 3-2)

1. Vibration exposure—driving screws
2. Vibration factors
   • the type of clutch used to regulate torque, e.g., air shut-off or slip-clutch
   • the alignment of the bit and the screw
3. 460 Exposures per hour

Poultry worker (see Table 3-3), no sig-nificant vibration exposure identified
Computer analyst (see Table 3-4)—no significant vibration exposure identified

CONTROL—INTERVENTIONS

Interventions can be designed after in-vestigating alternative ways of doing the job to eliminate stresses identified in the job analysis.[16,50,51,66] They may involve changing the process, materials, tools, work station, or methods or standard. The design of interventions is greatly facili-tated by working with members of the er-gonomic team who often have many years of experience with that technology.

Some ways of controlling posture in-clude the following:

• Automobile assembly—stressful pos-tures can be controlled by changing the tool or work station used in auto assembly (Fig. 3-12)
• Poultry processing—posture can be controlled by changing the knife used in poultry processing (Fig. 3-14)
• Computer analyst—posture can be controlled by placing the keyboard on an adjustable mount (Fig. 3-15)

It is not uncommon to introduce a new piece of equipment only to have it re-jected by the workers because it is not installed or adjusted properly or they do not understand how to use it. Education of the workers in the proper adjustment and use of new equipment is essential.

It is also essential that all interventions be evaluated to ascertain their effective-ness. Often, an intervention may work in one situation, but not in another. Possible evaluations strategies include doing a drawing-board analysis, making mock-ups or prototypes of the new design, and doing a re-analysis of jobs and surveil-lance as described above. Several modi-fications of interventions and evaluations may be required to control a given prob-lem.

SUMMARY

Upper limb cumulative trauma disor-ders are a major cause of worker impair-ment, disability, and compensation in contemporary work settings. Prevention of these disorders is best achieved by organizing an ergonomics program. This program should include surveillance to identify affected workers and jobs, medical evaluations and interventions, job analysis and interventions, and evaluation of all interventions. The ergonomics program should be managed by a team of people from medical, safety, management, supervision, labor, and engineering. Training should be provided to members of the team, workers, supervisors, and managers so that they can cooperate in the management of the program. Job analysis should include documentation and an ergonomic assessment of repeated and sustained exertions, forces, localized mechanical stresses, posture stresses, vibration, and low temperatures. Interventions may be designed to reduce or eliminate ergonomic stresses. Workers and supervisors must be trained in the proper use of the interventions. All interventions should be evaluated on an ongoing basis to evaluate and improve their effectiveness.

REFERENCES

1. Ramazzini B: Treatise on the Diseases of Workers. Translated by WC Wright. Hafner Publishing Co, New York, 1964
2. Dawson WJ: Reed-maker's elbow. Med Prob Performing Artists 1:24, 1986
3. Dobyns JH, O'Brien ET, Linscheid RL, Farrow GM: Bowler's thumb: diagnosis and treatment. J Bone Joint Surg 54A:751, 1972
4. Howell AE, Leach RE: Bowler's thumb. J Bone Joint Surg 52A:379, 1970
5. McCowann T: Spce-invaders' wrist, letter. N Engl J Med 306:751, 1982
6. Minuk GY, Waggoner JG, Hoofnagle JH, Hanson RG, Pappas SC: Pipefitter's thumb, letter. N Engl J Med 306:751, 1982
7. Moidel RA: Bowler's thumb. Arthritis Rheum 24:972, 1981
8. Neiman R, Ushiroda S: Slot-machine tendinitis, letter. N Engl J Med 305:1368, 1981
9. Parsons JS: Tobacco-primer's wrist, letter. N Engl J Med 305:768, 1981
10. Reinsein L: De Quervain's stenosing tenosynovitis in a video games player. Arch Phys Med Rehabil 64:434, 1984
11. Thurn JR: Wall washer's thumb, letter. Ann Intern Med 99:412, 1983
12. Waugh D: Cuber's thumb, letter. N Engl J Med 305:786, 1981
13. Campbell CS: Gamekeeper's thumb. J Bone Joint Surg 37B:143, 1955
14. Goldie I: Epicondylitis lateralis humeri (epicondylalgia or tennis elbow) a pathogenetical study. Acta Chir Scand, suppl. 339:1, 1961
15. Sandler SA: Racquetball wrist, letter. N Engl J Med 299:494, 1978
16. Armstrong TJ: Ergonomics and cumulative trauma disorders. Hand Clin 2:553, 1968
17. Hershenson A: Cumulative injury: a national problem. J Occup Med 21L674, 1979
18. McPhee B: Musculoskeletal complaints in workers engaged in repetitive work in fixed postures, p. 101. In Bullock MI (ed.): Ergonomics: The Physiotherapist in the Workplace. Churchill Livingstone, New York, 1990
19. Hymovich L, Lindholm M: Hand, wrist, and forearm injuries: the result of repetitive motions. J Occup Med 8:573, 1966
20. U.S. Department of Labor: Recordkeeping Requirements Under the Occupational Safety and Health Act of 1970. U.S. Government Printing Office, Washington, DC, 1978
21. Browne CD, Nolan BM, Faithfull DK: Occupational repetition strain injuries: guidelines for diagnosis and management. Med J Aust 140:329, 1984
22. Chatterjee DS: Repetition strain injury—a recent review. J Soc Occup Med 37:100, 1987
23. Ferguson DA: "RSI:" putting the epidemic to rest. Med J Aust 147:213, 1987
24. Kiesler S, Finholt T: The mystery of RSI. Am Psychologist 43:1,004, 1988

25. Bammer G, Blignaut I: More than a pain in the arms: a review of the consequences of developing occupational overuse syndromes (OOSs). J Occup Health Safety Aust NZ 4:389, 1988

26. World Health Organization: Identification and Control of Work-Related Diseases. Who Technical Report Series 714, 1985

27. Hadler N: Medical management of the regional musculoskeletal diseases. Grune & Stratton, New York, 1984

28. Goldstein SA, Armstrong TJ, Chaffin DB, Matthews LS: Analysis of cumulative strain in tendons and tendon sheaths. J Biomechan 20(1):1, 1987

29. Lundborg G, Gelberman RH, Minteer-Donvery M, Lee YF, Hargens AR: Median nerve compression in the carpal tunnel—functional response to experimentally induced controlled pressure. J Hand Surg 7:252, 1982

30. Armstrong TJ, Castelli WA, Evans G, Diaz-Perez R: Some histological changes in carpal tunnel contents and their biomechanical implications. J Occup Med 26:197, 1984

31. Szabo RM, Chidgey LK: Stress carpal tunnel pressures in patients with carpal tunnel syndrome and normal patients. J Hand Surg 14A:624, 1989

32. Sunderland S: The nerve lesion in the carpal tunnel syndrome. J Neurol Neurosurg Psychiatr 39:615, 1976

33. Feuerstein M, Papciak A, Hoon R: Biobehavior mechanisms of chronic low back pain. Clin Psychol Rev 7L243, 1987

34. Harms-Ringdahl K, Brodin H, Eklund L, Borg G: Discomfort and pain from loaded passive joint structures. Scand J Rehabil Med 15:205, 1983

35. Harms-Ringdahl K, Ekholm J: Intensity and character of pain and muscular activity levels elicited by maintained extreme flexion position of the lower cervical-upper thoracic spine. Scand J Rehabil Med 18:117, 1986

36. Daniel RK, Breidenbach WC III, Warren C: Tendon: structure, organization, and healing, p. 383. In The Musculoskeletal System—Embryology, Biochemistry, and Physiology. American Academy of Orthopedic Surgeons, Park Ridge, Ill, 1982

37. Gelberman R, Goldbery V, An K-N, Banes A: Tendon, p. 383. In Woo S S-L, Buckwalter JA (eds.): Injury and Repair of the Musculoskeletal Soft Tissues 1987

38. Cannon LJ, Bernack EJ, Walter SD: Personal and occupational factors associated with carpal tunnel syndrome. J Occup Med 23:255, 1981

39. Armstrong TJ, Fine LJ, Goldstein SA, Lifshitz YR, Silverstein BA: Ergonomic considerations in hand and wrist tendinitis. J Hand Surg 12A:830, 1987

40. Silverstein BA, Fine LJ, Armstrong TJ: Occupational factors of carpal tunnel syndrome. Am J Indust Med 11:343, 1987

41. Stock SR: Workplace ergonomic factors and the development of musculoskeletal disorders of the neck and upper limbs: a meta-analysis. Am J Indust Med 19:87, 1991

42. Basmajian JV, De Luca CJ: Muscles spared when ligaments suffice, p. 239. In Muscles Alive: Their Functions Revealed by Electromyography. Williams & Wilkins, Baltimore, 1985

43. Basmajian JV, De Luca CJ: Muscle fatigue and time-dependent parameters of the surface EMG signal, p. 201. In Muscles Alive: Their Functions Revealed by Electromyography. Williams & Wilkins, Baltimore, 1985

44. Chaffin DB: Localized muscle fatigue—definition and measurement. J Occup Med 15:346, 1973

45. Rohmort W: Problems in determining rest allowances. Part 1: Use of modern methods to evaluate stress and strain in static muscular work. Appl Ergonomics 4(2):91, 1973

46. Hagberg M: Work load and fatigue in repetitive arm elevations. Ergonomics 24(7):543, 1981

47. Hagberg M: Occupational musculoskeletal stress and disorders of the neck and shoulder: a review of possible pathophysiology. Int Arch Occup Environ Health 53:269, 1984

48. Viikari-Juntura E: Tenosynovitis, periteninitis, and the tennis elbow syndrome. Scand J Work Environ Health 10:442, 1984

49. Armstrong TJ, Silverstein BA: Upper ex-

tremity pain in the workplace–role of usage in causality, p. 333. In Regional Musculoskeletal Illness. Grune & Stratton, New York, 1987

50. Armstrong JT, Radwin RG, Hansen DJ, Kennedy KW: Repetitive trauma disorders: job evaluation and design. Hum Factors 28:325, 1986

51. Armstrong TJ: Ergonomics and cumulative trauma disorders of the hand and wrist, p. 1175. In Hunter, Schneider, Machin Callahan (eds.): Rehabilitation of the Hand: Surgery and Therapy. CV Mosby, St. Louis, MO, 1989

52. Kinser WH: Thumb neuroma: a hazard of ten-pin bowling. Br J Plast Surg 29:225, 1976

53. Hanrahan LP, Moll MB: Injury surveillance. Am J Publ Health, suppl. 79:38, 1989

54. U.S. Department of Labor: Ergonomics Program Management Guidelines for Meatpacking Plants, OSHA 3121. U.S. Department of Labor, Washington, DC, 1990

55. Fine LJ, Silverstein BA, Armstrong TJ, Anderson C: Detection of cumulative trauma disorders of the upper extremities in the workplace. J Occup Med 28:674, 1986

56. Buckle P: Musculoskeletal disorders of the upper expremities: the use of epidemiological approaches in industrial settings. J Hand Surg 12A:885, 1987

57. BNA Occupational Safety and Health Reporter. The Bureau of National Affairs. Washington, DC, 1990

58. Katz JN, Larson MG, Fossel AH, Liang MH: Validation of a surveillance case definition of carpal tunnel syndrome. Am J Publ Health, suppl. 79:38, 1989

59. Hennekens CH, Buring JE, Mayrent SL (eds.): Epidemiology in Medicine. Little Brown, Boston, 1987

60. Corlett EN, Bishop RP: The ergonomics of spot welders. Appl Ergonomics 3:23, 1978

61. Kuorinka I, Jonsson B, Kilbom, Vinterberg, Biering-Sorenson, Andersron G, Jorgensen K: Standardized Nordic health questionnaires for the analysis of musculoskeletal symptoms. Appl Ergonomics 18:233, 1987

62. Karlquist L, Bjorksten MG: Design for prevention of work related musculoskeletal disorders, p. 149. In Bullock MI (ed.): Ergonomics: The Physiotherapist in the Workplace. Churchill Livingstone, New York, 1990

63. Liker JK, Joseph BS, Armstrong TJ: From ergonomic theory to practice: organizational factors affecting the utilization of ergonomic knowledge, p. 563. In Hendrick HW, Brown O (eds.): Human Factors in Organizational Design and Management. Elsevier Science Publishers, Amsterdam, 1984

64. Ash RA: Job analysis in the world of work, p. 3. In Gael S (ed.): The Job Analysis Handbook for Business, Industry, and Government, 1988

65. Armstrong TJ, Foulke JA, Marin BJ, Rempel D: An investigation of finger forces in alphanumeric keyboard work. Proceedings of the 11th Congress of the International Ergonomics Society, Paris, July 15, 1991

66. Armstrong TJ, Punnett L, Ketner P: Subjective worker assessments of hand tools used in automobile assembly. Am Indust Hyg Assoc J 51:639, 1989

67. Snook SH: The design of manual handling tasks. Ergonomics 2:963, 1978

68. Herrin GD, Jaraiedi J, Anderson CK: Prediction of overexertion injuries using biomechanical and psychophysical models. Am Indust Hyg Assoc J 46:322, 1986

69. Armstrong TJ, Foulke JA, Joseph BS, Goldstein SA: Investigation of cumulative trauma disorders in a poultry processing plant. Am Indust Hyg Assoc J 43:103, 1982

70. Lundervold AJS: Electromyographic investigations of position and manner of working in typewriting. Acta Physiol Scand, suppl. 24: 1951

71. Buchholz B, Frederick LJ, Armstrong TJ: An investigation of human palmar skin friction and the effects of materials, pinch force, and moisture. Ergonomics 31:317, 1988

72. Armstrong TJ: Mechanical considerations of skin in work. Am J Indust Med 8:463, 1985

73. Phalen GS: The carpal-tunnel syndrome:

seventeen years' experience in diagnosis and treatment of 644 hands. J Bone Joint Surg 48A:211, 1966

74. Smith EM, Sonstegard DA, Anderson WH: Carpal tunnel syndrome: contribution of flexor tendons. Arch Phys Med Rehabil 58:379, 1977

75. Brain WR, Wright AD, Wilkinson ML: Spontaneous compression of both median nerves in the carpal tunnel. Lancet 2:277, 1947

76. Tichauer ER: Some aspects of stress of forearm and hand in industry. J Occup Med 8:63, 1966

77. Armstrong TJ: Upper extremity posture: definition, measurement, and control, p.

59. In Corlett N, Wilson J, Manenica I (eds.): The Ergonomics of Working Posture. Taylor and Francis, London, 1986

78. Shiefer RE, Kok R, Lewis MI, Meese GB: Finger skin temperature and manual dexterity—some intergroup differences. Appl Ergonomics 15:135, 1984

79. Flatt AF: Kinesiology of the hand. Am Acad Orthopoaed Surg Instructional Course Lectures SO: 902, 1961

80. Georgitis J: Extensor tenosynovitis of the hand from cold exposure. J Maine Med Assoc 69:129, 1978

81. Brammer AJ, Taylor W: Vibration Effects of the Hand and Arm in Industry. John Wiley and Sons, New York, 1982

4

The Legal Basis of Workers' Compensation

Edward M. Welch, J.D.

This chapter explores the legal and theoretical structure of the workers' compensation system in the United States. It examines briefly each important concept in the system and gives special attention to how disability is measured.

There is such great diversity among the state workers' compensation systems that no chapter of this size can give a specific explanation of how the system is applied to a given state. Readers will need to look to local resources to determine how the basic principles of workers' compensation have been applied in their jurisdiction.

THE GREAT COMPROMISE

The worker's compensation system is a trade-off, a compromise. Before its introduction in about 1911, persons injured on the job could only be compensated if they could show that the employer was in some way negligent or at fault and that they were completely free from fault. If workers could prove this, however, they could recover whatever damages a jury might grant, including compensation for pain and suffering and loss of enjoyment of life.

Workers' compensation was introduced in Wisconsin in 1911 and quickly spread to other states. Under this system workers do not need to prove that the employer was at fault or that they were free from fault. If they are injured on the job, benefits are paid regardless of who was to blame. It is thus what has come to be called a no-fault system. At the same time workers are now limited in the damages that they can receive. They can recover a specified amount of indemnity benefits, payment of their medical expenses, and usually some form of vocational rehabilitation. They receive these benefits and nothing more.

COVERAGE AND INSURANCE

Almost all employees in the United States are covered by workers' compensation. Most are covered under state laws, but some, such as employees of the federal government, are covered under special federal laws. Self-employed workers are not "employees" of anyone and thus are usually not covered. Therefore, disputes often arise over whether a person is an *employee* covered under workers' compensation or an *independent contractor* who is not covered.

If workers are covered, then workers' compensation benefits are the only damages that they can receive from their employer. With only a few exceptions they cannot sue the employer in a civil action. Workers' compensation is thus the *exclusive remedy* that workers have against their employer. If however, someone else—a third party—was responsible for the injury, that person can be sued.

All states require employers to provide some assurance that they can pay the benefits that they might owe to their workers. Most often this is in the form of an insurance policy. Usually the insurance can be purchased from a number of private insurance companies, but a few states have an exclusive state fund that is in effect the only insurance company allowed to write this kind of business. Most states also allow companies to be self-insured if they can convince the state that they are financially sound and large enough to undertake this risk.

ELIGIBILITY FOR BENEFITS

For a specific injury or disease to be covered it must *arise out of and in the course of* the employment. *In the course of* means that the injury must have occurred while the employee was at work as opposed to at home or doing recreational activities. Generally an injury occurring when a worker is going to or coming from work will not be covered unless he or she was "on the premises" when it

happened. Injuries that occur during lunch hours, when traveling, and while engaged in "horseplay" are troublesome and may or may not be covered, depending on the laws of a given state.

The *arising out of* requirement means that the work must have, in some sense, "caused" the disability. Usually the work does not have to be the sole cause of the disability. It is generally sufficient if the work contributed to the problem or aggravated a pre-existing condition. There is an old rule of law that is applicable to many areas, including workers' compensation, that a person "takes his victim as he finds him." Thus, it might be that two workers could perform the same repetitive motions with their hands, and only one would develop a disability. Presumably, this disability is related, at least to some extent, to a predisposition in one of these individuals to be susceptible to it. This predisposition is *not* a defense for the employer. In most states, a pre-existing condition will not result in a denial of benefits. In some states benefits will be reduced if it can be shown that the pre-existing condition in itself created a partial disability.

Originally most states had the requirement that, to be compensable, an injury must in some way have been an accident. The importance of this requirement has diminished over the years. Now it is usually sufficient that either the cause of the injury or the result of the event was unexpected. Thus, if a worker is injured as the result of an ordinary lifting incident, it might be said that, although the lift was not an accident, the injury was an accidental result of the lift.

In order to encourage employers to hire workers with a missing limb or the loss of sight in an eye, most states have set up a *second injury fund*. If a worker with one lost member loses a second, the worker receives the usual benefits payable to a person with two lost members, but the fund helps the employer pay the cost. Over the years the special funds have been assigned a variety of different responsibilities.

Some work-related disabilities do not in any way result from an injury or accident. They are the result of an *occupational disease*. These disabilities are nearly all now covered by workers' compensation, but this was not always the case and under many circumstances they still receive special treatment.

DISABILITY

The determination of who is disabled and the extent of disability is the heart of a workers' compensation system. It is also the area of most interest to physicians. At the same time, it is an area of great complexity and broad diversity among the various jurisdictions.

There is, in fact, so much variation among the jurisdictions that it would be beyond the scope of this chapter to describe the law as it applies to any particular state. Instead, this chapter describes the various alternatives that are used most frequently. Readers will have to determine which approach is used in the state where they practice. To put it differently, this chapter does not provide all of the answers, but does suggest the questions that should be asked.

There are three types of benefits. In general, *temporary disability benefits* are paid for less serious injuries and for a specified time period in more serious injuries. *Permanent total disability benefits* are paid to the most seriously injured workers. *Permanent partial benefits* are paid to workers who have some permanent residual from their injury, but who are not totally disabled. It is this last category that is the most costly and the most troublesome.

By far, the greatest number of cases receive only temporary total benefits. These are the workers who recover in a relatively short period of time and return to their prior jobs. The most costly individual cases, of course, involve permanent total disability. In most states, however, they make up only a relatively small portion of all cases. Cases involving permanent partial disability, although fewer in number than temporary cases and less costly than permanent total disability cases, are nevertheless the most problematic for workers' compensation. Their total cost is larger than either temporary total or permanent total disability cases, and because they are difficult to evaluate, they are the cases in which adjudicators most often seek assistance from physicians in making a determination.

For all three categories, benefits are based on a percentage of the workers' pre-injury earnings or average weekly wage. Most often workers receive benefits equal to two-thirds of the gross average weekly wage. A few states pay benefits equal to 80 percent of the after-tax value of the average weekly wage. In all states, the benefit is subject to some maximum cap. Most frequently, this is set in terms of the state's average weekly wage.

Assume for example that State X had a state average weekly wage of $400 and paid benefits at the rate of two-thirds of the gross pay, up to a maximum of 90 percent of the state's average weekly wage. If Mr. A was earning $300 when he was injured, his rate would be $200 ($300 × $\frac{2}{3}$). If Ms. B was earning $600 when injured, she would receive the maximum rate of $360 per week (the state average weekly wage of $400 per week × 90 percent = $360).

A few states provide cost of living increases for workers who have a permanent total disability. For the vast majority of workers, however, benefits are fixed as of the date of injury, and there is no adjustment for increases in the cost of living.

Temporary Disability

Temporary disability benefits are paid during the period immediately after an injury. This period lasts until either the worker recovers and returns to work or achieves as much recovery from the injury as can be expected. At this point it is said that the workers' condition has *stabilized*. This point in time is usually called the point of *maximum medical improvement*.

Some jurisdictions allow for temporary partial disability benefits. If workers are still recovering from their injury and return to work at a wage less than they earned before the injury, they receive a percentage of the difference between the preinjury wage and the current wage.

Fifteen states place a limit on the number of weeks for which an individual can receive temporary total disability benefits. The limit ranges from 208 weeks in West Virginia to 700 weeks in New Mexico.[1]

Although they comprise the largest number of cases, temporary disability claims are the least controversial. These are usually the cases in which there is an obvious injury, a clear period of disability, and an early return to work. Although more serious cases usually also involve a period of temporary total disability, it is the period during which parties generally agree that some disability exists that should continue to be compensated at least until maximum improvement is reached. Accordingly, there is not great controversy concerning this portion of workers' compensation systems.

Permanent Total Disability

One might think that the cases involving the most serious injuries would be the most troublesome part of the system. In general, however, this is not the case. The category of permanent total disability is reserved for workers with extremely severe injuries, and although there may be controversy as to who fits into that category, it is generally agreed that those individuals are entitled to substantial benefits.

In general, qualification for total and permanent disability requires a finding that such a severe disability is suffered that the worker will never be able to return to gainful employment. Even this seemingly clear standard can, however, be subject to interpretation and controversy. The most troublesome question is whether economic factors are considered when deciding whether a person can return to work.

Suppose Mr. X lives in the woods in northern Minnesota, has very little education, and injures his back. The only work available to a person in his area with his education requires very heavy lifting. He would claim that he is entitled to permanent total benefits because he has a condition that permanently prohibits him from doing the only work at which he can expect to make a living. His employer would argue, however, that if he lived in Minneapolis or had a better education, there would be many jobs that he could do in spite of his injury, and therefore his disability is only partial. States differ in the extent to which they consider geographical, educational, and economic factors in determining permanent total disability.

A few jurisdictions restrict the definition ever further and only award benefits in this category to individuals who have lost two limbs, both eyes, or some combination thereof. In those jurisdictions a situation can arise in which a worker is, for all practical purposes, completely unable to work and for whom there is no hope of improvement but who is still not considered to have a permanent total disability.

Generally, permanent total disability benefits are payable so long as the worker remains disabled. Six states, however, place a limit on the number of weeks of total permanent disability benefits that a worker may receive. The limit ranges from 260 weeks in Massachusetts to 700 weeks in New Mexico.[1]

Permanent Partial Disability

Permanent partial disability is the most difficult part of the workers' compensation system to describe. It accounts for a larger share of workers' compensation costs than any other type of disability. There is also a greater diversity among states in this area than in any other part of the system. The system for compensating permanent partial disability benefits in some states is extremely complex, and there is great controversy over these benefits. Workers argue that benefits paid are not adequate, employers argue that they are too costly, both complain that they are not delivered efficiently, and scholars points out that they are not distributed equitably.

The following discussion attempts to describe some of the considerations in the area of permanent partial disability and provides some examples of how these benefits are paid. Monroe Berkowitz and John F. Burton, Jr.,[2] both of Rutgers University, have written an excellent, in-depth analysis of this topic that should be read by those wishing to pursue the question of permanent partial disability benefits further.

There have been many attempts to categorize permanent and total disability benefits along one continuum or another. Different authors use different terms and sometimes different categories. These categories often overlap and interact. This chapter presents the various choices that are available in the way that per-

manent partial disability can be compensated. These choices are multidimensional and often interact with one another. No state has a "pure" system, as virtually all states employ some combination of the various approaches.

What Is It We Wish to Compensate?

Most commentators point out that, before we examine the specific compensation alternatives, we must look at the basic issue of what it is we wish to compensate. As discussed at the beginning of this chapter, there is a trade-off in the workers' compensation system. Workers are guaranteed the right to recover some benefits regardless of who was at fault. In return they give up the right to some damages for which an employer might otherwise be liable. The general formulation is that a person should be compensated for the work-related consequences of an injury, but not for its personal or social consequences.

Sometimes, however, this formulation seems too harsh. Assume Ms. X is a laborer and suffers the loss of both legs. Clearly, she will be entitled to a very large payment of compensation benefits. In many states she might receive benefits for the rest of her life. Suppose, however, that she was a clerk and that she returned to work in a few months. What should be the compensation? If we are limited to job-related consequences of the injury, this person has suffered only a few months of wage loss, and her compensation should be limited to a percentage of that loss. This however, seems like very little compensation for such a serious injury.

One way to deal with this dilemma is to pay compensation for the physical impairment that results from the injury. The clerk in the example above suffered a serious impairment and thus should receive substantial compensation, even though there was only a small wage loss. In fact, nearly all states pay at least some benefits based on the physical impairment, and for many it is a primary means of determining compensation. Sometimes it is said that impairment is used because a worker should be compensated for the physical loss. Sometimes it is said that impairment is used because it is a convenient way of measuring or predicting the wage loss and serves as a "proxy" for the wage loss. Thus, although the loss is measured by the degree of impairment, it is really the job-related consequences that are being compensated.

Impairment Versus Wage Loss
The most often used approach to analyzing permanent partial disability benefits distinguishes between impairment and wage loss, with loss of wage-earning capacity being seen as somewhere in the middle.

In a pure impairment system an assessment is made of the extent of the workers' physical or mental impairment at the point of maximum medical improvement. The assessment is made by physicians and is based entirely upon the functional limitations that resulted from the injury. Such an assessment might evaluate how much a person could lift, the limitation of motion in the back or a limb, or the capacity of the heart or lungs. It would *not* include such factors as the workers' age, the type of work performed, or the education or skill of the worker.

At the other extreme is a pure wage loss system, in which benefits are based entirely upon the extent of the workers' wage loss as a result of the injury. Benefits are ordinarily paid weekly, and the amount of the wage loss is assessed retrospectively. The payment could potentially be adjusted each week. So long as there is a wage loss related to a compensable injury, benefits are paid, and no

assessment is made of the degree of physical or functional impairment.

In both cases the calculation of the amount of benefits begins with a determination of the preinjury wages. This is usually based on a determination of the workers' average weekly wage. The benefit payment is some percentage of this preinjury wage. Usually this payment is a percentage of the gross wage (most frequently 66 ⅔ percent), but in some states it is based upon the after-tax wage (most frequently 80 percent).

In an impairment system, some arbitrary number of weeks is established as the value of a "whole person." Individual impairments are then assessed as a percentage of the whole person. For example, if a state set 700 weeks as the period of payment for a whole person, the loss of an arm might be rated as 50 percent of a whole person, and if Ms. A suffered such a loss she would receive benefits for 350 weeks.

Assume Ms. A had a rate of $200 per week. In a pure impairment system, she would receive $200 per week for 350 weeks regardless of whether or not she returned to work. If, however, she had only suffered an injury to one finger, the disability might only be rated at 5 percent. She would then receive benefits for 35 weeks (5 percent of 700). Once again these would be paid regardless of whether or not she returned to work. There then could arise a situation in which Ms. A was an attorney and returned to work shortly after the loss of an arm, but continued to receive benefits for 350 weeks even though she had virtually no wage loss; in contrast, Mr. B, a watchmaker who suffered the loss of only one finger, might never return to work, but would only receive benefits for 35 weeks.

Under a pure wage-loss system the extent of the physical injury would not be considered. Ms. A would only receive benefits for those few weeks that she was off, and Mr. B would receive benefits for the rest of his life. If Mr. B returned to work at a lower paying job, he could receive partial benefits. If he were earning $300 per week when injured and the state paid at the rate of two-thirds of the gross wages, he would receive $200 per week when he performed no work. If he returned to work at a job that paid $200, he would now have a wage loss of $100 ($300 − $200 = $100) and would be entitled to a benefit of $66.66 per week ($100 × ⅔ = $66.66).

Incentives are built into both the wage loss and impairment systems. In an impairment system, workers have an incentive to return to work since they can receive both wages and workers' compensation benefits. In contrast, in a wage loss system there is an incentive for the employer to offer workers a job since when they return to work, benefits stop. This is important because the vast majority of all successful rehabilitation occurs when the worker returns to work with the previous employer. Virtually all states following the wage loss system provide that, if a worker refuses an offer of reasonable employment, benefits may be reduced or terminated. Accordingly there is an incentive for the worker in a wage system as well.

There are other trade-offs. In a wage loss system, an employer can be forced to pay full compensation to an individual with a relatively minor injury who, for various reasons, does not return to work. In an impairment system, employers frequently pay substantial compensation to workers who have for all practical purposes recovered and returned to their old job.

Loss of Wage-Earning Capacity
Loss of wage-earning capacity is a concept that falls somewhere in between pure impairment and pure wage-loss. It

is, in fact, used in most systems to modify the extremes mentioned above.

In an impairment system the concept of loss of wage-earning capacity adds the consideration of vocational factors to the assessment of the degree of an impairment. Many states start with an assessment of the amount of physical impairment, but modify this by such vocational factors as the workers' education, skill, age, and the relationship of the particular impairment to the kind of work the person was performing. Thus, if Ms. Jones suffered an injury to her back that prevented her from doing heavy lifting, she would be given a substantially higher impairment rating if she was a dockhand unloading trucks than if she was a file clerk. Virtually all states using the impairment system give some weight to vocational factors. Some, however, give more weight to these factors than others, and some do it explicitly as part of the statute or by a formula, whereas others include these factors in an informal or subjective manner.

Commentators sometimes create two categories, one termed "impairment systems" and another termed "loss of wage-earning capacity systems." They mean that in both cases a prospective assessment is made of the workers' disability, and benefits are paid for a fixed number of weeks regardless of whether or not the individual returns to work. In one category, however, physical or mental limitations are the overriding criteria. In the other physical or mental limitations are explicitly modified by vocational factors.

In wage loss systems the concept of wage-earning capacity is also sometimes used to soften the extreme cases. In many such systems an employer can establish that individuals have a certain wage-earning capacity even though they are receiving no actual wages. In this situation the workers' loss of wage-earning capacity is less than their actual wage loss, but benefits are limited to the loss of wage-earning capacity.

For example, assume Mr. X was a heavy laborer earning $400 per week at the time he was injured. As a result of his injury he is now limited from performing very heavy work, but could perform a variety of medium and light duty jobs. In a pure wage loss system, his benefits would be based upon a wage loss of $400 per week unless he actually receives some earnings. Suppose, however, that his employer could establish by credible testimony that Mr. X had the capacity to perform a variety of jobs that would pay $300 per week. In other words, he had a wage-earning capacity of $300 per week and a loss of wage-earning capacity of only $100 per week. Many wage loss states would hold that his benefits are limited to a wage-loss of only $100 per week.

The factors that are taken into consideration in determining the worker's wage-earning capacity vary greatly by state. The most difficult question here is the extent to which general economic factors are taken into account. For example, why is it that Mr. X is not, in fact, earning $300 per week? Are there jobs that he could really obtain, or are these merely theoretical jobs? Is he simply too lazy to go out and get a job, or is here an economic downturn such that he has no real prospect of being hired? What if there are jobs that he could do and there are vacancies in these jobs, but no one will hire Mr. X because he has a history of having had a back injury? States that use the loss of wage-earning capacity to limit the application of the wage loss principle vary in the ways they answer these questions.

Some wage loss states require that workers demonstrate that they have performed a *job search*. That is, workers can only obtain wage loss benefits if it can be shown that they have attempted to obtain work and have been unable to do so because of the injury. States vary a great deal in how strictly they enforce this requirement.

Other Variations

There are numerous other ways in which states assess permanent partial disability. Some states use schedules, a listing of how many weeks are payable for specified disabilities. Some states restrict their schedules to the most serious injuries, such as an amputation or injuries that are the equivalent of an amputation. At the other extreme, some states have a schedule that purports to cover every conceivable disability. Some states apply their schedules to the extremities and perhaps the trunk, but not to internal organs or psychiatric conditions. In some states, a worker is paid impairment-based benefits if the disability fits on the schedule and wage loss benefits if it does not. The American Medical Association *Guidelines to the Evaluation of Permanent Impairment*[3] is the most frequently used "schedule." Some states by law adhere strictly to this rating. Other states use it as a guide, but allow variations from it.

Another important consideration is how the final determination is made. For example, Texas has passed a new law that requires that the final impairment rating be a rating given by a physician based upon the AMA Guides. If two physicians offer differing opinions, a third physician may be brought in, but the judge must ultimately choose one of the numbers suggested by one of the physicians. Most states allow a judge to compromise between numbers that are suggested by physicians. Some states specifically provide that a judge or a disability examiner will adjust the impairment rating given by a physician to take into consideration vocational and economic factors. In some states, the physician is required to base the rating on the AMA Guides or some other schedule. In a few states, the physician is allowed to make a completely subjective judgment about the percent of disability.

Finally, it is important to understand the extent to which a state allows *reopenings* or *settlements*. For example, Michigan appears to have a pure wage loss system, in which benefits are paid retrospectively based on the amount of wage loss. However, it allows a worker and employer to agree to a compromise lump sum "redemption." Some commentators have suggested that this provision essentially converts much of Michigan's system into a prospective impairment system, in which the impairment rating is not based on a medical assessment, but on a negotiation process between attorneys. On the other hand, a state that has a pure impairment system, but allows the parties to reopen and adjust an impairment rating, will generally give consideration to the actual wage loss in making readjustments, even though the original assessment was based entirely on the degree of physical impairment.

MEDICAL AND VOCATIONAL REHABILITATION BENEFITS

Under most circumstances an injured worker is entitled to have all medical expenses paid by the employer. Rules vary as to whether the employer or the worker can choose the physician. In rare instances benefits can be terminated for refusal to accept reasonable medical care. Recently, there has been much emphasis on efforts to control the cost of medical benefits.

Nearly everyone agrees that vocational rehabilitation is worthwhile, but there is a great deal of controversy over how it should be done and when it is appropriate. In some states it is mandatory; in oth-ers it is optional. Sometimes vocational rehabilitation involves nothing more than having the worker make phone calls to prospective employers. Sometimes it can lead to a college education.

ADMINISTRATION AND PROCEDURES

All jurisdictions have a commission, bureau, or other agency that is responsible for the administration of workers' compensation. How active this agency is varies among states. In some states it must approve the payments in virtually every case. In others, the agency only becomes involved when there is a dispute.

There are time limits within which a worker must report an injury and file a claim. These are often interpreted quite liberally.

Unfortunately, workers' compensation is an area fraught with many controversies. In some states attorneys are involved in a large percentage of cases. In some cases the worker and employer must agree on the outcome of a case, or it is automatically reviewed by the state agency. In others it is the responsibility of workers to file a dispute if they are not satisfied with what the employer pays. In nearly all states, workers' compensation cases are heard by special judges without a jury. There is a right to appeal to the courts, but this may be limited to legal and not factual disputes. Recently many states have begun emphasizing mediation and other forms of alternate dispute resolution.

WHO BEARS THE LOSS?

It is often said that workers' compensation is a system for shifting or spreading the cost of on-the-job injuries. It is the conventional wisdom that the loss is shifted to consumers. A few people complain about this shifting, but most consider it appropriate. It is said that, if a certain number of people are hurt for every car that is manufactured, then the cost of those injuries should be passed on to the people who buy the cars. In any event this assumption is widely held by lawyers, administrators, and politicians. There are however, reasons to doubt the validity of this assumption. These reasons are both practical and theoretical.

First, certain portions of the loss must necessarily be borne by the injured worker. Some physical and emotional consequences of an injury can never be shifted to anyone else, no matter how hard we try. Furthermore, the system does not even try to shift all of the loss from the worker. As mentioned at the outset of this chapter, it does not even attempt to compensate the worker for pain and suffering. Furthermore, it does not compensate the worker fully for the wage loss. Instead, approximately two-thirds of the lost wages are covered.

There are also many who doubt that the costs actually assigned to the employer can be shifted to consumers. In today's competitive global economy, a business cannot necessarily raise the price of its product or service merely because workers' compensation costs increase. Although some of the cost is undoubtedly passed on to the consumer, some is made up for by a reduction in wages paid to all workers. This reduction may not come immediately, but studies do indicate that, when workers compensation costs go up, wages tend to go down. Finally, it is likely that some part of the cost of workers' compensation comes out of profits. Some economists suggest that it is appropriate that workers' compensation losses should affect profits. This, it is suggested, will create an incentive for employers to implement safety and return to work programs.

REFERENCES

1. U.S. Department of Labor: State Workers' Compensation Laws. U.S. Government Printing Office, Washington, DC, 1990
2. Berkowitz M, Burton JF Jr: Permanent Disability Benefits in Workers' Compensation. W. E. Upjohn Institute for Employment Research, Kalamazoo, MI, 1987
3. American Medical Association: AMA Guidelines to the Evaluation of Permanent Impairment. American Medical Association, Chicago, 1991

5

A Practical Approach to Workers' Compensation

Edward M. Welch, J.D.

Chapter 4 described the workers' compensation system in legal terms. This chapter takes a much more practical approach to workers' compensation. It begins with a discussion of some research that has demonstrated that individual employers can exercise remarkable control over their workers' compensation experience. It then discusses the role of physicians in the workers' compensation system and concludes by looking briefly at the role of attorneys.

STRATEGIES THAT LOWER COST AND REDUCE WORKER SUFFERING

In the past, workers' compensation has been seen primarily as a legal problem. If workers did not receive the benefits that they thought they deserved, they hired a lawyer and sued the employer. If employers thought they were paying too much money in benefits, they approached the legislature and sought a change in the law. We need to take a new,

better approach to workers' compensation. There is evidence that some companies are treating workers' compensation as a human resource management problem and that they are being very successful in this approach. They are using new strategies designed by the employers primarily to save money. Remarkably, these same strategies also benefit workers.

The Michigan Research

Are there really strategies that both lower costs and reduce workers' suffering? The Michigan Bureau of Workers' Disability Compensation has conducted some research that suggests that indeed those two aims can be achieved at the same time.[1] The research shows great variability in workers' compensation experience among Michigan employers. In examining what accounts for these differences, it identifies factors that appear to benefit both the employers and workers.

It has been customary in workers' compensation to focus on interstate differences e.g., is it more costly in Michigan than in Indiana? Beginning in 1987 Michigan sought instead to examine the intrastate differences. Michigan's Bureau of Workers' Disability Compensation contracted with H. Allen Hunt, Ph.D., of the W. E. Upjohn Institute for Employment Research in Kalamazoo, Michigan, to study the variables accounting for these differences. Hunt in turn enlisted the aid of Rochelle Habeck, Ph.D, of the Rehabilitation Counseling Program at Michigan State University and later Michael J. Leahy, Ph.D., also of the Rehabilitation Counseling Program at Michigan State University.

The study examined the workers' compensation experience of approximately 5,000 Michigan firms with 50 or more employees. It compared the number of claims closed in 1986 with the number of workers employed. It was assumed that there would be substantial differences among employers in different industries. Accordingly the study focused on the differences among employers within the same industry.

The study found remarkable differences among employers in the same industry. In fact, it found that these intrastate differences were substantially greater than interstate differences. The National Commission on Unemployment Compensation and Workers' Compensation[2] reports that Michigan's costs are about two times those of Indiana. Maine's costs (the highest cost state) are about six times those of Indiana (the lowest cost state). Because of limitations in the data available, the study looked at frequency of claims, rather than their cost, but there is clearly a relationship between frequency and cost. The Michigan study found that the difference in frequency among employers within Michigan was about tenfold; that is, the "worst"

employers had ten times as many claims as the "best" employers.

The study examined 29 different industries and found this tenfold difference in each of those industries. For example, in the Transportation Equipment Manufacturing Industry, 6 percent of the plants had less than 1 injury per 100 employees, whereas 8 percent had 11 or more injuries per 100 employees. At the same time, 38 percent had less than 3 injuries per 100 employees, and 15 percent had 9 or more injuries per 100 employees.

These large differences among employers within the same state are obviously not attributable to differences in the law. What factors do account for the differences? To answer this question the researchers conducted a mail survey of the high and low frequency employers in four industries: food production, fabricated metals, transportation and equipment, and health services. The survey covered a number of areas, but special attention was focused of three factors:

1. safety and the prevention of accidents
2. management climate and culture
3. disability prevention and management.

The survey asked a series of questions in each category. When the responses from all of the questions in each category were analyzed together, each of the three categories was found to be a significant factor in differentiating between low and high frequency employers.

In summary, the study demonstrated that those employers that most frequently engage in safety and prevention efforts, tend to have an open managerial style and a corporate climate that shares decision making, and make the most effort to prevent and manage disability are the employers most likely to have a low frequency of workers' compensation claims.

How Is It Done?

In conjunction with the School of Labor and Industrial Relations of Michigan State University, Michigan's Bureau of Workers' Disability Compensation has conducted a series of conferences on "Strategies That Lower Cost and Reduce Worker Suffering." LRP Publications has published a book based on the first two such conferences.[3] The following is adapted from the introduction to that book and offers some suggestions on how such strategies can be implemented.

Safety is the first and most obvious factor. Those of us who are involved in workers' compensation programs sometimes overlook this obvious solution. If no one were ever injured, there would be no workers' compensation claims. The first and most important step in controlling workers' compensation costs and protecting employees is thus a comprehensive, effective safety program.

Ergonomics is another factor. For years, engineers have been using their talents to design plants that use as few people as possible. Now we must put these talents to work to design plants that use people in the most efficient way possible. Many employers are finding that the money spent on such changes is repaid in lower disability costs and increased productivity. Sometimes, it requires the expertise of a graduate engineer to design work stations ergonomically. Other times, however, even a minor change will prevent many injuries. Often, a physician is in a position to recognize the need for such changes and can help both employers and workers by offering suggestions along these lines.

Of course, much more than safety is involved. The relationship between the worker and the employer, both before and after an injury, has a great influence on whether an employer will be sued.

Why does someone who has been a loyal and devoted employee for many years decide to hire a lawyer and sue after suffering an injury? Consider the analogy of the football player. Think of what happens when a football player is injured. The action stops, and all attention is focused on the injured player. He is assured, "You'll be all right. We'll take care of you." He is applauded as he is taken off the field. Contrast this to what occurs in most industrial settings. The foreman is told, "Joe thinks he hurt his back." What does the foreman say? Most likely, something obscene. Now of course this scenario is not played out in all plants or with all supervisors. But where it is, it makes a big impression.

The satisfaction of employees with their preinjury work has a direct influence on their response to job-related injury. For example, one Michigan company has an index by which it measures the "quality of work life" in a plant. As one would expect, there is a direct inverse relationship between the quality of work life and workers' compensation costs: when quality of work life is high, costs are low.

Consider the return-to-work situation. The employee is released to return to work with restrictions, but is very scared, thinking, "They'll be out to get me. The least little thing that I do, they'll fire me." At the same time, the employer is afraid to take the worker back: "The least little thing that goes wrong, he'll holler 'comp.'" This is a classic example of a situation in which both parties would profit by the employee's returning to work, but both are afraid to try. Both think they are at a disadvantage.

One company in western Michigan has a different approach. When an individual is about to be released to return to work, the worker is called by the supervisor and invited to have lunch in the plant a few days before the release. The worker sees the old work station, talks with co-workers, learns what to expect, and is welcomed. Is it any wonder that this employer has a good record of getting people back on the job and keeping its costs down.

Employers should visit workers when they are homesick. During my years of practice, workers would often complain to me that, although they put in many good years for a company, when they were lying on their back for 3 months, no one came to see them. I used to reply that they could not expect to be visited by employers and that their companies indeed did not care about them. After becoming Director of Michigan's Bureau of Workers' Disability Compensation, however, I learned that there are companies that do care. They do send supervisors out to visit sick and injured workers. They do it, and they save money.

There are a very few cases in which the worker is lying about the injury, and the legal system deals with those few cases quite well. The claims handling system also deals very well with the large number of cases in which the injury is clear and the symptoms proportionate to what would be expected. The difficult cases are those in which the worker clearly has some injury, but the pain is greater or lasts longer than would ordinarily be anticipated. It is these cases that are challenges for the physicians, employers, claims adjustors, families, and workers themselves. We must examine every possible approach to healing these injured men and women.

Unions must also play a role in this process. Strict seniority rules can be a hindrance to finding lighter duty jobs for injured workers. One very large employer in Michigan for years had a policy that workers must be completely recovered and able to handle all their duties before returning to any job. At one point

the company recognized the futility of this approach and changed its policy to encourage the return to work of partially restricted employees. However, it announced both the change and immediate implementation of the new policy without consulting its union. The union resisted, and the change in policy was a complete failure.

The seniority system is very important to organized labor in the United States. At the same time, it has been my experience that most unions are genuinely concerned about workers who have been injured on the job. When approached within the framework of collective bargaining, unions are nearly always willing to work with an employer to help deal with this situation. The important element is that the union be part of the process.

Many of these ideas are not really new. Insurance companies have been aware of them for a long time. They have often made concerted efforts to influence their policy holders to adopt many of these practices.

There are many more successful strategies that both lower costs and reduce workers' suffering. More information is available from a variety of sources.*

These strategies are the trend of the future. The Michigan research shows that some employers are already using them and saving money. In order to be competitive, more companies will have to adopt them. Many insurance carriers offer "loss control" services, which will similarly be expanded and given more emphasis. State agencies will follow the lead

---

* More information is available in a newsletter and other publications of the author of this chapter. For information, contact *Ed Welch on Workers' Compensation*, 2875 Northwind Drive, Suite 205-B, East Lansing, MI 48823, 517-332-5266.

of Michigan and offer educational programs on these topics. The treating physician can play a very important role in helping employers, unions, and individual workers implement these strategies.

ROLE OF PHYSICIANS

This section focuses on the role that a physician can play in nurturing the employer-employee relationship and in providing information and testimony to the workers' compensation system.

Both individual patients and the workers' compensation system in general depend very heavily on the active participation and cooperation of physicians. Therefore, it is very important that physicians are actively involved with the workers' compensation system, particularly in making judgments about what benefits are to be paid.

Relationship between the Patient and the Employer

The research described earlier suggests that the employer-employee relationship can dramatically affect the number of injuries that occur and the potential recovery of an employee from an injury. This has important implications for physicians. On the one hand, it suggests that, if there is a good employer-employee relationship, treatment is much more likely to be successful. On the other hand, if there is a very bad relationship between the worker and the employer, it is unlikely that there will be a desirable outcome, regardless of how hard the physician works or how good a job is done. Physicians should not be discouraged by this situation. You must understand that there are simply some things beyond your con-

trol, and although you must make great efforts to do your best, you should not be discouraged if outside factors interfere with or frustrate your best efforts.

Yet, there are many situations in which the relationship between the employer and employee is neither clearly good, or bad, but can perhaps best be characterized as "fragile." The physician has a very important role to play in these situations. You have the potential to "heal" the employer-employee relationship, as well as the worker's body. Doing so will enhance greatly the likelihood that the treatment of the physical problem will be successful.

Work-related injury puts great strains on even the best employer-employee relationship. Sometimes even the best employers react in strange ways when a worker is injured. They "blame" the worker for getting hurt and resent the claim for benefits. Workers feel themselves in a vulnerable position. They feel the need to test their employer's loyalties. They are worried about what will happen to them and tend to overreact if there is any feeling that the employer will not support them. The physician is in a unique position to help this situation by facilitating communication of the things that both sides should know or that they do not seem to understand. Tell them what they should know or at least encourage them to talk to one another.

The return to work situation is the setting for the most typical example of misunderstanding. Most employers would like you to give them a simple one-line statement that defines the worker's limitations, e.g., "No lifting over 30 pounds," "One-handed job," "No repetitive motion with right hand," or "No lifting above the shoulder." Of course, the situation is rarely as simple as this, and what is needed is patience and flexibility. No one is going to be very happy with you if you write a report that says, "He could try using his right hand, but only until it gets painful. Then he should stop and rest," or "I would like to try having her use her hands for an hour or so, then rest until it feels better and try again.' Nevertheless, if this is the right advice in the situation, it is your responsibility to give it. The difficulty is in making people understand.

It is important that the physician realize the dynamics of the return-to-work situation. Some workers are desperate to return to their jobs and want you to give them the least restrictions as possible. Others want any excuse not to return and will be seeking the most restrictive limitations. Employees may have more subtle agendas. They may want those restrictions that would require the employer to place the worker on a job that they consider more desirable for reasons not related to the injury. What should you do in those circumstances? Is it best for the physician to adhere very strictly to the technicalities and only make recommendations that relate to the specific injury for which the patient is being treated? Or is it appropriate for the physician to consider the other dynamics? Might it be best in the long run to help the worker obtain the more desirable job for a short period of time? Is this the alternative that is most likely to result in the worker's complete recovery? Such judgments must be made by the physician in every case.

The return to work decision is also influenced by the employer's agenda. Optimally, the human resource manager realizes that the swift, complete recovery of the worker is in everyone's best interest and will work to arrange the job to facilitate this outcome. This is not always the case, however, The workers' compensation manager may want to do everything possible to reduce the company's short-run losses and accordingly will urge you to give the lowest restrictions possible. Or, you may be working with a human resource manager who is looking for the most appropriate restrictions and who is working in good faith to place the worker on the right job. Yet, the worker's first-line supervisor may be under great pressure to meet production demands and may feel at a great disadvantage in taking on the payroll of a worker who is not able to "carry the load." Such a supervisor can sabotage the best efforts of a well-meaning human resource manager. When this happens, the worker feels deceived and is quick to blame everyone involved in the process, including the physician.

Because of the complexities of such situations, it is important for the physician to have as much information as possible, to learn what is going on and to deal as best as possible with the situation.

In closing this section, I would encourage the physician to realize the importance of your role in workers' compensation situations. Even today, when many people are quick to file malpractice suits, physicians still play a very important role in our society. Many people, including injured workers and employers, see physicians as "healers" who can solve problems that go beyond traditional medical issues. Be sensitive to opportunities you have to help people in a variety of ways. Anything you can do to heal a breach in the employer/employee relationship will pay off by expediting the healing of the physical problems.

Reports and Testimony

Treating patients with work-related injuries poses problems for physicians because it places on them an extra burden of filling out forms, preparing reports, and providing testimony. Yet, such tasks are an important part of the help that both workers and employers need from treating physicians. This section offers some advice on making these tasks somewhat easier.

First and foremost, *be a doctor.* Do not try to be the lawyer or the judge. When physicians are embarrassed, when they become embroiled in disputes, or when their opinion is taken lightly, it is most frequently because they tried to play a nonmedical role. To the greatest extent possible, stick with your field of expertise by providing simple, straightforward medical opinions.

Of course, your opinions should be supported by the evidence that led to your conclusion; objective tests, laboratory data, or x-ray findings should be cited wherever possible. A few states require medical opinions to be based on "objective tests." In enacting such provisions, legislators must have assumed that there was some clear dividing line between what are often referred to as "objective" and "subjective" findings. In fact, this line is quite blurred, and in the ordinary practice of medicine, physicians continually rely on subjective complaints, patient histories, and other factors that cannot be quantified.

Although a workers' compensation case might require you to explain your decisions in greater detail than in other cases, you should not make those decisions in a different manner. You may be required to think through the basis of your decision, to put it in writing, and to explain it, but the judgments for injured workers should be made in the same manner that you make all other judgments about surgeries, treatment, or advice that you give.

Of course, workers' compensation cases are unique in that they often require the physician to provide an opinion about the cause of the disability and the extent of the impairment. Very often, the workers' right to benefits and, in some cases, the question of how much income they will have for the rest of their life depend upon the physician's opinion. Many physicians do not see this judgment as part of their primary role. It is nevertheless an obligation that society has placed on physicians.

The role of the physician varies greatly from state to state. In some states the issue will simply be deciding whether a worker can do a specific job. In many states the physician is asked to provide some kind of impairment rating, which is often based upon the *AMA Guidelines to the Evaluation of Permanent Impairment.*[4] In other states it is based on some other set of criteria, and in a few states it is left to the physician's subjective judgment. The degree to which the physician's opinion is binding also varies greatly from state to state. A few states base the award entirely on the physician's impairment rating. In many states, however, it is only one factor in the final determination of the amount of disability. It is important for physicians who frequently offer opinions in workers' compensation cases to do the necessary research to understand the workers' compensation laws applicable to their state.

Filling out Reports

Physicians receive many requests to fill out forms and write reports. What is a lawyer looking for when requesting a medical report from a physician? What do employers or insurance companies want on the forms they send?

The precise question asked on these forms varies from state to state and will depend on the particular circumstances of the case. It may concern causality, the degree of impairment, or whether a worker can return to a specific job. The request for a report or form should indicate the type of question being asked.

The answer should be a simple straightforward opinion, supported by the information that formed its basis—x-rays, laboratory results, objective findings, etc. Attorneys, claims examiners, and adjudicators are also very frequently interested in the history you received for several reasons. First, the law tends to assume that workers and others will give an honest account of their history when they expect it could be used in their treatment. Two, if you obtain the history immediately after the injury, it is assumed that the person's recollection will be most accurate. Finally, in some circumstances when formal litigation is involved, the attorney for the insurance company may have no access to the worker. The worker's own attorney may shield the worker from answering questions directly to the company's lawyer. In these circumstances, attorneys and claims examiners sometimes use examining physicians as their only means of learning how the worker is describing the history of the injury.

Many physicians anticipate requests for reports when they are creating their regular office notes. The initial history and physical examination results, as well as later office visits, are maintained in such a fashion that they can be easily reproduced and mailed to requesting parties as part of a report. It is my experience that doing so is most often acceptable to attorneys, claims adjusters, and courts. If a party has asked specific questions that are not addressed in these documents, you may wish to write a simple paragraph answering those questions and then refer to your other reports as the basis for your conclusion.

Although many of those who deal with workers' compensation, including lawyers, judges, and claims assessors, have considerable experience reading medical records and consider themselves "experts" to some degree or another, you are well advised to state your conclusions in clear terms that are understandable to a layperson, as well as supporting that opinion with the more sophisticated medical findings.

Physicians must, of course, always be conscious of their responsibility for confidentiality. This responsibility is placed on physicians both by the very trusting nature of the patient-doctor relationship and by the law. In general, you should never release information about a patient unless that patient has signed an authorization allowing you to do so. When the employer or insurance company has paid the physician's bill, and especially when it has referred the patient to the physician, it is often assumed that it is permissible for the physician to release information. There is a simple way for the physician to be protected under these circumstances. When you first begin treating such a patient, have the person sign a simple statement that says something to this effect:

> I understand that I have been referred to Dr. _____ by my employer and/or its insurance company. My employer and/or its insurance company will be paying my medical expenses. Accordingly, I hereby authorize Dr. _____ to release to my employer and/or its insurance company information concerning my medical condition and treatment.

The legal necessity for such an authorization may vary from state to state. It is, however, a very simple process and one that I would recommend in every case.

Generally, workers "waive" or give up their right to confidentiality when they file a lawsuit against another party and take medical testimony as part of that case. When you receive an order or subpoena from the court to provide your records, you no longer need to be concerned about whether the information is privileged or confidential. Someone else, an officer of the court, has now taken the responsibility for that determination. If they are wrong, it is they, not you, who will be blamed for the decision.

Offering Testimony

Physicians are often asked to testify in workers' compensation claims. The frequency with which this happens and the form it takes vary from jurisdiction to jurisdiction. In some states written medical reports are admitted into evidence. In others, the opinion of an expert witness, such as a physician, can only be admissible if the other party has a chance to cross-examine the witness. In some jurisdictions physicians regularly come to court to testify. In others, most medical testimony is presented by way of *deposition*. That is, the lawyers for all the parties go to the physician's office and question him or her as if they were in court. The testimony is recorded either electronically or by a stenographer. This process has obvious advantages. First, the deposition can be scheduled at the convenience of the physician, rather than at a time that is subject to the delays that are so common in court hearings. In addition, a deposition that might take an hour to give can usually be read by a judge in much less time. Yet, there is an advantage for the witness in the court situation. If questions or disputes arise, a judge is present in court to monitor the proceedings, respond to objections and, in a sense, to "protect" the witness. In a deposition, objections are placed on the record and ruled upon by the judge at a later time. This sometimes leaves the witness more vulnerable to the tactics of the attorneys.

When is it appropriate for a physician to express his or her personal opinion on a topic as opposed to a medical judgment? This can occur in two situations. The first is the physician's opinion about the law or the entire workers' compensation system. If a physician feels that in general the system is unfair or one-sided, it is best to set aside those feelings to the greatest extent possible when providing information about a given patient. Of course, every citizen who sees problems with our judicial or legal systems should work through the legislative and other political processes to make people aware of those

problems and to seek a solution. However, it is unfair to a given worker or employer to let those feelings change the testimony given in a specific case. If you feel so strongly about the unfairness of a system, it might be best to decline to participate in a case.

A different standard should apply when the physician has a strong feeling about an individual case. It is important that that opinion be placed on the record. For example, a situation might arise in which using the *AMA Guidelines* would result in a specific impairment rating, but the treating physician feels it would be grossly unfair to give that much (or that little) rating to the patient in question. Under those circumstances, it is perfectly appropriate for the physician to express a personal opinion. That opinion, however, should be clearly distinguished from the physician's judgment about the impairment rating. In other words, the physician might say, "Under the *AMA Guidelines* I come up with a rating of 20 percent in this case. But it seems to me there are considerations in this case that make that rating unfair."

It is quite likely that, if a physician offers such an opinion in a deposition, one of the attorneys will object. Yet, the other attorney will ordinarily give the physician an opportunity at the right time to express these feelings and the reasons for them. Some courts may give great weight to these special feelings, and in others they will be ignored totally. In either case, that is a judgment to be made by the judges and the legislature. I believe that it is the physician's role to put his feelings on the record.

Often, physicians encounter problems when they try to discern the reasons for an attorney's questions. Once again, do not try to be the lawyer or judge. It is very hard to outguess an attorney's questions. Indeed, sometimes their purpose is to lead you into a "trap." Other times, questions are phrased in a certain way because of the technicalities of the rules of evidence. Do not rule out the possibility that the attorney is asking questions in a strange way simply out of ignorance of how to phrase them any better. If the question is unclear, ask the attorney to clarify it. In deciding how to respond to a question, do *not* try and figure out what the lawyer is getting at, but rather offer the most simple, common sense reply. It is most likely that the judge, the appeal panel, or whoever reads the record will make the same kind of common sense judgment that you will. Judges tend to doubt the credibility of physicians who are trying to outsmart lawyers, but are very much impressed by physicians who give common sense answers. Never overlook the persuasive power of simple common sense.

Spending a few moments of preparation before giving testimony will pay off in the long run. Read your file over carefully. Pay special attention to reports that you have written concerning this case. It is only reasonable for the attorneys to expect you to remember the opinions you have previously offered. In a deposition, the attorneys may be rustling their papers in your waiting room and acting impatient for their turn. I would encourage you, however, to go into your private office, close the door, review the file, and think about the case. Do not think "What are they going to be asking me?" or "What will they really be trying to get at?" Remember, instead, that you are a person specially trained in dealing with medical problems. You have had years of experience in this area and have undoubtedly seen many patients similar to the one in question. Ask yourself, "What do I think is really going on with this person?" Then ask, "What are the things that lead me to this conclusion?" A few minutes of thinking along this line will prepare you to deal with even the most difficult lawyers.

The rules of evidence have evolved over many years, some for reasons that are not clearly apparent. In some jurisdictions, the strict rules of evidence are not applied to administrative hearings, such as workers' compensation. In some jurisdictions, however, they are applied very strictly. Although a complete discussion of these rules is far beyond the scope of this chapter, there are two areas about which every witness should have a basic knowledge: leading questions and the hearsay rule.

A *leading question* is one that suggests to the witness the answer that should be given. A question that is somehow "tricky," such as, "When did you stop beating your wife?," is not a leading question. Rather, an attorney representing an injured worker who called you as a witness could not ask you, "You think this person is disabled, don't you?" That attorney would be "leading" you into the desired answer. Attorneys are prohibited from asking a leading question of their own witness although during cross-examination of another party's witness, they may do so. This prohibition can sometimes be escaped by calling a person as "an adverse witness."

Hearsay is the statement of a person who is not present and subject to cross-examination and that is given for the truth of the statement. Thus, Ms. X cannot testify, "Dr. Y told me that my work caused by disability." Only Dr. Y can testify about things that he or she knows or believes to be true. The hearsay rule is more famous for its exceptions than for its general application. Many exclamations do not come within the rule. Ms. X could testify that she heard Mr. Y holler "Ouch!" because Mr. Y is not saying "Ouch" to establish the truth of anything. Histories given to physicians for the purpose of treatment are also generally considered exceptions to the hearsay rule, as are many business and hospital records kept in the ordinary course of business. The hearsay rule is, however, used in some states to prohibit the admissibility of medical records in which a physician offers an opinion about the cause or extent of disability. In states that apply the rule strictly, the opinion of a physician is not admissible unless the other party has an opportunity to cross-examine.

How do you deal with an attorney who is being abusive? If the testimony is in court, the judge or hearing officer should provide guidance. This problem is more difficult to deal with in depositions where no judge is present. There is, of course, a point at which you could simply say, "This is too much, I won't put up with this," and leave. In general, however, civility and common sense are rewarded. If the witness joins the fray and descends to the level of the squabbling attorneys, the judge's assessment of the witness will also be lowered. If, on the other hand, the witness can rise above these tactics, remain calm, and give sensible answers, the judge is likely to be highly persuaded by those answers. It is unfortunate that there are many attorneys who stoop to these practices. Yet, you are not alone in finding it offensive. Many lawyers are themselves complaining that their colleagues are exceedingly abusive. There have lately been a growing number of articles in legal journals calling for a return to civility and professionalism.

ROLE OF LAWYERS

Some suggest that many of the problems in workers' compensation are attributable to the role played by attorneys. In most states, attorneys who represent workers are paid a contingent percentage fee. In other words, they are paid a percentage of the benefits that they recover for the individual workers. This is the most appropriate approach for several reasons. First, most workers could not afford to hire competent attorneys if they were required to guarantee the payment of an hourly fee. Second, by having the amount of the attorney's fee coincide with the benefits obtained there is an incentive for attorneys to do the best possible job for their clients.

However, this approach creates an incentive for attorneys to maximize the amount of benefits that a worker will receive when that may not be in the best interest of the system or even of the worker. In some instances individuals are able to return to work but are advised against doing so by their attorney because returning to work will diminish the appearance of disability and thus probably reduce the amount of benefits awarded. In many of these cases, it would clearly be to the long-term advantage of the worker to return to work as soon as possible, even though doing so might result in a lower amount of benefits being paid. How widespread is this practice among attorneys? There is no way to tell us. There have been no studies that attempt to quantify this practice in any way.

Many attorneys do take a more reasonable approach. Most of the referrals an attorney receives are from friends or associates of previous clients. This creates an incentive for attorneys to do what is best for the worker in the long run. Most ethical attorneys realize that it is in their client's best interest to return to work as soon as possible. They also realize that helping their client in this way will, in the long run, be to their benefit, even though it might result in a slightly diminished award and fee in a given case. In recent years, the United States Supreme Court ruled that states may not prevent attorneys from advertising. Advertising has undoubtedly changed the way in which many workers now find attorneys and may have an adverse effect upon the incentive for attorneys to consider their clients' best interest in the long run.

The trial bar plays a very important role in any legislation dealing with workers' compensation. In many states, the debate concerning legislative amendments to workers' compensation pits the business community against organized labor. Very frequently, unions have no independent expertise about workers' compensation and rely on advise from the trial bar. In other states, the trial bar is itself a powerful lobby. The bar argues, of course, that it is only advocating for the rights of injured workers and that is undoubtedly true. That advocacy, however, is usually combined with a point of view that places a great deal of value on formal dispute resolution procedures. It thus often happens that attorneys oppose amendments designed to simplify the dispute resolution process and that might reduce costs significantly. In recent years, a package of workers' compensation amendments that had the support of both business and labor, but that were opposed by the trial bar, has been developed in several states. In general, the bar has not been successful in blocking the passage of such legislation, but it has often jeopardized its success and sometimes forced compromise. In some jurisdictions, such as California, the bar has been joined in its opposition by certain segments of the medical profession.

There will always be some need for lawyers in a workers' compensation system. We are dealing with matters that are very difficult to quantify and situations in which there are temptations on both sides for deceit. This results in both good faith disputes and outright lies, which must be handled by the legal system. Yet, some changes can be made to reduce the reliance upon attorneys. Workers' compensation systems were originally designed to be simple, informal methods of resolving disputes. Over the years, these methods have grown more complicated. Consideration should be given to simplifying the dispute resolution procedure where possible.

In the long run, however, the real promise lies in reducing the number of disputes. The strategies discussed in the first part of this chapter are the real tools that employers have for reducing their workers' need for the assistance of attorneys.

REFERENCES

1. Habeck RV, Hunt HA, Leahy MJ, Welch EM: Differences in Workers' Experience Among Michigan Employers. Michigan Bureau of Workers' Disability Compensation, Lansing, MI, 1988
2. The Bulletin, June 15, 1988
3. Workers' Compensation Strategies for Lowering Costs And Reducing Workers' Suffering. Fort Washington, PA, LRP Publications, 1989
4. American Medical Association: AMA Guidelines to the Evaluation of Permanent Impairment. American Medical Association, Chicago, 1991

6

Employers' Response to Occupational Disorders

William W. Eversmann, Jr., M.D.

Increasing specialization in the work place has required workers to use their hands and upper extremities in the same few movements for hours at a time. The growing use of computers and video terminals in concert with other office automation has also produced a group of work injuries with a vague onset, uncertain pathology and confusing treatment. These disorders are generating increasing costs for the employer and insurance company.[1]

By providing goods and services, employers engage in business to make money with which they satisfy the needs of their employees, their owners, or even their stockholders. Rising health care expenses due to worker injuries increases the cost of doing business and inevitably attracts the full attention of the employer. Cumulative trauma disorders have received such attention recently. According to recent statistics released by the Occupational Safety and Health Administration, these disorders account for 50 percent of workers compensation injuries.[1,2] Although industry has accepted acute in-juries in the work place as its responsibility, particularly when a definitive date location, and type of injury can be documented by plant health or safety personnel, cumulative trauma disorders, because their onset is less precise, their pathology less certain, and their cause illusive are more problematic. The States Supreme Court has dictated the date of onset of cumulative trauma disorders as either the day the employee first complained of symptoms to health and safety personnel of the employer or first reported for treatment to a medical facility.

The successful treatment of patients by the physician alone or by a more complex, occupationally oriented medical team requires an understanding of the response and reaction of employers to these occupational disorders. It is the purpose of this chapter to review the responses and reactions of employers to occupational disorders, suggest some solutions in dealing with difficult employer problems, and outline an appropriate physician response as the health care provider is approached by industry.

IDENTIFICATION OF INJURIES BY INDUSTRY

An increase in the number of injuries is often first recognized by the health and safety representative to the personnel department of a business.[3] Normally injuries are categorized, as required by the federal government, as diseases or injuries, then further subdivided by the employer as slips or falls, cumulative trauma disorders, cuts or bruises and medical emergencies such as heart disease, arthritis, or pulmonary emergencies.

Plants of a sufficient size have a full-time or part-time nursing office that provides, in addition to the administration support of recording of injuries, a limited amount of first aid to plant employees who are injured on the job. In plants in which several thousands employees work, a physician is often on duty either part- or full-time to provide consultation for work-related injuries, to do triage for their continued care, and to administer initial care for acute lacerations and injuries.

In recent years, the greatest increase in plant injuries has been in cumulative trauma disorders,[4] with many plants noticing a three- to fivefold increase. When injuries are recorded in a nursing office, they can be traced to working areas of the plant and when localized provide the employer with an efficient clue as to the direct cause. In the face of an increasing incidence of injuries within their company, executives may bypass their medical and nursing personnel in favor of outside consultants. Doing so is almost always counterproductive since the outside consultants most often must rely on the in-plant personnel as they begin to survey the facility to determine the incidence and cause of injury.

When an increase in work injuries recorded by a facility occurs over a longer period of time or is more subtle or possibly when the plant itself has a limited ability to record and act upon that increase, the initial response might well come from the carrier of the workers' compensation insurance policy. This response may come in two forms: an alert to the company of an increasing incidence of injury or a cancellation of the workers' compensation policy. Since most states require that businesses carry workers' compensation insurance, the second method of notification will evoke an immediate and sustained response by the employer.

However, worker injury alerts by the insurer are often sufficient to gain the employers' attention. They typically require a response within a limited period of time by the employer to the insurance company. The employer normally contacts consultants either within the insurance industry itself or occasionally from an independent source to address the increasing incidence of injury. Outside consultants are required to submit a report to the insurance company or have their analytical and ergonomic methods reviewed by the insurance company during the course of the consultation. The insurer then in a de facto sense assumes secondary control of medical or injury consultation within the plant. If it finds the response of the employer to be inadequate, it will often cancel the company's workers' compensation insurance.

When the workers of a facility are represented by a labor union, the labor union itself may call attention, either directly or indirectly, to an increasing incidence of injury to their members working in the plant. In many cases the plant records are not directly available to the union except through legal subpoena. Accordingly, the first sign of the union's concern for its members may well be a subpoena or request for records of injuries from the personnel office or the nursing office of the plant. When such requests are ignored by the employer or when that information is not forthcoming, the administration of the union may seek to obtain these records by requesting a review of the plant by either the state or federal Occupational Safety and Health Administration (OSHA). After either the state or federal OSHA has been contacted according to the usual procedures of that organization, the plant manager or executives in charge of the company will receive either an unannounced visit or announced survey of the plant facilities. Although it would be unusual for an unannounced survey by a state or federal OSHA to be the initial notification to company executives of an increasing injury problem within the facility, it may be the first event that will elicit action to address that problem.

Ultimately, regardless of the initial event that attracts attention, the employer will be impressed with the expense of treating these injuries. That expense involves not only the cost of medical treatment for the injuries, which may be significant, but also increasing premium costs of workers' compensation insurance, the cost of unemployment and disability insurance should the worker not be able to return to work, the cost of workers' compensation payments while the injured worker is away from the work place, which is usually a percentage of the worker's wage, and finally the cost of hiring another employee to perform the worker's job during his or her absence. These multiple expenses together may add up to $20,000 over an approximate 6-week period for an employee earning approximately $8.50 an hour, with the medical care representing no more than $3,000 to $4,000 of this amount.

RESPONSES OF EMPLOYERS TO AN INCREASED INCIDENCE OF INJURIES

The responses of an employer to an increasing incidence of worker injuries depend more on the type of injuries than on the increase in those injuries and the number of employees affected.[5]

Acute Injuries

Responses to an increase in acute injuries are straightforward. When employees working with machines are injured, employers have learned over the years that appropriate guards on those machines may prevent injuries, shutoff devices on the machines will reduce the severity of those injuries, multiple switches to operate the machines may preclude an employee's hand or arm being caught in a machine, and areas of water or wetness on the floor need to be removed to prevent slipping and falling. With acute injuries, employers are usually able to identify the cause of the injury and to take appropriate, direct action to eliminate the cause of injury for other employees.

Corrective action for acute injuries thus has an immediate effect, one that can be immediately measured and sustained. Employers are so accustomed to this approach to work-related injuries that the corrective action after the injury is often contained on the injury report itself, justifying for the insurance company or OSHA the fact that corrective action has been taken immediately following the injury to the worker.

Cumulative Trauma Disorders

Cumulative trauma disorders, in contrast to acute injuries, are refractory to immediate correction by the employer.

Many employers attribute the multiple, vague complaints that accompany cumulative trauma disorders to a lack of motivation on the part of their employees. Indeed, after having symptoms of cumulative trauma disorders or overuse syndrome for a long period of time with no diagnosis or a treatment, employees may become depressed. Seeing this depression, usually through the eyes of their supervisory personnel, employers may interpret it as a lack of motivation. In addition, employers who have difficulty understanding the nature and cause of cumulative trauma disorders will in all likelihood have an even greater difficulty appreciating the abstract nature of motivation.

Incentive Pay

Predictably, such employers will attempt to "cure" motivational inadequacies by providing incentive pay to their employees. The workers, even while experiencing the symptoms of cumulative trauma disorders, will then not seek appropriate medical treatment, thereby increasing their injuries, further complicating their medical problems, increasing the cost to their employers, and possibly risking permanent disability. Thus, the administration of timely and effective treatment for cumulative trauma disorders is often negated by the incentive pay system.

Companies that employ such a system are often seasonal in nature, using incentive pay to obtain the maximum number of workers on a seasonably adjusted basis to meet the needs of the larger industries that they supply. The most typical example of such business is the automotive parts industry, which supplies parts for the assembly of vehicles.

Those businesses that have an extremely high turnover of personnel also use the incentive pay system to their advantage. A plant that replaces its entire work force every 4 to 6 months will attempt to retain an integral portion of its work force for the training of new employees through an incentive pay system.

Using the incentive pay system in the face of increasing numbers of cumulative trauma disorders can only lead to disaster for both the employer and the employee by increasing costs; increasing the employee's time away from the work place, impairment, and disability; and ultimately preventing the employee from participating in the work force often on a permanent basis.

Wellness Programs

The most common reaction of employers to the increasing incidence of cumulative trauma disorder is denial. There can be no more frequently heard response from an employer, when told of the increasing incidence of cumulative trauma disorders in the work place, than "it couldn't possibly be due to the work we do here." Cumulative trauma disorders by their nature require employers, whether they be a plant manager, health and safety officer, or personnel director, to reconsider their thinking about work injury, which traditionally meant acute injuries. They must come to realize that the repetitive use of muscles and muscle-tendon units and repeated pressure on nerve and nerve trunks can produce over a period of time an increasing incidence of tendon irritation and muscle tendon dysfunction, as well as neuropathy. Initially still following the acute injury model, employers will look for an immediate solution to the problems of cumulative trauma.

This immediate solution may take the form of a so-called wellness program. Through a wellness program, either one engaged in before, during, or after the work day, the employer hopes to reduce the incidence of cumulative trauma by physical conditioning of workers or by increasing their resistance to disease and injury through a general program of more healthful living. Such a program may also include dietary controls, smoking cessation programs, and weight reduction.

Exercise programs that interrupt the work day have a subtle benefit of providing the employee a break from the motions and muscle activities that are often the primary cause of the cumulative trauma syndrome. Providing these 10- to 15-minute breaks from the activities instrumental in causing the cumulative trauma disorder may well reduce muscle stress. Wellness programs that promote healthful living also benefit the worker and the work place by reducing absenteeism and improving motivation and employee well-being. However, other than the side effect of providing breaks during the work day, wellness programs have little direct effect on the number of cumulative trauma disorders within a work place.

Within the last several years some employers have used psychologists to systematically develop peer pressure, within the work place under the titles such as "team work group." These methods which can reduce absenteeism and lost work days through peer pressure techniques can also prevent the worker from seeking medical care and consequently have the same effects as an incentive pay system.[6]

Altering the Duties of Affected Workers

The employer who does not wish to address the causes of cumulative trauma disorder by evaluating the work place ergonomically may attempt to reduce the costs of workers' compensation by altering the responsibilities of workers with cumulative trauma disorders. Recognizing that the employee who is not working increases the cost of business not only by increasing the premiums for workers' compensation insurance but also by being paid while not being productive,

employers may have the worker return to the work place either in a light duty or alternative job position sooner than is recommended by good medical practice and before the worker can return to full duty. Some workers have been forced to return to the work place in almost a nonwork capacity, often doing little more than reading a book in the front office of the business just to lower the employer's workers' compensation costs. Having the employer return to the work place reduces the number of lost work days due to injury, thereby making it appear to the insurance company who provides workers' compensation insurance to the employer that the employer has in fact reduced the rate of injury and lost work days. Occasionally, health care professionals may be manipulated by the employer into contributing to this mishandling of patients by giving workers who are otherwise unable to return to the work place a mandate to return to work in what they believe to be an altered capacity. However, these new capacities are often not sufficiently altered to allow healing during the treatment program and, as a consequence, contribute further to injury, disability, and increased cost.

One example of an altered duty is the one-handed job to which a patient returns after the operation on the other hand. Unfortunately, if there were a significant number of one-handed jobs in industry, the incidence of cumulative trauma disorders would be far lower, since the worker could alternate from one hand to the other in performing work activities. The experience of many hand surgeons indicates that there are very few positions in either production or service-related industry that allow a worker to use a single hand and at the same time protect the hand that is receiving treatment during work place activity. Even if an employee can use one hand for the majority of the work activity, the other hand is neglected and often not elevated. Therefore, even with reduced or no use during the course of the work day, the hand under treatment, by being dependent, will swell, thereby complicating its care.

Ergonomic Evaluation of the Work Place

There is no doubt that detailed ergonomic analysis of the work place, with the resulting reorganization of space, redistribution of jobs, and enlargement of jobs, will provide the employer with cost-effective solutions for cumulative trauma disorders.[4,7,8] However, some employers seek ergonomic analysis only to reinforce their denial of the existence of working conditions that create cumulative trauma. These employers' denial of the existence of cumulative trauma causation within their work place may well contribute to litigation between the employees affected with cumulative trauma disorders and the workers' compensation insurance carrier.

PHYSICIANS' RESPONSES TO AN INCREASED INCIDENCE OF INJURY

The single most important factor in determining the effectiveness of a physician's response to an increased incidence of injury in the work place is the motivation of the employer when faced with that problem. There is little, if anything, that a physician can provide of use to industry if the employer is merely seeking a "quick fix" response to the increasing problem of worker injury. This is particularly true when the employer's motivation is to satisfy an unnamed, often belligerent third party with the appearance, but not necessarily the commitment to addressing the problem of worker injury.

Having been cited by either a state or federal Occupational Safety and Health Administration, the company that seeks a physician's help simply to meet the needs of the OSHA complaint without addressing the primary cause of the citation—that is, increasing worker injury—will be impossible to satisfy since the third party is likely to be satisfied only by a comprehensive approach to the problem.

The response to work injury problems of course depends on the type of problem. An acute injury problem is amenable to direct action; for example, replacing guards on a machine, altering handles, modifying the work station, adding turn-off switches, or altering the clothing that employees wear so that it does not get caught in the machinery.

The response to an increased incidence of cumulative trauma disorders requires a detailed health survey designed to address the particular symptoms of the workers, a detailed ergonomic analysis of the work area and work stations within the plant, and a comprehensive treatment program for injured workers as they are identified.[3] A comprehensive approach to cumulative trauma disorders also includes a detailed plan of preventing them since it is only through prevention, not through the treatment of injured workers, that control can be gained and the number of disorders reduced.[3] The prevention plan must include a method of monitoring their existence within the work place.[4,5,7,9] Such monitoring can detected the disorders when they are mild and will respond to conservative treatment. Treating these patients conservatively will increase the chances of avoiding permanent disability.

It is desirable for the physician to participate in this monitoring program, either directly or through a plant task force whose work[3] is designed specifically to reduce cumulative trauma disorders. Such a task force should include representatives from the engineering department; the administration of the plant, including health and safety personnel; worker-supervisors; and even workers themselves. The participation of the physician in these regular task force deliberations is essential in the management of workers who are injured. The physician should also be able to identify those common uses of the upper extremities within the work place that may be the mechanism causing the cumulative trauma disorder.

Treatment of Injured Workers

The other major role of the health care provider, usually the treating physician, is the treatment of patients who have been injured in the work place. Although the treatment of patients should be specific to their injury, several principles should guide treatment.

No single service is more important to the workers returning to the work place than rehabilitation for work. Rehabilitation may take several forms, depending on the type of work that the employee performs. For any manual worker, whether one at a keyboard or on an assembly line, it is important to simulate the patient's work as part of the rehabilitation process. Such rehabilitation is sometimes called *work hardening*. The importance of work hardening lies not in strengthening those muscles that the worker uses repetitively in the work place, which actually matters very little. Rather, it is in simulating the worker's day-to-day activity, which enables the physician to know exactly what the injured worker does in the work place.[10] This information can be gained either through video tape analysis of the job simulation or by direct observation of the

workers performance.[11] Gaining a familiarity with the injured worker's exact activities at the work station is by far the best way for the physician to be educated about the needs of the worker during the rehabilitation process.

Just as it is the responsibility of the physician returning a worker to the work place to be aware of the work that that injured employee will perform, so it is the responsibility of the employer to inform the physician of the activities to which the worker will return. Most physicians' practices are replete with workers returning to them with descriptions of activities that they have been required to perform that are very different from the physicians' expectations. Therefore, the coordination of the physician's knowledge with the employer's needs and the worker's capabilities upon return to work is essential to the successful recovery of the worker and eventual re-entry into the work place.

The use of the term "light duty" has caused more confusion among physicians, employers, and workers than any two words in the workers' compensation process. Undoubtedly, appropriately altered activities, particularly those changed to prevent reinjury of the worker, can be a most useful modality in enabling re-entry of the worker into the work force. Altered work activities shortens the period of time that the worker is away from the work place, reduces the cost of the workers's compensation system in several ways, and can, if well designed, continue the work hardening and rehabilitation process for the injured worker.[5] It is unfortunately just as true that poorly designed light duty or light duty that is not monitored and adhered to by the employer can be one of the most detrimental situations to which an injured worker can be returned and can increase worker injury, impairment, and disability. The physician is often caught in the middle between an employee who may be less than eager to return to work and an employer who may or may not be using a light duty environment to punish the injured worker. Only close and continuous communication and coordination among the worker, employer, and physician can resolve this situation.[10]

Job Analysis

If the health care provider is unfamiliar with the job to which the worker will return, the physician or an assistant, often a hand therapist, should prepare a detailed analysis of that job.[10] Such an analysis should include the job's work objective, work standard, and work method; the layout of the work place, the equipment with which the work is performed and the materials used in the product or function; these subsections are described below. This method of job documentation has been widely discussed by Armstrong and others[4,10] and remains the standard of job analysis in the work place.

The work objective describes the reason why the job is performed and is often contained in the title of the job. The work standard expresses the quantity or quality of work that is to be performed; it may be couched in terms that are applicable for a majority of the work force or may be based on individual performances or on a performance of a group of workers.[10]

The work method simply describes the procedures and techniques that are used to accomplish the work objective. These techniques may often be described as a sequence of motions or activities of the arms, hands, and wrists. Because these motions may differ significantly among workers, a number of workers must be observed individually or on occasion a group of workers analyzed to assess accurately the work method.[10]

The work place layout describes the arrangement of the equipment for the job within the work place and the relationship of the worker to this equipment. The work equipment is those tools, devices, machines, and other implements that are used by the worker in performing the work objective. Work materials are those objects and products that may be assembled or united in some way, such as parts, dividers, packing, or inserts.

The enactment of the Disabilities Act of 1990 lent new importance to the use of detailed job descriptions and their coordination with pre-employment and pre-placement physical evaluations.[3] Using the detailed elements of job design and job evaluation to prevent the inappropriate match of the worker's capability to the necessities of the job may reduce worker injury, impairment, and disability. Preplacement physical evaluations could include screening tests for neuropathy, including detailed sensory evaluation of one or more modalities of sensibility. It may be undesirable to use invasive techniques to evaluate nerve function. Noninvasive techniques, however, are useful, dependable, and repeatable and have been used in industry successfully.[3] A single measurement of static group strength may be of small value in the determination of a worker's ability to grip and grasp, but repeated grasp with maximum strength can help elucidate an occult weakness of repetitive motion grip.[7] Just as a work hardening facility was useful in the rehabilitation of an injured worker before returning to the work place, so the same equipment and facility can be useful in the pre-employment and preplacement physical evaluation of a prospective worker.

SUMMARY

The increasing specialization of industry has produced a unique set of injuries known collectively as cumulative trauma disorders. The physician and staff, using well-designed work evaluation facilities, must be willing to assist industry in the rehabilitation of injured workers, the evaluation of new workers, and the design and institution of programs to prevent workers injuries. Through these programs focused on the work place, physicians, supported by a staff of ergonomists, hand therapists, and occupational health care providers, can assist both the worker and employer by reducing the costs and numbers of injuries.

REFERENCES

1. Kilborn PT: Department of Labor Report: rise in worker injuries is laid to the computer. New York Times, November 16, 1989
2. Mallory M, Bradford H, Freundlich N: An invisible work place hazard gets harder to ignore. Business Week January 30, 1989, pp 92–93
3. Rystrom CM, Eversmann WW: Cumulative trauma intervention in industry: a model program for the upper extremity. p 489. In Kasdan ML (ed): Occupational Hand and Upper Extremity Injuries and Disease. Hanley & Belfus, Philadelphia, 1991
4. Armstrong TJ, Radwin RG, Hansen DJ, Kennedy KW: Repetitive trauma disorders: job evaluation and design. Hum Factors 28:325, 1986
5. Iserhagen SJ: Work Injury Prevention and Management. Rockville, MD, Aspen Publications, 1988
6. Milbank D: Companies turn to peer pressure to cut injuries as psychologists join the battle. Wall Street J 72:B1, 1991
7. Browne CD, Nolan BM, Faithful DK: Occupational repetitive strain injuries: guidelines for diagnosis and management. Med J Aust 140:329, 1984
8. Fine L, Silverstein BA, Armstrong TJ, Anderson CA: Detection of cumulative trauma disorders of the upper extremities in the work place. J Occup Med 28:674, 1986
9. McKenzie F, Storment J, Von Hook P, Armstrong TJ: A program for control of repetitive trauma disorders associated with hand tool operation in a telecommunications manufacturing facility. Am Ind Hyg Assoc J 46:674, 1985
10. Armstrong TJ: Ergonomics and cumulative trauma disorders of the hand and wrist. In Hunter JM, et al (eds): Rehabilitation of the Hand. CV Mosby, Philadelphia, 1990
11. Hadler NM: Industrial rheumatology: clinical investigations into the influence of the pattern of usage on the pattern of regional musculoskeletal disease. Arth Rheumatol 20:1019, 1977

SUGGESTED READINGS

Brown PW: The Role of motivation in the recovery of the hand. p 1. In Kasdan ML: (ed): Occupational Hand and Upper Extremity Injuries and Disease. Hanley & Belfus, Philadelphia, 1991

Hall DT, Bowen DD, Lewiciki RJ, Hall FS: Experiences in Management and Organizational Behavior. 2nd Ed. John Wiley, New York, 1982

Liker JK, Joseph BS, Armstrong TJ: From ergonomic theory to practice: organizational factors affecting the utilization of ergonomic knowledge. In Hendrick HW, Brown O Jr (eds): Human Factors in Organizational Design and Management. Elsevier North-Holland, Amsterdam, 1984

Moody L, Arezzo J, Otto D: Screening occupational population for a symptomatic or early peripheral neuropathy. J Occup Med 28:975, 1986

National Institute for Occupational Safety and Health: A proposed strategy for the prevention of musculoskeletal injuries. p 17. In Proposed National Strategies for the Prevention of Leading Work-Related Diseases and Injuries, pt 1, Association of Schools of Public Health, Washington, DC, 1986

7

The Australian Experience with Cumulative Trauma Disorders

Damian C. R. Ireland, M.D.

Before addressing the specifics of the Australian experience with work-related arm pain, this chapter gives a brief summary of the categories of arm pain and the consequences associated with placing patients in those categories. Although there are differences between the Australian and American legal and welfare systems, what is of interest is the striking similarities in the epidemiology of cumulative trauma disorders (CTD) in both of these industrialized nations.

EVALUATING OCCUPATIONAL ARM PAIN

Before one can treat arm pain effectively, accurate diagnosis of the cause of the pain is necessary. Making the diagnosis is aided by the following broad etiologic classifications:

1. Pain caused by the work task, e.g., rotator cuff tendinitis, tennis elbow, cross-over bursitis, deQuervain's stenosing tenosynovitis
2. Pain aggravated by but not caused by the work task, as in a pre-existing (symptomatic or asymptomatic) conditions, e.g., carpometacarpal joint (CMC) arthritis, chronic scaphoid non union with posttraumatic arthritis
3. Pain that is unrelated to the work task, but that develops serendipitously during work, e.g., Dupuytren's contracture
4. Pain that is unrelated to the physical work task but is related to the psychological stress of the work task and conditions and the patient's personality, e.g., occupational cervico brachial disorder (OCBD), regional pain syndrome, repetitive strain injury (RSI)
5. Pain that is unrelated in any way to the work task but is dishonestly attributed to it, e.g., Bennett's fracture, fractured fifth metacarpal neck, fractured scaphoid

Of course, some diagnoses can fit into more than one etiologic grouping for example, tennis elbow can be caused by work or may be a pre-existing condition that is aggravated by work. The contentious diagnosis of carpal tunnel syndrome (CTS), can fall into etiologic groups 1, 2, or 3; its diagnosis is discussed in Chapter 13. The etiologic classification of these diagnoses continues to be a subject of debate.

Classifying occupational arm pain into one of these five categories carries great responsibility, because it will determine (1) the effectiveness of treatment, (2) liability for the costs of treatment and the future employability of the patient, and (3) the outcome of any litigation.

Effectiveness of Treatment

In Australia charges are now being leveled against some industrial rehabilitation specialists for treating a nonphysical and psychosomatic condition occurring in the work place with understandably ineffective physical treatments, such as splinting, physiotherapy, and anti-inflammatory medication. These charges have been made by the patients who have been managed incorrectly and denied effective treatment while experiencing worsening symptoms because of the erroneous assumption that they were suffering from a physical condition caused by an injury. In a recent industrial accident tribunal in South Australia, the defendant, the Commonwealth Government, was held partially responsible and assessed damages for retiring a keyboard operator on disability for what was subsequently accepted as a nonphysical condition. The rationale was that the employer incorrectly reinforced the notion that the plaintiff was suffering a physical injury caused by keyboard operation, thereby making her unemployable.

Liability for Costs of Treatment and Future Employability of the Patient

The physician's diagnosis often determines who will be financially liable for the costs of treatment. Obviously, those patients in category 1 whose condition, whether acute or chronic, has been caused by work and who had no pre-existing predisposition to the condition could have all costs, including treatment and time away from work, paid by the employer and retain the right to sue the employer if an unsafe work place caused the injury or condition. Category 2 patients could arguably have the cost of treatment paid by the employer and share the cost of lost pay during treatment with the employer, but forfeits the right to sue the employer for negligence. Category 3 patients should obviously pay for their own treatment and time away from work. The costs of treatment and time away from work and employer culpability for category 4 patients will depend on the relative putative role of the patient's premorbid personality in causing the resultant psychological condition. Category 5 patients should be handled in the same manner as any one who fraudulently deceives an insurance company.

The diagnosis will also determine whether the worker will be paid during the absence from work or will possibly be fired. Consider the not uncommon scenario of a boiler maker/welder, with chronic scaphoid non-union and with no recollection of a prior injury at or away from work, who develops the insidious onset of progressive wrist pain in the course of his normal work. He may be unable to return to his normal work for 6 months after surgical treatment aimed at scaphoid osteosynthesis. If this condition is deemed noncompensatable, his employer may dismiss him in anticipation of this prolonged absence from work. If the patient then contests his firing, his unsettled claim places him in limbo and renders him virtually unemployable until his dispute is settled, because his workers' compensation claim history may follow him as a prison record follows an ex-convict.

Outcome of Litigation for Residual, Permanent Disability

The physician's answer to the worker's quite legitimate question—"Did my assembly line process work cause the carpal tunnel syndrome, or has it just aggravated the condition that I would otherwise have developed?"—will often determine whether the matter goes onto litigation and how expeditiously it is settled. Succinct and early advice to the patient and employer will often spare the patient the dehumanizing "medicolegal merry-go-round" instigated by multiple, conflicting medical opinions or, worse still, by lawyers or other vested interest groups. Once having filed a claim, the patient may lose all control of the situation, and become bitter, recalcitrant, anxious, and neurotic. The longer this prevails, the less likely is successful rehabilitation and return to work (even after effective treatment). We must also be mindful of the considerable legal costs to the potential plaintiff, whether the case is spurious or legitimate.

REPETITIVE STRAIN INJURY

As orthopaedic surgeons dealing with upper limb problems, it is therefore essential for us to debate the issue of diagnosis and etiology and to form a consensus that will give informed direction to our patients, their employers, insurance companies, and lawyers. However, there is a group of symptoms that we are unable to diagnose accurately. These symptoms are either (1) hitherto unrecognized new physical illnesses, injuries or diseases; (2) nonphysical or psychological conditions; or (3) combinations of recognized physical conditions and/or new physical conditions and/or psychological disorders.

Recognizing that some symptoms cannot be diagnosed accurately is a more rational and scientific approach than simply calling all occupational arm pain "repetitive strain injury" or "cumulative trauma disorder." These terms are confusing and misleading and are not based on sound scientific logic when attempting to extrapolate aged cadaveric muscle/tendon stress/strain in vitro preparations.[1,2] They have done much to hinder our understanding of the true nature and origin of occupational arm pain, by including with them: rotator cuff tendonitis, lateral epicondylitis, CMC arthritis, and carpal tunnel syndrome. To the untrained general practitioner and to many industrial physicians these terms imply that occupational arm pain is an injury caused by repetition or that it is caused by the trauma of work that is cumulative. These remain conjectural hypotheses that have certainly not been proven.

Therefore, we should use the established diagnostic terms—arthritis, periostiotis, myostis, bursitis, tendonitis, tenosynovitis, and nerve entrapment—when the following diagnostic criteria for these conditions are met:

- Clearly defined and distinguishable subjective clinical symptoms
- Reproducible, objective physical findings
- Recognizable gross and microscopic pathologic findings
- Response to accepted and proven forms of effective physical treatment

Although prolapsed intervertebral disc (which was first described in 1934) may have few reproducible, objective physical clinical findings and carpal tunnel syndrome (which was first described in 1947) may have symptoms without signs and vice versa, the other two diagnostic criteria are usually positive in both these conditions. The notion that a new physical condition has emerged is presumptuous, as work practices have not changed significantly over the last three decades in many occupations where RSI and CTD are now diagnosed, e.g., machinist clothing and shoemaking. However, if a new physical condition has arisen, it should by now have fulfilled all four of these diagnostic criteria. The logical conclusion then is that symptoms, which do not fulfill any of the four diagnostic criteria of a physical condition, are manifestations of a nonphysical condition.

THE AUSTRALIAN EXPERIENCE

In the early 1980s Australia experienced an epidemic of occupational arm pain, which became known as RSI. RSI was a hitherto unseen (in Australia) upper limb pain that is attributed to rapid, repetitious use, initially on a keyboard. It is a collection of symptoms affecting the upper limb, including weakness, paresthesias, swelling, and pain, which is the most prominent. This pain, although often consistent in a given patient, is not consistent among patients and does not conform to any known neurologic pathway, anatomic structure, or pathophysiologic pattern. There are no primary objective physical findings in the upper limb other than tenderness, which is frequently of equal severity at any randomly selected point on the limb. Clinical investigations, including biochemistry, radiography, electromyography, nerve conduction studies, radioisotope bone scanning, thermography and hematology, are negative.

The condition commonly affects young to middle-aged, predominantly female employees engaged in low-paying, monotonous, low-prestige occupations. The symptoms fail to respond to any form of physical treatment, including rest, splinting, symptomatic physical therapy, and anti-inflammatory medications. Moreover, such treatment is often accompanied by a deterioration in symptoms.

The epidemic of RSI spread to involve a wide spectrum of occupations, including data processors, process workers, typists, clerks, cashiers, bank tellers, musicians, packers, and textile industry machinists whose manual tasks and productivity had not changed significantly for decades. It then spread to workers who were not engaged in repetitive movements, such as retail sales assistants. This implied that repetitive use and motion of the upper limb were *not* the common denominator of RSI. In fact Hocking's[4] 1987 study of Telecom (the government-run national telephone company) employees revealed the highest incidence of RSI was in telephonists (34%) who had the lowest keystroke rate, followed by clerks (28%). Keyboard operators, who had the most repetitive tasks and highest keystroke rate, had the lowest incidence at 3.4%.

Strain implies deformation of tissue, but there is no evidence of morphologic gross anatomic or histologic abnormality in RSI. Dennett and Fry's[5] 1988 muscle biopsy study failed to preserve anatomic muscle fiber length before preparation for histologic and electron microscopy analysis, had a small sample size, and lacked adequate matched controls, thereby invalidating many of their conclusions. Ancillary investigations, such as electromyography and nerve conduction studies, thermography, and most other forms of radiologic imaging, also fail to show any abnormality.

There is no history of physical injury having occurred and there are no sequelae of localized tissue trauma, such as swelling, bruising, redness, or increased temperature.

RSI therefore differs from those conditions in etiologic categories 1 and 2, which are commonly attributed to "overuse" in the upper limb, in the following ways: it does not have clearly defined and distinguishable clinical symptoms, there are no reproducible objective physical clinical findings, it is not accompanied by any recognizable gross or microscopic pathologic changes; and it does not respond effectively to accepted and proven forms of physical treatment.

In my opinion, RSI fits into category 4—pain related not to the physical work task but to the psychological stress of the work task. If RSI is classified as category 1 or 2,[6,7] serious consequences may follow physical treatment, including surgery, for a nonphysical condition not only fails to alleviate the symptoms but usually results in a steady chronic deterioration, with the patient believing that the surgical scar attests to the underlying "injury." Moreover, the patient is denied appropriate nonphysical treatment, and the longer this treatment is delayed, the more fixed the symptoms become, making the patient's rehabilitation a futile task.

This failure of RSI to respond to physical treatment in Australia was accompanied by a meteoric rise in incidence until it assumed epidemic proportions. The implied physical etiology of RSI requires those affected to avoid the alleged cause, whether it be a repetitive job, such as data processing, or the nonrepetitive task of sales assistant. The estimated cost of lost work from July 1984–June 1985 in the Australian Commonwealth Public Service (excluding state public servants and private enterprise employees) was $24.13 million.[8] In June 1985 26% of Commonwealth Public Service employees in the Australian Capital Territory suffered from RSI, and most of them were certified unfit for work in the year 1984–1985. From December 1983 till November 1984, the Commonwealth Banking Corporation saw a 275% increase in the incidence of RSI.[8]

RSI is preventable, but only after acceptance of its psychological origin. There are historical precedents for this condition. In 1713 Ramazzini,[9] in a treatise on "Diseases of Clerks and Scribes,'" described the same symptoms of modern-day RSI, implicating "continuous sitting, repeated use of the hand and strain of the mind."

In 1830 Sir Charles Bell[10] described "writers' cramp," which differs from RSI only in the high incidence of "hand spasm." Gowers[11] in 1888 further elaborated on writer's cramp, terming it an "occupational neurosis" in his extensive monograph, *Diseases of the Nervous System*. He logically dismissed it as being a peripheral physical condition and upheld the "primarily and essentially central nervous system origin, the result of 'a deranged action' of the centers concerned in the act of writing." He also noted that writer's cramp sufferers frequently "are of distinctly nervous temperament, irritable, sensitive, bearing overwork and anxiety badly" and that it "is a disease easily imagined by those who have witnessed the disorder." He reckoned that 50 percent of writer's cramp occurred bilaterally.

Gowers[11] also mentioned other similar occupational neuroses of the time: "piano forte player's cramp," "violin player's cramp," "seamstress cramp," and "telegraphist's cramp." The similarity of "telegraphist's cramp" to "writer's cramp" was noted in 1882 by Robinson,[12] and telegraphists' cramp was again mentioned in 1888 by Gowers.[10] After the addition of "telegraphists' cramp" in 1908 to the schedule of diseases covered by the British Workman's Compensation Act, its incidence steadily increased to affect 60% of operators. The Great Britain and Ireland Post Office Departmental Committee of Enquiry[13] in 1911 concluded that "telegraphists cramp" was a "nervous breakdown due to nervous instability and repeated fatigue." Its incidence subsequently declined, though as late as 1971 Ferguson[14] described cramp in Australian keyboard telegraphists. The clinical presentation was similar to today's RSI. The widely varying incidence in different regions—25% in Sydney and 4% in Melbourne—had no physical explanation and recalls Gowers' description of writer's cramp as "a disease easily imagined by those who have witnessed the disorder." A parallel between this autosuggestion and the mass hysteria about witchcraft portrayed in Arthur Miller's[15] "The Crucible" in 1968 presents itself here.

The clinical symptoms and work circumstances of occupational cervicobrachial disorder (OCBD) in Japan, Switzerland, and Sweden; "tension neck" and "occupational disorder" in Finland; and "occupational complaint number 2101" in West Germany[8] are also similar to those of RSI. The Australian experience differs only in its epidemic spread and high incidence. These conditions share employee targeting, repetitive stereotyped upper limb exertion, and mental stress.[16] Physical injury has not been described preceding either RSI or OCBD.

Hadler[17] and Lucire[18] have drawn attention to the prevalence of neck and arm pain in the normal activities of daily living. Lawrence's[19] 1969 study, based on a random sample of over 1,000 working-aged people in the north of England re-

vealed that, at any point in time, 9% of men and 12% of women had arm or neck pain sufficiently severe to consult their physician. Also relevant to the Australian RSI epidemic is Horal's[20] 1969 low back pain study that comprised two groups of 212 patients each, matched for age, sex, and occupation. One group presented to their family doctor complaining of low back pain, and the other group complained of symptoms other than low back pain. However, on direct questioning 60% of the second group had low back pain that was identical to the first group in symptoms, signs, and x-ray findings. Why then did the second group not complain of low back pain while the first group did, converting their symptom to an illness and a subsequent work incapacity based on the physician's interpretation of the clinical presentation? The answer is provided by the later research of Magora,[21] who in 1973 revealed that the two correlates linking the symptom of low back pain and work incapacity were (1) a belief by patients that their work had injured their back and (2) job dissatisfaction.

However well-intentioned the early medical proponents of RSI may have been, their concept was misleading and irresponsible. The climate having been established for the apparent creation of a "new disease," RSI gained in popularity as an occupational disease diagnosis. Although arm pain is a common accompaniment to the normal activities of daily living, potential RSI sufferers lacking fulfillment in their work came to believe that their pain was due to the repetitious tasks of their work. This notion was reinforced by the press, trade unions, and legal and medical professions. Physicians, ergonomists, social workers, physiotherapists, and occupational therapists who operate Industrial rehabilitation clinics have developed a commercial symbiosis with their clients who request and receive periodic certification of their work incapacity so they can continue to receive expeditious payment by the workers' compensation insurer, a point noted by Hadler[22] in 1985 when in Australia to investigate RSI.

The increased public awareness of RSI has been further fueled by the print media that publicized widely the notion that repetitive tasks in the work place cause injury.[23] The predictable effect on the RSI sufferer or potential sufferer has been to raise emotions and cause anger, preventing an otherwise spontaneous resolution. The futility of physical treatment leaves the sufferers with the only palliation remaining—in addition to not working—in the form of compensation through court awards which vindicate the plaintiff's belief in the employer's culpability.[24] Such publications as the 1984 "Sufferers Hand Book: R.S.I."[25] by the Australian Public Service Association and the 1986 English publication by the General, Municipal, Boilermakers and Allied Trades Union[26] expound the same view.

This barrage of misinformation has paradoxically, in the case of the Australian Public Service, been extended by the employers who, rightfully concerned for the welfare of their employees, have in some instances insisted on 15-minute breaks every hour and appointed staff specifically to police this edict. In addition, the employers have directly questioned unaffected employees about the possible emergence of RSI symptoms. The vested interest of the legal profession in RSI as an injury with residual permanent disability, requiring the pursuit of workers' compensation and common law claims, is obvious.[27]

Patients who have diagnosed themselves as having RSI are aware of the treatment recommended by some physicians—total rest from work lest RSI progress from stage I through stage III, which, according to Browne et al.,[28] "may

last years." Similarly, Fry[29] characterized five grades of RSI, with progression either ending or seriously threatening the working careers of sufferers. These patients then present to the family doctor requesting confirmation of the diagnosis and certification to be absent from work. Pressure is placed on the medical practitioner to comply with the patient's request in a free market, which is determined largely by supply and demand, rather than the quality of the service. The validation of the patient's request then adds further credibility to the unproved claim that repetitive tasks cause injury.[30] In addition, the Australian family doctor was not exposed to debate on RSI until 1985 when its psychological aspects were first presented in the *Medical Journal of Australia*.[18,31,32]

RSI has brought ergonomists and their costly ergometric redesign of the work place, work furniture, and equipment to prominence based solely on the unproven assertion that RSI is a physical condition. Undoubtedly, ergonomists and their industry have provided a more comfortable and less arduous work place and have lowered the incidence of many of the so-called overuse conditions by recommending changes in work practices, work stations, and work tools. However, their claims to have lowered the incidence of RSI have not been verified. Hocking[4] in 1987 reported an increased incidence of RSI after ergometric intervention at the work station. Enforced 10-minute work breaks from keyboarding every hour were also paradoxically accompanied by an increased incidence of RSI.

Why did RSI develop in the early 1980s in Australia? It came at a time of relative prosperity in a country with as many physicians and pharmacists per capita as any industrialized nation and one in which more patent medicines are consumed per capita than in the United States. The inability to work due to a physical ailment became socially acceptable.

Most importantly, the epidemic occurred at a time of technological change—the computerization of clerical tasks. This change has increased a worker's worth in terms of increased productivity, but threatened those less adaptable to change who then had to compete with younger, computer-educated job applicants.

Similarly, the increased incidence of writer's cramp was accompanied by a change from the feather quill to the more productive steel nib, and telegraphists' wrist developed with the introduction of the Morse key. "Miner's nystagmus," which bears no relationship to the upper limb, affected up to 34 percent of British underground coal miners[32] at a time when battery-operated helmet lamps and mechanized coal extraction were introduced early in this century. These two innovations increased coal productivity enormously. It was only when the nonphysical nature of miner's nystagmus was established and accepted that the condition disappeared. In much the same manner, telegraphists' wrist disappeared following a departmental committee of inquiry in 1911[13] that concluded that telegraphist's cramp was "a nervous breakdown due to nervous instability and repeated fatigue."

The incidence of RSI has plummeted in Australia since 1986 following two Victorian Supreme court decisions (*Zabaneh v. Commonwealth of Australia*, 1985; *Cooper v. Commonwealth of Australia*, 1987) that found the defendant (employer) not guilty of negligence and the plaintiff (RSI sufferer) not having suffered an injury. Damages were assessed to the RSI-affected plaintiff. Subsequently, many suits pending by RSI sufferers against their employers have been withdrawn on the advice of their trade union leaders and sections of the legal industry.

RSI should be classified as a sociopolitical phenomenon, rather than a medical condition. The responsibility for its prevention does not rest with the medical profession, but with those authorities capable of changing the milieu that has been conducive to RSI. Prevention will require public education and acceptance of RSI as a multifactorial, occupational, socioeconomic problem with a major psychological basis, rather than a physical condition resulting from injury.

The key to effective treatment of RSI is the accurate clinical and investigative assessment of patients complaining of occupational upper limb pain. Such an assessment should clearly differentiate physical conditions from nonphysical occupational neuroses. Once the nonphysical nature of these conditions is established and accepted, thereby obviating any significant secondary gain, the condition rapidly disappears.

The treatment of established RSI is unrewarding as it requires the patient's acceptance of the psychological basis of the condition. Many patients are hostile to this suggestion even when it is described to them in lay terms, such as "muscle tension." The majority of RSI patients experience the symptoms of which they complain and are innocent victims of circumstances, rather than seekers of secondary gain. Most express a genuine wish to return to work, but always on the preconditions of cessation of symptoms and transfer to a different occupation, believing that the physical work has caused their RSI.

Those few patients who accept the psychological basis of their RSI should then undergo treatment in the form of instruction in coping mechanisms both at and away from home and in relaxation therapy under the nonthreatening care of occupational therapists trained in these techniques. It is surprising how often unsatisfactory social, family, marital, and economic circumstances are expressed as job dissatisfaction. The third prerequisite for cure of RSI is the patient's willingness to return to work, as absenteeism only reinforces the incorrect and misleading notion that the physical aspect of work has caused the symptoms. Patients often find the initial resumption of work in a different job more acceptable than a return to the same task, and it is in this avenue that occupational rehabilitationists are able to apply their skills effectively.

In this chapter the term "RSI" has been used only to expose its deficiencies and for convenience. The two terms that best describe the clinical presentation of these symptoms are "regional pain syndrome" and the preferable and more descriptive "occupational cervicobrachial disorder". If indeed cumulative trauma disorder is the same or a variant thereof, then this confusing terminology would be better replaced by "occupational cervicobrachial disorder" as well.

propriate treatment. RSI and CTD may be trans-Pacific counterparts.

The scientific basis of modern medicine demands that disease be caused by a pathologic process that if not identifiable, has an rational hypothesis, thus enabling formulation and instigation of appropriate management. Although such conditions as carpal tunnel syndrome and lumbar disc protrusion causing sciatica were only described as recently as the mid-twentieth century, a physical basis for RSI has not yet been discovered. RSI now bears the hallmarks of a sociopolitical phenomenon, rather than a medical condition, and its incidence has declined since this formulation has become generally accepted in Australia.

Medical practitioners with a major interest in upper limb complaints are in a responsible position to enter the R.S.I. debate to prove or disprove its physical or psychological basis, and thereby to prevent its occurrence and propagation elsewhere.

CONCLUSION

The self-generating term RSI is misleading, for there is no scientific evidence proving that repetitive work causes either tissue strain or injury. As with most new conditions, RSI has an historical basis. A similar condition has been described, as long ago as 1830, as "writers cramp," which, like telegraphists' wrist, which was described between 1882 and 1971, is an occupational neurosis. Its' latter-day model in clinical presentation is occupational cervicobrachial disorder, a term that accurately describes what is known as RSI. The classification of RSI with the commonly acknowledged overuse conditions of the upper limb is similarly confusing and misleading and has in many cases denied those affected with RSI ap-

REFERENCES

1. Armstrong TJ, Castelli WA, Evans FC, Diaz-Pepez R: Some histological changes in carpal tunnel contents and their biomechanical implications. J Occup Med 26:P197, 1984
2. Goldstein SA, Armstrong JJ, Chaffin DB, Matthews LS: Analysis of cumulative strain in tendons. J Biomech 20:P1, 1987
3. Ireland DCR: Psychological and physical affects of occupational arm pain. J Hand Surg 13:P5, 1988
4. Hocking B: Epidermiological aspects of repetition strain injury in Telecom Australia. Med J Austr 147:P218, 1987
5. Dennett X, Fry HJH: Overuse syndrome: a muscle biopsy study. Lancet 1:23, 1988
6. Stone, WE: Repetitive strain injuries. Med J Aust, 2:616, 1983
7. Fry HJH: Physical signs in the hand and

wrist seen in the overuse injury syndrome of the upper limb. Aust NZ J Surg 56:47, 1986

8. Task Force: Repetition strain injury in the Australian Public Service. Canberra: AGPS, 1985.

9. Ramazzini, B: Diseases of Workers. Translation by Wilner Cave Wright. Hafner Publishing Co, New York, 1964

10. Bell C: Partial Paralysis of the Muscles of the Extremities. The Nervous System of the Human Body. Duff Green, 1833

11. Gowers WR: A Manual of Diseases of the Nervous System. Vol 2. Churchill, London, 1888

12. Robinson E: Br Med J, November 4th, 1882

13. Great Britain and Ireland Post Office: Departmental committee telegraphists' cramp report. H.M.S.O., London, 1911

14. Ferguson D: An Australian study of telegraphist's cramp. Br J Indust Med 28:280, 1971

15. Miller A: The Crucible. Penguin Books, New York, 1968

16. Maeda K, Hunting W, Grandjean E: Localized fatigue in accounting machine operators. J Occup Med 22:810, 1980

17. Hadler NM. Illness in the workplace: the challenge of musculoskeletal symptoms. J Hand Surg (Am) 10A: 451, 1985

18. Lucire Y: Neurosis in the workplace. Med J Aust 145:323, 1986

19. Lawrence JS: Rheumatism in cotton operatives. Br J Indust Med 18:270, 1961

20. Horal J: The clinical appearance of low back disorders in the city of Gothenberg, Sweden—comparisons of incapacitated probands with matched controls. Acta Orthoped Scand 118:1, 1969

21. Magora A: Investigation of the relation between low back pain and occupation. V. Psychological aspects. Scand J Rehabil Med 5:191, 1973

22. Hadler NM: Repetitive strain syndromes—Definition of Causality and Disability. International Congress of Rheumatology, Sydney, May 20, 1985

23. McIntosh P: "The Age" November, 21, 1984, p. 17

24. Worrall JD, Appel D: The wage replacement rate and benefits utilization in workers' compensation insurance. J Risk Insur 3:361, 1982

25. Australian Public Service Association: Sufferer's Handbook—Repetition Strain Injury. Union Media Services, September, 1984

26. General Municipal, Boilermakers and Allied Trade Union: Tackling Teno—1986

27. Macmillan, J: What you must know about repetition strain injury. Law Inst J, 11:1305, 1984

28. Browne CD, Nolan BM, Faithful DK: Occupational repetition strain injuries. Guidelines for diagnosis and management. Med J Aust 140:329, 1984

29. Fry HJH: Overuse syndrome of the upper limb in musicians. Med J Aust 140:329, 1986

30. Kuorinka I. et al: Occupational rheumatic diseases and upper limb strain in manual jobs in a light, mechanical industry. Scand J Work Environ Health, suppl. 3:39, 1979

31. Awerbauch M: RSI or "kangaroo paw." Med J Aust 142:237, 1985

32. Morgan RG: RSI. Med J Aust 144:56, 1986

33. Wright P, Teacher A (eds): The Problem of Medical Knowledge. Edinburgh University Press, Edinburgh 1982

8

Managed Care Programs

Gail F. Brain, R.N., B.S., CRRN, CIRS

An injury does not have to be catastrophic to produce devastating results for the injured worker. Whether it is a spinal cord injury resulting in paralysis or a laceration of a finger tip, the events that take place within the first few days can often determine how the injured worker will respond to treatment and whether the employee will return to the work place. Although the preinjury attitude of the worker is important, the events after the injury often determine whether there will be a successful resolution to the injury or resultant long-standing disability with significant costs for the worker and society.

Worker's compensation premiums have increased dramatically in recent years, and in 1988, on-the-job accidents cost American companies $47.1 billion.[1] It is estimated that 30 percent of every workers' compensation dollar goes toward medical costs, and the remaining 70 percent is spent on indemnity expense or the costs of lost time.[2] Faced with skyrocketing workers' compensation costs, employers are now recognizing the need for programs that will assist them in reducing the incidence of work-related injuries and controlling the costs of treating those injuries once they have occurred.

The purpose of this chapter is to discuss an alternative approach to the traditional workers' compensation system, which is often inadequate and lacks controls in many areas. Managed care programs for workers' compensation claims are gradually being recognized as a viable alternative to the current system. Through the cost-effective management of the work-related injury, with emphasis on reducing the amount of lost work days, the managed care technique has been shown to produce savings for the employer. At the same time, it offers the injured worker guidance and emotional support, as well as accessible, appropriate medical treatment.[2]

The success of any managed care program depends upon the immediate referral of the injured worker by a designated person at the work site to a case manager. The case manager is usually a registered nurse who directs the worker through the acute injury phase and rehabilitation process and monitors a rapid return to work. This approach can prevent or minimize the often adversarial scenario that develops from mismanagement of these injuries.

REVIEW OF THE TRADITIONAL SYSTEM

In order to understand better how a managed care program can be effective, it is necessary to examine the traditional workers' compensation system and how it works. Each state has a governing agency that oversees injuries sustained by workers, and laws vary from state to state. An employer is either self-insured or obtains workers' compensation coverage through an insurance carrier. Once a lost time injury occurs, a report must be filed by the employer, and notice is sent to the party handling the claims administration. Under the current system, it is not unusual for the First Report of Injury to be filed in an untimely fashion, not reaching the insurer or claims administrator until a week after the occurrence of the injury. In most states, the insurer is obligated to respond within a certain time frame; in Massachusetts, the insurer must respond within 14 days of receipt of the first report. A decision must be made at that time whether to accept or deny the claim.

Conceivably, it could be as long as 3 weeks before injured workers are contacted by anyone about their injury. During that time, they have been left to their own resources to seek appropriate treatment, to cope with their injury and newly acquired free time, and to establish a course of action. If the injured workers have had no contact by the employer since the injury, feelings of confusion and isolation may develop. The longer the disability continues, the greater the possibility that they will experience feelings of anger and resentment toward their employer and insurer. Unless the insurance carrier has a rehabilitation nurse within the office assigned to the claim or contracts out to a private rehabilitation company for medical management, workers, more often than not, must find a physician on their own. Many physicians refuse to treat workers' compensation injuries because of the extremely low reimbursement rates, particularly in states with fee schedules. In addition, many physicians have not been trained to understand the complex issues often associated with work-related injuries, primarily the socioeconomic and legal issues that often interfere with recovery. Therefore, workers may be unable to gain access to good quality medical care in a timely fashion, which can clearly influence their recovery, as well as the cost of the claim.

While waiting for their employer to contact them, the injured workers may begin to feel neglected and may consult an attorney at the advice of friends or coworkers. The attorney would advise them of their rights and benefits due, which would include reimbursement for lost wages based upon a percentage of the average weekly wage and coverage for medical expenses relating to the injury. These benefits would continue until the physician determines that the worker is capable of returning to work. The interests of the attorney may differ from those of the employer and insurer if the attorney's primary means of financial reimbursement is a percentage of the lump sum settlement, rather than a fee for service.

If the injury prevents the worker from returning to the employer or if the worker chooses to seek employment elsewhere, then a lump sum settlement may be obtained as a means of resolving the claim. The lump sum settlement is based upon future disability, and the cash value is determined by the extent of disability. It is not uncommon for the value of the settlement to be 1–3 years of compensation.

For example, depending upon the weekly compensation rate, the amount of the settlement could be between $20,000 to $60,000. The attorney would then receive a percentage—generally around 20 percent of the lump sum settlement. If a worker has no savings and has always had a dream of buying a home or a luxury item, the thought of a $50,000 settlement can appear most attractive and could be equated to a chance of winning a lottery. The attorney may feel that it is in the client's best interest not to return to the work place once the client is medically cleared to do so because of the vehicle of a lump sum settlement. Generally, if an insurer agrees to a lump sum settlement, the decision and the amount of settlement offered are based upon the assumption that the injured worker is unable to return to the job performed at the time of the injury.

In the traditional system, the worker is paid a percentage of the average weekly wage in weekly compensation benefits. For some workers, the weekly compensation check may equal or be very close to the amount of their take-home pay, since this benefit is nontaxable; for others, a substantial financial loss can be experienced.

In many families, a role reversal occurs after the injury. If the head of the household is unable to work, then the spouse may take a job outside of the home and leave the care of the house and children to the injured worker. If the injured worker is a single parent, child care expenses are eliminated when the parent is at home, which may be a disincentive for the worker to engage in return to work efforts.

A worker's attitude toward the job and employer plays an important role in determining the response to an injury. If the workers were unhappy with the job or if previously voiced concerns that the job was causing discomfort were ignored, they may have a negative attitude about returning to work. Experts in the field of workers' compensation report that the claim begins long before the injury and is based on the employee's mindset about the employer's attitude concerning the injured worker.[3]

In addition to these factors, there is also the psychological impact of the disability. The injured worker begins to lose self-confidence, and self-esteem diminishes. The worker's sense of connection to the work place and society in general is altered, and it is not uncommon for the injured worker to feel anger and resentment toward the employer. Domestic problems often arise, and the abuse of chemical substances is commonly encountered. Depression comes to play a major role in the continuation of disability, and unless recognized and appropriately treated, it can cause significant problems in the management of these patients.

MANAGED CARE PROGRAMS

In order to prevent this scenario of anger, frustration, and depression and to avoid long-standing disability, a team approach is necessary. Such an approach is ideally provided in a managed care program that is staffed by professionals who understand not only the mechanics of the work-induced injury but also the plight of the injured worker.

For more than a decade, managed care techniques have been used in health care to reduce costs without compromising the quality of care. Health maintenance organizations are successful examples of managed care programs in the health field.

Within the past few years, experts have begun to recognize that managed care programs in the workers' compensation system could be effective in reducing both medical costs and lost work days, as well as in offering quality and timely treatment for the injured worker.[4] A medical care access study in Massachusetts recently reported that a number of employers and managed care companies have begun to take steps to assure successful therapeutic outcomes and faster return to work for injured workers. These companies have developed specialized relationships with medical providers to assure both access and availability of service for injured workers and cooperation with return to work planning.[5]

A managed care program coordinates the services of a network of medical specialists—qualified physicians, therapists, social workers, psychologists, and rehabilitation professionals who understand work-related injuries. The cornerstone of the program is the case manager who directs the worker through the sometimes complicated and frustrating medicolegal system. By providing information, emotional support, and reassurance throughout the recovery process, the case manager develops a trusting relationship with the worker and is able to direct the employee through the maze of paperwork, appointments, and bureaucracy. Such guidance can often prevent the worker from developing feelings of anger and frustration, which would only trigger a series of even further negative events.

The program can be housed either in an acute care facility in conjunction with an occupational health program or in a rehabilitation setting. Some innovative employers have developed on-site rehabilitation centers that include occupational and physical therapy programs, as well as on-site case managers to oversee return to work programs. Providers enter a contractual agreement with prearranged fees. The employer can also contract with a risk management company to provide this program, or it can be provided through the insurance carrier.

The goal of the treatment team is coordination of medical care to maximize a rapid return to work and prevent the development of long-term disability, which has often been caused by the problems associated with the workers' compensation system. The role of each participant may vary, but the objective is to minimize the effects of the injury and the amount of lost time incurred.

The protocol of any managed care program should require that the first report of injury be completed immediately after the incident by the worker's supervisor and be reported within 24 hours to the claims administrator or the case manager. The case manager, who is generally a registered nurse with a background in occupational health or rehabilitative nursing, is then assigned to the case. The first step is to advise the injured worker that the case manager has been asked by the employer to assist with his or her medical care. Depending upon the seriousness of the injury and the magnitude of the socioeconomic issues, the degree of assistance will vary. At the very least, a message of interest and concern is conveyed to the worker, along with reassurance that timely and appropriate treatment will be provided. The case manager also discusses what the worker can expect to happen after the injury and addresses any questions or concerns. The case manager evaluates the extent of injury and suggests the names of appropriate physicians. Assistance is provided in obtaining appointments, and the case manager should attend the initial visit. When appropriate, a return to work date is established depending upon the extent of the injury.

Throughout the process, the case manager is in contact with both the employer and physician, advising the physician about light duty or modified work programs. Ideally, the physician is familiar with the employer's industry and is aware of the physical requirements of specific jobs. If not, the case manager should discuss with the physician various jobs that are available, emphasizing the physical demands of each one. If this is not feasible, then a written job description should be made available to the physician; it should include descriptions of physical demands, as well as information regarding the availability of light duty positions.

The case manager keeps in close contact with the injured worker either by telephone or visits to the home. This contact is vital to the proper management of the claim. The worker is psychologically tied to the place of employment by the frequent contact of the case manager, as well as by contact from the employer.

Accompanying the worker to physician or therapist appointments is also very helpful. Doing so ensures that the worker receives accurate information about the diagnosis and necessary treatment plan and, most important, has a return to work target date upon which to focus.

Injured workers must have a clear understanding of their responsibilities in following through with the recommended treatment plan. They must recognize that a cooperative effort must take place among all participants in order to realize a return to the work place. They are encouraged to focus on the concept that they will recover quickly and will return to the employer, rather than the notion that they are now disabled.

It is true that the managed care system does not provide the injured worker with the opportunity to choose a medical provider. However, experience in the medical insurance industry has shown that when an attractive voluntary provider network is established, approximately 75 to 80 percent of the population will take advantage of it. Within that system, pa-

tients' right to use the provider of their choice is preserved.[5] In addition, injured workers who are not familiar with the workers' compensation system need guidance to find appropriate treatment. If employers do not take the initiative to direct their workers toward appropriate medical treatment, then the workers will find someone else to direct them in order to make certain that their needs are met.[5]

The worker must be given time to understand what has happened as a result of the injury and be given the opportunity to accept any loss that has resulted from it. This may include the inability to return to the previous level of functioning; retraining in another line of work may be required. With a managed care system in place, the period of disability can be minimized with the provision of timely and quality medical treatment. If it is determined that return to the employer is not feasible as a result of the injury, then early referral can be made to a vocational counselor to begin exploration of vocational options.

No doubt there exist workers whose intent is not to return to work but rather to seek as much monetary gain as possible. However, the number of workers who share this avaricious attitude are few. The majority of workers want to get well and are looking for direction through an often confusing and frustrating process. A managed care system provides a comprehensive means of giving that direction.

ROLE OF THE PHYSICIAN

Traditionally, physicians have been trained to treat a diagnosed condition or disorder and to focus primarily on the injured body part, rather than on the person as a whole entity. In addition, physicians traditionally have not been involved with complex return to work issues. However, today's physician must not only be expert in treating the musculoskeletal condition but also needs to understand how the disability will affect the patient's life in general. The physician needs to determine whether the injury is creating financial hardship and whether the worker has a job to which to return. Such variables as attorney representation and the patient's attitude toward the employer can dramatically affect the patient's response to treatment and desire to return to the work place. Physicians need to be aware of the problems that injured workers can face as a result of becoming caught up in a system that often fosters disability.

The physician is the key player in this entire process and is in a position to influence greatly the injured worker's attitude and ability to return to work. This author has repeatedly heard injured workers say, "It is up to my doctor to advise me when I can return to work, and I have no idea of when this will be. I guess I will just have to wait and see what happens." Unfortunately, it is this wait-and-see attitude that promotes a feeling of uncertainty and negativism about returning to work as the worker is unable to visualize a clearly defined plan that will conclude with a return to gainful employment. The most important period for charting the course of treatment is during the immediate postinjury days. Whether the worker has a 4-day convalescence from an easily controlled infection or 3 months of treatment for a ruptured disc, the initial patient/physician encounter is crucial in controlling the amount of time lost from work.[6]

Physicians need to become familiar with the basic workers' compensation laws in the state in which they practice. In additional to practicing their own speciality, they need to be aware of the overall occupational and socioeconomic issues that can complicate the diagnosis. Just as diabetes can cause complications

in a patient's recovery, so too can the psychological and socioeconomic issues associated with the work-related injury. If the physician is able to recognize these nonmedical factors, referral can be made to the appropriate professional, such as a social worker or psychologist, to assist in the management of these patients. Since the case manager is in frequent contact with the worker and the physician, the case manager can assist the physician in identifying problems as they develop and arrange for referrals as needed.

Experience has shown that, if all of the worker's needs are addressed, then the recovery can take place in a more expeditious manner and the length and amount of residual disability can be minimized. The worker needs to feel confident that the physician understands the impact of the injury on his or her life, and a sense of trust needs to be established between the physician and the worker.

ADVANTAGES FOR PARTICIPATING PHYSICIANS

Many physicians are unwilling to treat workers' compensation patients because of the low reimbursement rates established by fee schedules. In addition, a recent study showed that the medical specialist perceives work-related injuries as much more difficult and much less desirable to treat because of the number of nonmedical players, such as lawyers, insurers, and employers, who interfere with treatment. The level of motivation of the injured worker and the amount of paperwork involved were also mentioned as deterrents to the care of injured workers.[5]

Treating the patient with a work-related injury can be extremely frustrating and difficult. For various reasons, recovery is often delayed in comparison to those patients with the same conditions that were not work induced. Recent studies have shown that work-injured individuals were found to be out of work for an average of 8.3 months compared to 1.25 months for the non-workers' compensation population.[5] One reason for this great disparity may be that the specialty medical provider community is not organized to serve the unique needs of the work-injured individuals, which call for great coordination among employee, employer, insurer, and provider.[5]

One of the primary reasons why physicians choose medicine as their profession is that they enjoy enabling their patients to get better. Being part of a managed care system provides the physician with the opportunity to see patients respond in a positive way, perhaps because of their attitude is somewhat influenced by the way they are being treated. The case manager can often attend to the details that the physician does not have time to handle and can deal with attorneys, insurers, and employers, thereby freeing up the physician's time. The role of the case manager is to coordinate the efforts of all of the participants in the compensation system, and the physician has the opportunity to work closely with the case manager, who can really be viewed as an extension of the physician.

The managed care system allows physicians to be involved immediately in planning the injured worker's care before the mindset of disability has developed. The worker is given the sense that the health care team members—the physician, the therapist, and the case manager—are working in concert to minimize the effects of the injury and subsequent period of disability. As a result, the patient presents with a more positive attitude, having been treated fairly by the employer and case manager from the outset and been given the sense that he or she is a valued human being. Physicians take a great deal of pride in being able to identify the patient's diagnosis, recommend a surgical or nonsurgical approach, and implement the appropriate treatment plan. They are then able to witness the patient's recovery in an expected time frame and eventually see the patient discharged to resume work activities. Physicians can provide the type of incentives that place the injured worker on the road to recovery.

ADVANTAGES FOR THE INJURED WORKER

Perhaps the most significant benefit of a managed care program for the injured worker is the sense of validation it conveys, in contrast to the suspicion that is often seen in the traditional system. The injured worker is guided through the process and supported along the way, provided with quality medical treatment, and is promptly made eligible for workers' compensation benefits as the injury is reported to the carrier or claims administrator in a timely fashion. The worker's financial, emotional, and medical needs are being met concurrently. Workers experience peace of mind and a feeling of security knowing that they are receiving benefits and will return to the work place in a designated time frame.

Research into the factors that cause some employees to seek attorneys has revealed that the major reason for attorney involvement was the employee's lack of understanding of the benefits and how the system worked.[5] The overall theme of a managed care program is treating the worker with respect and honesty. The employer, along with the case manager, is available to provide information on such matters as the workers' compensation law and medical issues. By being given adequate information and reassurance, the worker may be less likely to feel the need to seek attorney representation.

ADVANTAGES FOR EMPLOYERS

The advantages for employers who use a managed care program are many. The most obvious advantage is a reduction in lost time work days, which translates into cost savings.

As workers' compensation costs have skyrocketed, employers are now taking a more active role in examining how their workers' compensation dollar is being spent. "Five or six years ago, companies considered high disability claims part of the cost of doing business. Today, they are beginning to see these claims as the cost of not managing business."[1] For example, the cost of a carpal tunnel syndrome claim that does not involve surgery is approximately $3,500. With surgery, it averages around $20,000, if the individual returns to work. If the injured worker is unable to return, the cost for one carpal tunnel syndrome claim could be as high as $100,000.[7] Obviously, prevention for this and other cumulative trauma disorders is the best treatment. However, once the injury has occurred, putting disabled employees back into the plant or office as soon as possible has been a major cost saver for companies.[1] Employers can no longer rely solely on the insurance carrier to handle their losses, but must take a participatory approach to help contain their workers' compensation costs. The fact that the traditional system lacks controls at both the work site and with the insurer further supports the need for a more controlled system.

A managed care program provides the employer with more control and input into the handling and outcome of their claims. It allows the employer to monitor the progress of the worker through frequent contact with the employee. A disability management strategy in place before the injury occurs will help curtail claim disputes.[1]

LIGHT DUTY PROGRAMS

Along with managed care programs, employers must recognize the value of light duty programs and incorporate them into their loss management efforts. To maximize the benefits of the managed care system, employers must provide light duty positions for the injured workers. The longer an individual remains out of work, the more difficult it is to achieve a return to the work place. Light duty programs promote both faster psychological and physical healing. Unfortunately, in union companies, because of seniority and the need to bid on particular jobs, it remains extremely difficult if not impossible to bring a worker back in a light duty position. However, some unions are beginning to recognize the value of light duty work programs.

Light duty programs translate into savings by eliminating the need to bring in temporary workers and the expense of training new workers to assume the injured worker's duties. A light duty program can enable the employer to continue to benefit from their experienced workers by placing them temporarily in modified duty positions, thereby not having to compromise quality.

It is essential that light duty assignments be meaningful. Workers should not be expected to return to work to perform such demeaning tasks as counting how many paper clips are in a box or how many times the office telephone rings.

They need to feel productive and should be given the opportunity to contribute to the company's productivity within their physical limitations.

With cumulative trauma disorders, the physician and therapist need to review carefully the job descriptions of light duty assignments. The physician must be informed of the number of repetitions involved, duration of activity, and the like of a particular assignment. Light duty assignments need to be monitored closely so that the performance of the tasks remains within the worker's level of comfort. In addition, once assigned to light duty, the employee's rehabilitation progress must be closely monitored as if the employee was on a temporary disability and a return to work date must be set. The employee, the doctor, and the physical therapist have to be strongly encouraged to meet that return to work date. Otherwise, the injured employee can stay too long on the light duty assignment.[8] Light duty programs must be managed by someone with compassion and sensitivity for people.

In a managed care program, the case manager is available to monitor the light duty assignment and to relay information to the physician regarding the progress that is being made. The case manager must continue to follow the worker throughout the duration of the light duty assignment to assess adequately its effectiveness. The value of work hardening programs is discussed in Chapter 18; they should be used in conjunction with light duty assignments when appropriate.

Returning to work on a part-time basis initially is often recommended and has proven to be a successful way to ease the worker into the work place. The financial advantage to the employer is that the weekly compensation check can be either discontinued or reduced substantially. Since wage compensation is the largest expense resulting from a work-related injury, substantial dollar savings can be realized.

ADDITIONAL LOSS MANAGEMENT TECHNIQUES

In addition to a managed care program and light duty assignments, employers can also use pre-employment physicals as a means of reducing their workers' compensation expenses. Pre-employment physicals are helpful in identifying workers who may be at risk for injury. The employer can then avoid giving them a work assignment that may aggravate a predisposition to a particular disorder.

Using loss prevention techniques can also help the employer realize further savings. The use of loss control specialists, safety engineers, and ergonomic consultants is recommended. Ongoing education on safety issues and a common sense approach to decreasing the incidence of injury in the work place should take place with management and supervisory staff, as well as all employees.

Communication with workers needs to be encouraged, and suggestions by the workers regarding ways to perform a job more effectively need to be acknowledged. Employers must become more open to recommendations from employees at all levels. Offering such incentives as cash bonuses or paid days off for a reduction in the incidence of work injuries is an effective way to encourage workers to see that positive results can be achieved through a cooperative effort. The goal of all employers must be the creation of a safer work environment, which can be achieved by the use of continuous loss control activities.

Employers must enable all levels of staff, beginning with the corporate level to develop an awareness that the employee is not only a worker, but is indeed the employer's greatest asset. There is anecdotal evidence that workers' compensation claims increase when there is antagonism between employees and management.[9] Employers must recognize that the injured worker is a human being with a family and the aspirant of hopes and dreams for a successful life. One employer known to this author invites injured workers to lunch once a week at the plant and expresses interest and concern for their medical condition. During this visit they also explore the availability of light duty positions and discuss the possibility of returning the worker to positions appropriate to their physical limitations. The response has been positive, as workers have been given the sense of remaining connected to the work place.

REFORM PROPOSALS

Recently in Massachusetts, the Division of Insurance approved several workers' compensation reform proposals that are designed to help control workers' compensation costs. One proposal offers a 5 to 10 percent discount on premiums for employers in the high-risk pool who utilizes a loss management program.

In addition to the reform proposal, the Medical Care Access Study[5] recommended the promotion of education for employees, employers, and medical providers on the types of medical provider networks that exist, how to use them, and their benefits. The study results indicated that the employer and the employee are the parties most capable of coordinating the return to work process with the medical provider, because the employer has complete control over the decision to provide modified duty programs.[5]

Certainly, the reform proposal and the recommendations of the recent study are a step in the right direction and are evidence of the trend toward a more effective and human-oriented approach to the worker injury. However, the solution to the workers' compensation crisis does not lie with legislative reform alone. Employers need to take a more proactive role in ensuring a safe work environment for their employees, and if an injury does occur, there must be a system in place to provide quality medical care to the worker in a timely fashion.

SUMMARY

A managed care program can be instrumental in reducing the number of lost work days, thus producing dollar savings. The physician's approach to the treatment of the patient with job-related injuries is key to the successful outcome of the treatment plan.

The physician must be aware of the numerous nonmedical issues that can influence the patient's recovery and ability to return to work. For instance, one orthopaedic surgeon often asks patients who are well enough to return to work but have not done so if they would be back to work were they self-employed. An affirmative response is obtained more often than not, which often initiates a discussion about why the patient has not returned to work. Often after thinking this through, the patient goes on and makes the decision to return to work with the encouragement and support of the physician.

The physician who is sensitive to the needs of the injured worker and committed to treating this often complex patient can contribute significantly to the achievement of a positive end result for all involved. Employers who acknowledge that the work environment encompasses not only the physical surroundings but also the attitudes created by management in their approach to handling workers' compensation issues, will begin to realize a reduction in their workers' compensation costs. Rather than expending energy on the expectation that the traditional system will change, the opportunity exists for all participants to bring about a change from within. It is hoped that this type of effort can evolve into a more humanistic and successful approach to the workers' compensation problem.

REFERENCES

1. McDonald M: You can control your disability costs. Business Health, p 28, May, 1990

2. Ford M: System cuts workers' compensation costs. South Shore Business J, p 13, September, 1989

3. Howard L: Care cuts compensation cost. Experts, National Underwriter, p 32, May 21, 1990

4. Tufts Associated Health Plans: Managed Comp.—the solution to runaway workers' compensation costs. The Tufts Associated Health Plans, Boston, 1990

5. Lynch Ryan/Boylson Group: Medical care access study Massachusetts Workers' Compensation Advisory Council, 1990

6. Conway R: Treating workers' compensation patients right. New England Insurance Times. 6:29, 1988

7. VPS Case Management Services Inc: Carpal tunnel syndrome: case management concepts. Fall, 1988

8. McIntyre KJ: Light duty programs a must. Business Insur, p 8, April 16, 1990

9. Connors N: Staying in control of workers' compensation claims. CFO Magazine, pp 47–48, August, 1990

9

Clinical Evaluation of the Injured Worker

Lewis H. Millender, M.D.

Physicians are asked to evaluate patients with occupational disorders for different reasons. They may be the treating physician or may be asked to carry out an independent medical evaluation for the employer, insurance company, or attorney. The role is different depending on whether they are the treating physician or only the examining physician, and this difference must be clearly understood. As the treating physician the doctor's role is to treat the patient's medical problem and work closely with allied health professionals attempting to return the worker to the job market. The role of an independent evaluator is to examine the patient and make determinations regarding return to work, end result, permanent impairment status, or causal relationship of the condition to the job. If the patient's recovery has reached an end result the physician will be asked to state if the worker is able to return to the previous job, if modified work is necessary, or if rehabilitation is needed.

Additionally, the physician will be asked to determine the degree of physical impairment. The distinction between physical impairment and disability must be clearly understood. Impairment measures functional loss based upon deformity, loss of motion, weakness, and other physical determinations. The percent of impairment is based upon the *AMA Guidelines to the Evaluation of Permanent Impairment* (see Chapter 20). Physical impairment is determined by physicians. In contrast, disability is a legal determination and is based on such factors as education, job skills, and other socioeconomic considerations. Disability is rewarded by judges or other legal authorities.

Regardless of who requests an independent medical evaluation, the physician's job is to render honest, unbiased, dispassionate reports. When physicians become labeled as either "insurance doctors" or "attorney doctors," their reputation becomes tainted and their reports lose all credibility.

PATIENT CATEGORIES

When considering work-related disabilities there are three groups of patients who are seen (this excludes acute traumatic injuries which are treated by conventional orthopaedic methods and are not covered in this book). These groups are (1) acute onset at work, (2) unresolved, chronic upper extremity problem, and (3) chronic pain with return to work unlikely.

Acute Onset

This group presents with relatively acute onset of pain occurring at work. The condition is usually a tendinitis, myositis, bursitis, joint inflammation, or nerve entrapment. In these cases the history is usually straightforward, the etiology and relationship to the job are easily determined, and the condition is treated by conventional methods with a fast resolution and rapid return to work. Depending on the specific situation, a course of therapy or a short time with job modification may be indicated. When these conditions become chronic or recurrent, the physician then must evaluate the patient's job to determine whether a permanent job change or surgical intervention is appropriate.

Unresolved Chronic Upper Extremity Problem

The second type of patient is the worker with an unresolved chronic upper extremity problem who has not been able to return to work. This group is characterized by having few secondary gain issues, there is a high motivation level, and the employment issues are favorable. The physician must evaluate the disorder and the job to determine whether surgical intervention is reasonable or if job modification or rehabilitation is preferable.

The surgical judgment in these cases is critical and often difficult. The physician has traditionally been called upon to make a decision regarding surgery to alleviate pain or improve function. When treating the worker the physician must

consider not only whether the surgery will relieve pain, and improve function, but also whether it will allow the patient to return to work. If this outcome is questionable, the physician must be cautious in recommending surgery. Patients should be informed of the anticipated outcome of surgery, especially when there is doubt that it will allow them to return to their prior job. The alternative approach of job change or rehabilitation should be explained carefully so the patient can evaluate this alternative. A major cause of long-standing chronic disability is ill-advised or inappropriate surgery that leaves the worker disabled and unable to return to work.

Chronic Long Standing Disorders with Pain

The third group of injured patients have chronic and often long-standing occupational disorders that are usually associated with pain. In some cases the injury or condition will not allow the patient to return to employment, and in other cases complicated psychosocial or legal issues impede successful rehabilitation. The treating physician in these cases must direct the rehabilitation process and work with all the other allied health professionals either to rehabilitate the worker or recommend settlement to the case.

Although opinions vary regarding physician involvement in legal issues, such as vocational rehabilitation, or complicated return to work issues, physician involvement can be both appropriate and helpful. In cases where there is conflict between the insurer, employer, or attorney, the physician is often best qualified to advise the worker. When there is mutual trust between physician and worker, the patient can voice fears, frustrations, and anger. Whereas the employer, insurer, and attorney often have specific agendas, the physician's one concern is the total welfare of the patient. The authors in Chapter 5, 8, and 19 emphasize the importance of the physician's involvement in these difficult socioeconomic issues and how helpful the physician can be in resolving them.

APPROACH TO EVALUATING PATIENTS WITH OCCUPATIONAL DISORDERS

The complexity or thoroughness of the occupational history will vary depending upon the specific case and its requirements. When there are few occupational issues and minor impairment the evaluation is straightforward. However, when issues, such as causality, return to work, and the degree of impairment, arise, the history becomes very important. There are several components to the occupational history.

The initial history should be accurate and detailed because of the many issues that will need to be considered. Obviously, if an acute injury has occurred, the history should focus upon the events that caused the injury. If the worker developed an acute tendinitis, or sustained a laceration or crush injury to the hand, the details of the event should be recorded and a copy of the emergency room visit obtained if possible. In addition to the obvious questions regarding the mechanism of the injury and the type of instrument that caused the injury, one should inquire about the machine or the work factors that were responsible. This information might be important later from a legal standpoint, and it is wise to have an initial detailed record. Such a record

may be necessary when determining return to work issues and when causal relation issues are raised.

In chronic work-related disorders the history should be detailed, and many specific pieces of information must be obtained. In long-standing cases there are often a plethora of reports from other treating physicians, therapists, evaluating physicians, and lawyers. The patient may have had physical capacity evaluations, psychological evaluations, and multiple consultations. The physician must allow adequate time to study these reports. A frequent problem occurs when a worker comes in for a visit with a large folder of medical reports that must be evaluated and inadequate time has been scheduled. One's office staff should determine the complexity of the case before the patient is seen so that adequate time is allowed for consultation.

In complicated situations, having the rehabilitation specialist present at the initial visit can be very helpful. In addition to assisting the physician in understanding the complicated physical, social, and employment issues, the rehabilitation specialist facilitates the development of a strong and positive doctor-patient relationship, which is so important in these complicated cases. Although some physicians and patients are resistant to working with rehabilitation specialists, thinking that they represent the employer or insurer, I have found them invaluable in resolving difficult cases. Not only do they help coordinate the myriad bureaucratic issues, but they also aid physicians by explaining and reinforcing their recommendations. In difficult and long-standing work-related disorders I now refuse to treat the patient unless a rehabilitation specialist is assigned to the case.

It is important to allow the patient time to describe the injury and job in detail. This can be time consuming and seemingly nonproductive, depending on the patient's articulateness. Additionally, when the job is technical and the worker uses unfamiliar terms it is difficult to get a good feel for its demands. However, if the physician takes the time to listen insight will often be gained into the day to day task that the patient is required to perform. Patients also like to have the opportunity to describe in detail what caused their disability; when the physician takes the time to listen, positive relationship is established and the patient feels the physician really cares. One must realize that the history is often embellished because of the need for the patient to emphasize or prove a point, but this gives the physician an opportunity to understand some of the emotions surrounding the injury. It is wise to inquire about the patient's personal life as well. A simple question, such as "How are things at home?", may release a flood of emotion and sometimes tears due to the frustration and depression associated with the injury, as well as the confusion and anger with the worker's compensation system.

After the patient has described the injury, some specific facts need to be ascertained, such as how repetitive the job is and whether it is associated with a high degree of force. Cycle time is also an important factor. One needs to understand which joints are subjected to overuse and whether the worker is placed in awkward positions. Does the job require twisting motions, wrist flexion-extension, repetitive elbow flexion, or a significant amount of overhead work?

In addition to understanding the specific job, one needs to learn if there are opportunities to adjust the job. Is job ro-tation, job enlargement, or light duty work available to the worker? If the job is incentive pay or machine paced, can this be adjusted? What is the company policy regarding injured workers, and what other job opportunities exist for alternate work in the company? How long has the worker been employed there, and does he or she like it and wish to return to the same company? The rehabilitation specialist is valuable in providing answers to these questions.

In complicated return to work situations additional information should be obtained. Job descriptions are available that outline the work requirements very specifically. Therapists are trained to evaluate jobs and help determine with the physician if the worker can return to certain jobs. In difficult return to work issues the physician must consult with hand therapists trained in job evaluation or with vocational rehabilitation counselors. Together with these specialists, appropriate job recommendations can be made. However it is essential to emphasize that the treating or evaluating physician [in cases of independent medical evaluations (IME)] directs the multiple parties to help the patient.

The following chapters provide an approach to treating specific job-related upper extremity disorders. In addition to discussing specific treatment we have tried to emphasize those conditions for which surgery has not always provided the desired result for the worker and we describe alternate approaches. In many of these situations the options are controversial, and the scientific literature does not always provide clear answers.

10

Occupational Disorders of the Hand and Digits

Barry P. Simmons, M.D.
Mark J. Koris, M.D.

Obviously, this chapter cannot and should not be a comprehensive text of disorders of the hand and fingers. As are other chapters it is oriented toward the disorders that mostly commonly cause workers to seek medical attention. It focuses on the following subjects: trigger fingers, osteoarthritis of the proximal and distal interphalangeal joint, ligamentous/capsular injuries of the digital joints, amputations, Dupuytren's disease, sesamoiditis of the thumb, fingertip injuries, and the vibration syndrome.

TRIGGER FINGER/THUMB: STENOSING TENOSYNOVITIS

Clinical Picture

Patients with trigger fingers may present with a variety of complaints. The classic picture is painful "locking" of the digit in flexion whereby the patient has difficulty extending the proximal inter-phalangeal joint. Extension can be accomplished passively using the other hand and produces a moderate amount of discomfort and a palpable painful "snap." Any finger can be involved, but the ring finger and thumb are the two most common. Patients often complain of the pain and snapping at the proximal interphalangeal joint. On occasion they have triggering without pain or pain, usually in the palm at the base of the affected digit, without triggering. Triggering seems to be more common at night, but also can be seen in the worker intermittently during the day.

Triggering is most commonly seen in the over 40 age group. Although it can certainly occur without an inciting activity it occurs more frequently in workers who have to do multiple repetitive motions and/or grasp hard, cylindric objects firmly.

Examination discloses tenderness in the palm at the base of the digit at the level of the first annular pulley where a nodule in the tendon can also be palpated. If triggering does not occur spontaneously, it may be elicited by putting pressure on the pulley with the examiner's own finger. The examiner should check the range of motion carefully; fixed flexion deformities or diffuse flexor tenosynovitis can be a common complication of prolonged triggering and may be an indication for earlier surgical intervention. A limited range of motion in flexion and/or extension also implies osteoarthritis, which should be considered in the differential diagnosis in this age group.

Confirmatory Tests

An x-ray should be obtained if patients have a limited range of motion. Otherwise, no tests are necessary.

Treatment

NSAIDs may be tried, but rarely yield significant results. Injections of depo-steroid into the flexor tendon sheath alleviate complaints in 92 to 97 percent of patients with nodular disease and is the treatment of choice.[1,2] In fact a steroid injection is sufficiently successful that one may be reluctant to alter the patient's usual job requirements during the course of treatment. Occasional nighttime splinting in 30° of proximal interphalangeal flexion may also be indicated. If patients fail the initial injection, it can be repeated once or twice. A period of rest from their usual job may also be indicated. The results of a surgical release of the pulley are so good that the patient may opt for that treatment, rather than prolonging the course with several injections and a period of disability.

Prognosis

The prognosis is excellent for a complete recovery barring the occurrence of multiple trigger fingers and/or significant osteoarthritis.[3] In these cases the course is usually prolonged. Patients tend to question their ability to return to their old job and, on occasion, any job. In general, workers should be able to return to heavy work, although it may take somewhat longer after surgery because of a tender palmar scar.

OSTEOARTHRITIS OF THE PROXIMAL INTERPHALANGEAL JOINT

Clinical Picture

After the distal interphalangeal and thumb carpometacarpal joint, the proximal interphalangeal (PIP) joint is most commonly affected by osteoarthritis.[4] It is seen in patients over 45 years of age, except in rare cases. It is considerably more common in women than men over 50 years-old, but is slightly more common in men than in women in the younger age group. There is a real question of causality, especially in patients who do not perform heavy, manual labor, because it occurs fairly commonly in the population at large. Patients present with complaints of pain, deformity, and/or stiffness. On examination there may be synovitis with swelling, Bouchard's nodes, limitation of motion, and deformity that occurs frequently in the ulnar direction.

Confirmatory Tests

X-rays are usually all the tests are necessary. Especially in the younger age group or if there are systemic symptoms, it is wise, however, to obtain an arthritis screen to rule out rheumatoid arthritis or other systemic disorders.

Treatment

Initial treatment should consist of NSAIDs, which often yield good pain relief. Patients are referred to rehabilitation for instruction in the proper use of the hand at work, range of motion exercises, as well as intermittent splinting. None of these modalities will correct the deformity. If the symptoms are sufficiently severe, job modification to eliminate heavy lifting and/or repetitive motion will be necessary. If patients remain symptomatic in their job but are able to cope with their activities of daily living adequately, then either job modification or permanent partial disability should be suggested as the best course of action. On occasion workers may be able to return to their previous job after surgery.

If the patient is sufficiently symptomatic or the rehabilitation consultant, patient, and physician feel that surgery may enable a return to the job, it should be undertaken. The surgical alternatives include arthrodesis or arthroplasty. Generally, the former procedure has been suggested for the border digits, but arthroplasty in those fingers can also be considered; it depends on the age of the patient, the job, and the status of the other joints.[5] Although arthroplasty is effective in relieving pain, deformity may persist or recur, and the range of motion will still be limited.

Prognosis

The prognosis is guarded, although there are many variables to be considered. A patient who fails medical treatment is unlikely to return to work after surgery, especially if the job entails heavy labor.

OSTEOARTHRITIS OF THE DISTAL INTERPHALANGEAL JOINT

Clinical Picture

The distal interphalangeal (DIP) joint and the thumb interphalangeal joint are the joints of the hand most commonly involved with osteoarthritis.[4] The clinical picture is the same as seen at the proximal interphalangeal joint level, but the disorder at this level is known here as Heberden's nodes. Mucous cysts are commonly seen.

Confirmatory Tests

X-rays and an arthritis screen are sufficient.

Treatment

Conservative treatment is the same as for the PIP joint. When patients fail medical treatment, arthrodesis should be considered. It is excellent for relieving pain and correcting deformity, obviously at the cost of motion. However, patients rarely complain of stiffness. Small mucous cysts need no treatment. If they are large and the skin over them is thin, the potential for rupture is high. With rupture, infection can occur and may involve the DIP joint.[6] It is best to treat these cysts surgically to avoid more significant problems.

Prognosis

One can be somewhat more optimistic about the results of treatment for osteoarthritis of the DIP joint than for the PIP joint. Medical treatment may help a great deal, and if it does not, the results of surgery are sufficiently good that the worker may return to the job with minimal, if any, job modification.

LIGAMENTOUS/CAPSULAR INJURIES OF THE DIGITAL JOINTS

Clinical Picture

Soft tissue injuries of the digital joints are sufficiently common at the metacarpophalangeal (MCP) and PIP level that they can be discussed together. Acute injuries occur considerably more commonly at the PIP joint level than at the MCP joint. They are produced by a hyperextension mechanism that results from "jamming" the tip of one's finger. Patients present with pain, swelling, and/or stiffness; the joint is usually stable on lateral stress. At the MCP level the disorder is generally chronic in nature. It occurs from repeated stress in a lateral, usually ulnar direction. Tenderness can be located either over the base of the proximal phalanx or the metacarpal head. Pain can also be elicited by stressing the radial collateral ligament, which is most efficiently done with the MCP joint in full flexion. In the thumb, especially if there is a history of an old injury, instability is more common. The hallmark for all of these injuries is the slow rate of resolution. It is not uncommon for the pain to take 3 to 6 months to abate, and the patient may still be left with some swelling and stiffness, especially at the PIP levels.

Confirmatory Tests

X-rays are all that are necessary. Although one may wish to do a stress view to document the instability, the clinical examination is usually sufficient.

Treatment

Treatment for these disorders is usually mechanical. Although NSAIDs may occasionally help in chronic disorders, they generally are not useful. Rehabilitation in the form of edema control, intermittent splinting, "buddy" taping to the adjacent finger, joint protection, and range of motion exercises is the best approach. If chronic instability is present in the thumb, then ligamentous reconstruction or arthrodesis may be indicated.[7-9]

Prognosis

The prognosis is good as long as the patient and employer realize that resolution may take several months. The time lost from work may be minimized if the worker can tolerate mild discomfort, and/or the job can be modified to eliminate significant complaints.

AMPUTATIONS

Clinical Picture

Needless to say, there is nothing subtle about making the diagnosis on patients with amputations. This section addresses substantial tissue loss, not fingertip injuries, which are addressed later in the chapter. Patients who sustain amputations have many problems that go well beyond the loss of tissue. These include limited flexion, either due to trauma proximal to the amputation site or flexor tendon injury (the quadregia effect); neuroma pain; tissue durability problems; cold intolerance; and emotional problems. It is remarkable to see how often patients with amputations, regardless of their occupation, return to work. In fact, one of the cogent arguments for avoiding replantation of a single digit (except the thumb, which should always be replanted if possible) is the prolonged recovery time.[10] Patients who will have or have had prolonged disability because of their impairment are less likely to return to work.

Patients with cold intolerance may or may not have a demonstrably cold finger; findings can often be elicited by exposing the hand to a cold environment, such as ice water. However, there is rarely any need to perform this test as the patients are usually sensitive to lesser stimuli.

Patients with neuroma symptoms can present in many ways. They may have nothing more than an annoying paresthesia or positive Tinel's sign. However, they may present with symptoms of such severity that the examiner is not permitted to even touch the hand. Often, one should simply observe attempted active flexion/extension for evidence of dyssynchronous movement.Complaints and physical findings should be localized within the digit or upper extremity. Are the findings at the neuroma site? Do they radiate distally or distally and proximally, or do they involve the whole extremity?

Patients with problems relating to the loss of a body part may also present with varied emotional reactions. Some patients are forthright and acknowledge the ongoing grief, whereas others do not discuss it. Treatment plans must include social and psychological mechanisms to help the patient cope with the loss.

Confirmatory Tests

Stump pain may be an indication to obtain an x-ray to rule out either infection or a bony exostosis. Neurogenic pain may be an indication to obtain electrodiagnostic testing and/or Semmes-Weinstein evaluation.

Treatment

Treatment obviously depends on many factors. Stump pain may respond well to a local revision. Infection requires debridement and antibiotics. In the patient with limited flexion, rehabilitation exercises and/or surgery may be helpful. There is essentially no treatment for cold intolerance; it may resolve spontaneously after 1 to 2 years. Removing the worker from a cold environment is essential. The authors do not feel that medication either in the form of beta or calcium channel blockers is of any great value. Surgical sympathectomy is not indicated. Surgery is also rarely beneficial for neuromas. A patient who has not had previous neuroma surgery and who either has a locally painful nerve stump or limited antegrade paresthesias, may benefit from burying of the neuroma or simple resection.[11] Failed previous surgery and severe antegrade pain are good indications for referral of the patient to a chronic pain clinic.

The emotional result of an amputation, although not tangible, may be addressed easily. Patients who have nightmares about the accident and an extended grief period may benefit from counseling. These patients rarely return to their previous job and, in some cases, to the same or any work place. They are often quite forthright in their feelings, and any attempt to convince them otherwise is foolhardy. On occasion they may adjust better to the loss of a digit or a more extensive amputation with a cosmetic prosthesis. Some prostheses available now are quite excellent.

Prognosis

The prognosis is variable, depending on the injury. Surgery to correct limited motion, with the proper indication, may be successful. Patients with cold intolerance should be retrained and not placed in a cold environment. Although everyday cold intolerance may abate eventually, the condition may still be precipitated by working in a cold environment for a prolonged period. Prolonging a worker's absence from the work force while waiting for cold intolerance to resolve is usually counterproductive. The painful neuroma is unpredictable, but generally does not have a good prognosis. If emotional problems are the major factor, again one should not be too optimistic about the outcome.

DUPUYTREN'S DISEASE

Clinical Picture

Dupuytren's disease is seen most commonly in white men of Northern European extraction over the age of 50.[12] Patients seek medical advice for their condition for many reasons. Early in the course of the disease, patients may have no more than a thickening in their palm along the course of the pretendinous band or a nodule at the level of the distal palmar crease. This nodule occurs most commonly at the base of the ring finger. It may be tender. Patients may have minor difficulty in their work if their job involves grasping hard objects in their palm. The complaints of pain abate with time, usually in about 6 months. Other than painful nodules, Dupuytren's disease is usually painless. Another source must be looked for if pain is the reason for presentation to the health facility. Contractures occur in some patients with time. After the ring finger, the small, middle, and index fingers are the most likely to be involved. Obviously, the degree of contracture varies among patients. Significant radial-sided involvement is un-

common, although some thickening of the fascia in the first web space or base of the thumb might occur.[13]

This disorder is seen far more commonly in men than women and is usually found, except for the isolated nodule that may not progress to contracture, in the over 50-year-old age group. A group of patients have factors predisposing to a more aggressive Dupuytren's disease with significant contractures and extensive involvement of the skin by the diseased fascia.[14,15] These factors include a positive family history; such chronic diseases as epilepsy or juvenile/brittle diabetes; alcoholism; early age of onset of nodules and contractures; the presence of ectopic foci on the dorsum of the proximal interphalangeal joints, the penis (Peyronie's disease), or the plantar aspect of the foot; bilateral hand involvement, radial as well as ulnar-sided disease; and recurrence after previous surgery.

The findings on physical examination differ with the stage of the disease. A solitary nodule is usually firm and tender and is located at the level of the distal palmar crease at the base of the ring finger. The extent and distribution of thickened tissue both in the palm and digit vary with the contracture. Because flexion is not affected, absence of full flexion means that another disorder is present. Osteoarthritis is most likely in the older age group. Recurrent cases of Dupuytren's disease after partial facectomy should be evaluated for patency of all digital arteries.

Confirmatory Tests

No tests are necessary unless a patient complains of pain or has limited motion. In that case a routine x-ray of the involved fingers, especially a lateral view, is indicated.

Treatment

Nonoperative treatment for Dupuytren's disease is ineffectual. The indications for surgery vary depending upon the age of the patient, the degree of contracture, and the functional disability. Generally, flexion contractures at the metacarpophalangeal joint can be released at any time. The proximal interphalangeal joint presents greater problems, as prolonged contractures are associated with lower success rates. There is a greater indication for surgery in the younger patient with aggressive disease. Unfortunately, the recurrence rate is also higher, up to 80 percent.

Prognosis

The prognosis again is extremely variable. It is good in the older patient with less significant disease, especially if the job does not involve heavy labor. There is an unusually high percentage of complications from the surgery, including skin slough and reflex sympathetic dystrophy. An extended period of temporary impairment may be necessary. However, the worker can be expected to return to the original job.

There is a good deal of debate as to whether Dupuytren's disease is causally related to work; obviously, the only possibility would be in the worker who does heavy labor.[12] The authors have some misgivings about including it in this text; however, since a number of insurance carriers do accept workers' claims, it has been included. This is not meant to imply that Dupuytren's disease is definitely work related. At best, the judgment should be made individually. The young worker who has all the parameters of the aggressive form of Dupuytren's mentioned above is not felt to have the work-related disorder. Furthermore, if the disease occurs in the most common group (i.e., over 50-year-old men), one would be likely to consider it work related.

SESAMOIDITIS

Clinical Picture

Sesamoiditis is an uncommon disorder involving the two sesamoids at the metacarpophalangeal joint level in the thumb. Seen generally in those over 40 years old, it may occur spontaneously or as a result of trauma, either hyperextension of the joint or a direct blow. Patients complain of diffuse pain in the thumb, although they may localize it more to the palmar aspect of the joint. The diagnosis is often overlooked.

Physical examination discloses tenderness to palapation of the sesamoids. Either or both can be involved, but the ulnar sesamoid seems to be symptomatic more commonly. Crepitance may be elicited by direct pressure.

Confirmatory Tests

X-rays may be negative or show degenerative joint disease between the sesamoids and the metacarpal head. One has to order specifically a true lateral view of the thumb metacarpophalangeal joint. Negative films are more likely to be seen in younger patients who have had a discrete episode of trauma, especially, if no crepitance is present on exam. Local injection of Lidocaine in the region of the sesamoids can facilitate the diagnosis.

Treatment

Initial treatment should consist of rest, immobilization, and possibly NSAIDs. The degree of immobilization depends on the severity of the complaints. If the symptoms are mild, a short opponens splint might be sufficient; if they are more severe, especially in the younger age group where trauma has been the inciting factor, a short arm thumb spica cast may be necessary. Very little time out of work may be necessary if the worker can use the orthosis. Sesamoidectomy yields good results if conservative treatment fails. Both sesamoids should be removed even if only one is symptomatic.

Prognosis

The prognosis is variable, depending upon the same factors noted in previous sections. The results can be excellent, and a return to the original employment can be anticipated. However, it may take 3 to 6 months after the surgery for a patient to return to the original job if it involves heavy work.

FINGERTIP INJURIES

Clinical Picture

The literature is replete with extensive descriptions of complex operative procedures employed to treat fingertip injuries.[16-19] The initial treatment should not include such procedures unless the surgeon is quite familiar with their indications and complications. A cleansed, dressed fingertip can be referred to the hand surgeon for treatment within 24 to 48 hours. Often, spontaneous healing or a simple split thickness skin graft suffice.

After the initial injury is healed, patients' complaints may vary depending upon the extent of the injury, the digit involved, and the type of employment. Symptoms can vary from numbness in jobs that involve precision handling to cold intolerance. The examination should confirm the symptoms. One looks for lack of sensibility, tenderness of the tip, or stiffness of the proximal joints induced by overzealous splinting of the finger. If there has been a significant dorsal injury, nail problems can occur. An absent nail can make picking up small objects difficult and a split and/or nonadherent nail may catch or objects that the employee is required to handle. The therapist is extremely helpful in analyzing digital dexterity necessary for the patient's job and in training the worker to use the hand in alternative patterns.

Confirmatory Tests

Confirmatory tests are unnecessary except when there is a question of the validity of the response to evaluations of sensibility. A Semmes-Weinstein evaluation may determine this response more accurately.

Treatment

Assuming that the initial injury is healed when the physician sees the patient, minimal treatment is necessary. If numbness is a significant complaint, skin flap advancements or rotations may be indicated. If frequent skin breakdown occurs, then revision and bony shortening may be necessary.

Prognosis

Patients may have a variable course after a fingertip injury. Even if the injury is insignificant in comparison to an amputation, the worker may still have all the phobias seen in more significant amputations about returning to the same job or even the work place. These emotional factors have to be considered. Perhaps, other than in amputations where there has also been tissue loss, there is no other injury where a return to the workplace depends so much on the multiple, nonmedical parameters discussed in Chapter 9. One cannot generalize; some employees may return to work the day after injury and some not at all.

VIBRATION SYNDROME

Clinical Picture

Vibration syndrome, also known as vibration-induced white finger, white finger disease, dead hand syndrome, or occupational Raynaud's disease, was described as early as 1918.[20] Seen in workers involved in construction, farming, metal working, the steel industry, lumbering, furniture making, mining, auto manufacturing, and foundaries, the common denominator is the use of hand tools, chain saws, and pneumatic tools.[21] Although the actual numbers of workers with this disorder is small, it is estimated that as many as 1.2 million workers per year are potentially exposed to hand-arm vibration.[22]

Temporary tingling or numbness during or soon after use of vibrating tools is *not* considered vibration syndrome. To be diagnosed as vibration syndrome, these symptoms must be more persistent and/or occur without provocation by immediate exposure to vibration. Other symptoms include blanching, pain, and flushing, These symptoms usually appear suddenly and are precipitated by exposure to cold. With continuing exposure to vibration the signs and symptoms become more severe, and the pathology may become irreversible. The severity of the vibration syndrome is usually measured by a grading system developed by Taylor[23] (Table 10-1):

Objective findings on examination may be absent. Usually the history, including an accurate description of the worker's type of job, is essential to making the diagnosis.[24] Digital blood pressure after cooling, vibrogram testing, depth-sense ethesiometry, or somatosensory evoked

Table 10-1. Vibration Syndrome Grading System

Stage	Condition of the Fingers	Work and Social Interference
00	No tingling, numbness, or blanching of fingers	No complaints
0T	Intermittent tingling	No interference with activities
0N	Intermittent numbness	No interference with activities
TN	Intermittent tingling and numbness	No interference with activities
01	Blanching of a fingertip with or without tingling and/or numbness	No interference with activities
02	Blanching of one or more fingers beyond tips, usually during winter	Possible interference with nonwork activities; no interference at work
03	Extensive blanching of fingers during summer and winter	Definite interference at work, at home, and with social activities; restriction of hobbies
04	Extensive blanching of most fingers during summer and winter	Occupation usually changed because of severity of signs and symptoms

(From Taylor,[23] with permission.)

potentials may help establish the diagnosis.[25–27]

Confirmatory Tests

Differential diagnosis includes Raynaud's disease, connective tissue disease (e.g., lupus, rheumatoid arthritis, scleroderma), trauma to extremity or vessels (e.g., frostbite, hypothenar hammer syndrome, thoracic outlet syndrome), occlusive vascular disease, dysglobulinemia, toxic exposure, or neurogenic compromise.[28] Proper evaluation begins with a complete history and physical examination, including an Allen test. Noninvasive vascular tests, a full hematologic evaluation, and a toxic screen may be necessary.

Establishing the proper diagnosis is essential. Although early on the complaints are reversible, they can progress to be irreversible in as short a time as 1 year after exposure begins. Histologically, these patients have been shown to have thickened arterial walls, periarterial fibrosis, demyelination and loss of nerve fibers, and destruction of elastic fibers.[29]

Treatment

To decrease the incidence of vibration syndrome, both government and industry have made an effort to manufacture tools that produce less vibration and to maintain them well. If the worker develops these symptoms in spite of using proper tools, then a change in the work schedule to allow a 10-minute break every hour is indicated. Other suggestions include wearing warm clothes when working in a cold environment, grasping tools less firmly, and substituting manual tools where applicable.

Perhaps the best way to treat vibration syndrome is to avoid it. A preplacement history and examination to rule out Raynaud's disease or other disorders that predispose patients to the disorder would seem to be indicated.

Prognosis

Vibration syndrome is a sufficiently uncommon disorder that no large series reports the outcome of treatment and the number of patients that return to modified jobs that still can potentially produce the disorder. If the recommended job modifications are not possible, then retraining will be necessary. Once the disease becomes irreversible the worker no longer has the potential in return to the old job and may become permanently unable to perform any work.

REFERENCES

1. Freiberg A, Levine R: Nonoperative treatment of trigger fingers and thumbs. J Hand Surg 14A:553, 1989
2. Marks MR, Gunther SF: Efficacy of cortisone injection in treatment of trigger fingers and thumbs. J Hand Surg 14A:722, 1989
3. Stellbrink G: Triggering finger syndrome in rheumatoid arthritis not caused by flexor tendon nodules. Hand 3:76, 1971
4. Swanson AB, Swanson GD: Osteoarthritis in the hand. J Hand Surg 8:669, 1983
5. Swanson AB, Maupin BK, Gajjar NV, Swanson GD: Flexible implant arthroplasty in the proximal interphalangeal joint of the hand. J Hand Surg 10A:796, 1985
6. Ramgarathnam CS, Linscheid RL: Infected mucous cyst of the finger. J Hand Surg 9A:245, 1984
7. Binton RI, Margles SW, Lumseth PA: Small joint arthrodesis in the hand. J Hand Surg 11A:678, 1986
8. Sakellarides HT, DeWeese JW: Instability of the metacarpophalangeal joint of the thumb. J Bone Joint Surg 58A:106, 1976

9. Smith RJ: Post-traumatic instability of the metacarpophalangeal joint of the thumb. J Bone Joint Surg 59A:14, 1977

10. Brown PW: Less than ten—surgeons with amputated fingers. J Hand Surg 7:31, 1982

11. Tupper JW, Booth DM: Treatment of painful neuromas of sensory nerves in the hand: a comparison of traditional and newer methods. J Hand Surg 1:144, 1976

12. Early PF: Population studies in Dupuytren's contracture. J Bone Joint Surg 44B:602, 1962

13. Tubiana R, Simmons P, DeFrenne HA: Location of Dupuytren's disease on the radial aspect of the hand. Clin Orthop Rel Res 168:222, 1982

14. Watson KH, Lovallo J: Salvage of severe recurrent Dupuytren's contracture of the ring and small fingers. J Hand Surg 12A:87, 1987

15. Wheeler ES, Meals RA, Dupuytren's diathesis: A broad spectrum disease. PRS 68:781–3, 1981

16. Chow SP, Ho E: Open treatment of fingertip injuries in adults. J Hand Surg 7:470, 1982

17. Sturman, MJ, Diman, RJ: Late results of fingertip injuries. J Bond Joint Surg 45A:289, 1963

18. Porter RW: Functional assessment of transplanted skin in volar defects of the digits. J Bone Joint Surg 50A:955, 1968

19. Brody GS, Cloutier A, Woolhouse FM: The finger tip injury—an assessment of management. PRS 26;80, 1960

20. Hamilton A: A study of spastic anemia in the hands of stonecutters. US Bureau Labor Stat 19:53, 1918

21. Wasserman DE, Badger DW, Doyle TE, Margolies L: Industrial vibration—an overview. Am Soc Safety Eng J 19:38, 1974

22. National Institute for Occupational Safety and Health: Current Intelligence Bulletin, March 29, 1983

23. Taylor W (ed): The Vibration White Finger. London, Academic Press, 1974

24. Pike J, Arons MS: Vibration syndrome: a new test and rating system for disability compensation. Contemp Orthop 20:203, 1990

25. Ekenvall L: Clinical assessment of suspected damage from hand-held vibrating tools. Scand J Work Environ Health 13:271, 1987

26. Haines T, Ching JP: Peripheral neurological assessment methods for workers exposed to hand-arm vibration. Scand J Work Environ Health 13:370, 1987

27. Murata K, Araki S, Aona H: Assessment of central and peripheral nerve functions in chainsaw operators: a study of short-latency somatosensory evoked potentials. Tohoku J Exp Med 151:25, 1987

28. Taylor W, Pelmear PL: Vibration White Finger in Industry. Academic Press, London, 1975

29. Takeuchi T, Fatatsuka M, Imanishi H, Yamada S: Pathological changes observed in the finger biopsy of patients with vibration induced white finger. Scand J Work Environ Health 12:280, 1986

11

Evaluation and Management of Occupational Wrist Disorders

Andrew L. Terrono, M.D.
Lewis H. Millender, M.D.

The purpose of this chapter is to present a practical approach to the diagnosis and treatment of work-related wrist disorders. Since patients usually present with either radial-or ulnar-sided wrist pain the problems are grouped this way to facilitate diagnosis. The clinical approach to diagnosis is described, with a strong emphasis on treatment and prognosis for returning the worker to the original job.

Disorders localized to the radial side of the wrist are common industrial complaints (Table 11-1). The radial side of the wrist, including the thumb and radial digits, is subject to constant abuse in the work place. Acute injuries occur from direct blows to the hand and from falls on the outstretched hand; acute or chronic disorders occur from forceful pulling or grasping, as well as repetitive activities incurred in work and everyday activities (Fig. 11-1). These disorders are usually easily diagnosed and, depending on the specific condition, are generally treated successfully. However, some of the chronic radial-sided wrist disorders cannot be repaired completely, and the physician must be aware of the prognosis for the various disorders when making recommendations regarding return to regular or modified work or undergoing surgery.

SOFT TISSUE DISORDERS

Tendonitis

Clinical Findings

Any tendonitis disorder can cause pain and disability.[1] The condition may come on acutely after performing a new job task or stressful activity, or it can have a gradual onset (Fig. 11-2). In any tendonitis disorder, the pain is localized to the area, exacerbated by use, and generally im-

Table 11-1.   Radial-Sided Wrist
Disorders

SOFT TISSUE DISORDERS

Tendonitis
   de Quervain's tenosynovitis
   Abductor pollicus longus tenosynovitis
   Intersection syndrome
   Extensor indicis proprius or extensor dig-
      torium longus tenosynovitis
Ganglions
   Dorsal wrist ganglions
   Volar wrist ganglions

LIGAMENTOUS AND JOINT
DISORDERS

Trapezio-metacarpal joint
   Instability
   Arthritis
Scapho-trapezial-trapezoid arthritis
Wrist joint
   Scapholunate dissociation
      Static
      Dynamic
   Scapholunate advanced collapse
   Scaphoid fractures
   Keinböck's disease

proved with rest. Depending on the degree of inflammation, the tendon involved, and the patient's pain threshold, the disorder can cause differing degrees of impairment.

The diagnosis is established by careful physical examination. By far the most common condition is de Quervain's tenosynovitis, a well-known disorder characterized by pain on active radial abduction of the thumb and passive stretch of the abductor pollicus longus (Finkelstein test).[2] The pain extends proximally from the radial styloid along the dorsoradial aspect of the wrist. The most important confirmatory sign is tenderness over the distal radius where the abductor pollicus longus and extensor policus brevis enter the fibro-osseous sheath. Uncommonly, crepitation is noted as the thumb is abducted.

Less frequently, the disorder can be a tendonitis of the abductor pollicus longus

at its insertion into the base of the first metacarpal. In this condition the tenderness is located at the abductor pollicus longus insertion. Again pain is associated with active thumb abduction and sometimes with passive stretch. A grind test for symptomatic carpometacarpal joint degenerative arthritis is normal.

Less commonly, tendonitis or sprains of the thenar intrinsic musculature can cause pain at the base of the thumb. Patients present either with vague diffuse discomfort associated with activity or with more acute and localized pain either in the thenar region of the thumb or the thumb-index web space. Resisted opposition and pinch motions cause pain, and sometimes tenderness can be located to the muscle group. This diagnosis is often one of exclusion following a negative evaluation for other, more well-defined and common problems.

Tendonitis or tenosynovitis of the extensor carpi radius longus and brevis has been referred to as the intersection syndrome, because initially it was felt to be due to inflammation at the intersection of the abductor pollicus longus and extensor pollicus brevis tendons and the wrist extensor tendons. Patients have pain along the dorsum of the wrist slightly proximal and dorsal to the area of de Quervain's tenosynovitis. Swelling of the tendon sheath may be noted, and pain is associated with active wrist flexion and extension.[3]

Patients can also present with a painful tenosynovitis of the extensor pollicus longus, extensor indicis proprius, or extensor digitorum communis tendons. When this condition is associated with definite dorsal tenosynovitis, the diagnosis is easily established. However, sometimes there is only pain on active digital extension without other signs of inflammation. In these cases the diagnosis is one of exclusion. There is an uncommon conditional called drummer's palsy, which is a rup-

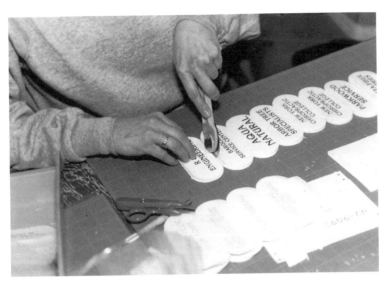

Fig. 11-1. Repetitive activities can precipitate occupational wrist disorders. (From Dawson et al.,[53] with permission.)

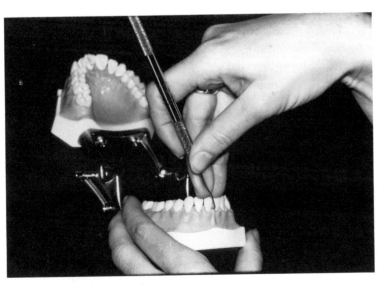

Fig. 11-2. Occupations associated with extreme positioning and repetitive motions such as a dental hygienist, may cause tendinitis. (From Dawson et al.,[53] with permission.)

ture of the extensor policis longus associated with repetitive wrist motions as would be seen with drummers.[4]

Confirmatory Tests
Radiographs should be negative unless there is a calcific tendonitis. There can certainly be radiologic findings of incidental carpometacarpal degenerative arthritis or wrist joint degenerative arthritis when the patient's pain is related to the tendinitis. If the tenosynovitis is secondary to rheumatoid arthritis, a rheumatologic work-up might be positive, and sometimes bone scans may be slightly positive in these conditions.

Treatment
Most of these conditions are treated conservatively with good results. Splinting, NSAID (nonsteroidal anti-inflammatory drugs) and steroid injections, and temporary job modification are often effective. For recurrent episodes of tendonitis, permanent job modification may need to be considered.[5]

Surgical release of the first extensor compartment is a safe, reliable operation to correct recurrent tenosynovitis. In cases unresponsive to nonoperative treatment, often a separate compartment for the extensor policis brevis is seen.[6] After this procedure most workers should be able to return to work except for those who do significant repetitive, uncontrolled assembly line work.

Surgical release of the second, third, or fourth extensor compartments is uncommonly needed, but for persistent disability from these conditions exploration of this option is appropriate.

Prognosis
Most patients do well after conservative treatment. The prognosis after de Quervain's release is usually excellent. Permanent job modification may be neces-

sary for patients with recurrent or chronic tendinitis. However, treatment failures, complications, and other conditions have been seen and been associated with a poor outcome.[7]

Ganglions

Dorsal Wrist Ganglions
Dorsal wrist ganglions are common work- and non-work-related problems that present as prominent cystic masses of varying sizes located over the dorsum of the wrist (Fig. 11-3).[8-9] Usually seen in women and often associated with ligamentous wrist laxity, the cystic mass invariable arises from the dorsal scapholunate interosseous ligament. The ganglion may be asymptomatic or associated with dorsal wrist pain that is usually activity related.

The physical examination in patients with dorsal wrist ganglions shows an obvious smooth, firm mass usually located over the dorsoradial side of the wrist. However, the mass can present any place on the dorsum of the wrist and still be

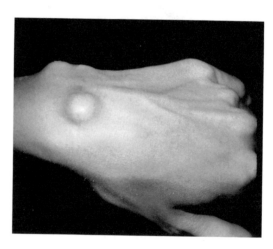

Fig. 11-3. Dorsal wrist ganglion may be multiple or recurrent.

attached to a stalk that arises from the scapholunate ligament. When the ganglion is symptomatic, both forced wrist flexion and extension cause pain, as well as direct pressure over the mass. Some patients have lax wrists and demonstrate a positive scaphoid instability test.

In addition to the obvious prominent dorsal wrist ganglion, small or occult dorsal wrist ganglion is a cause of unexplained dorsal wrist pain.[10,11] Patients present with dorsal wrist pain exacerbated by activity, particularly unusual activity. They demonstrate dorsal wrist tenderness located at the scapholunate capitate interval. On careful palpation the examiner may feel a small, firm, ballotable, smooth, tender cystic mass that represents the ganglion. As with patients with dorsal wrist ganglions, those with occult dorsal wrist ganglions are often women with lax wrists. Other entities that mimic dorsal wrist ganglion are anomalous extensor muscle bellies, lipomas, neuromas of the posterior interosseous nerve, synovial cyst secondary to rheumatoid arthritis, plexiform neuroma, and even malignant tumors, such as synovial cell sarcoma and clear cell sarcoma.[12] Although these causes are rare, one must at least think of the other possibilities.

Confirmatory Tests. Routine radiographs are usually normal, as are stress radiographs looking for scapholunate instability. Bone scans are sometimes hot, and wrist arthrograms may show dye entering the ganglion. In general the diagnosis is a clinical one.

Treatment. Asymptomatic ganglions require no treatment unless the patient is concerned with their appearance. Symptomatic prominent or occult ganglions sometimes recede with splinting or job modification. An important diagnostic fact to help confirm that a mass is a wrist ganglion is a history of the ganglion getting bigger or smaller with activity and rest, respectively.

Recommended conservative treatment is aspiration and installation of cortisone, which can be done by several techniques. One safe method is to puncture the sack with a 20 or 21 gauge needle and then instill several cubic centimeters of 1% xylocaine and cortisone into the ganglion. The wrist is then splinted for several weeks. Cure rates of up to 78 percent have been reported with this technique. Splinting for 3 weeks may help increase the cure rate.[13]

An excellent diagnostic test for a suspected occult painful dorsal wrist ganglion is to attempt injection. Often one can then appreciate a pop, signifying rupture of the ganglion. When this occurs the patient is often cured temporarily or permanently.

For persistent or recurrent dorsal wrist ganglions, surgical excision is recommended. To prevent recurrence, the ganglion must be disected to the scapholunate interosseous ligament, which should be scraped or curretted. After this technique recurrence should be low, approximately 5 percent.[9,13]

Prognosis. Prognosis for recurrence after injection is approximately 25 to 80 percent.[13] Surgical excision is often successful, and workers should be able to return to most occupations. However, if the patient has wrist ligamentous instability, wrist pain might recur with certain types of jobs that cause excessive wrist stress; additional, repeated stresses to the wrist may cause recurrence of the ganglion. In these cases, job modification is appropriate.

Volar Wrist Ganglions

Clinical Findings. The second most frequent ganglion is located over the volar radial side of the wrist.[8] It either protrudes from the radiocarpal joint, the trapeziometacarpal joint, or the scapho-trapezial-trapezoid joints. In the latter two cases it dissects along the flexor carpi radialis tendon sheath and presents adjacent to this tendon.

The signs and symptoms are similar to those for dorsal ganglion, with onset after a wrist injury or noted after a change in activity. These ganglions also may be asymptomatic and change in size depending on the patient's activity. The differential diagnosis is similar to the dorsal wrist ganglion, as well as radial artery problems.

Confirmatory Tests.   Routine radiographs are usually normal; however, ganglions can be associated with arthritic conditions, which will be confirmed by radiograph. A wrist arthrogram may communicate with the volar wrist ganglion.

Treatment.   The treatment is similar to that for dorsal wrist ganglions and includes splinting, job modification, and injection. Surgical excision is required for persistent symptomatic ganglions. However, surgery is not without complications. The radial sensory nerve, palmar cutaneous nerve, and terminal portions of the lateral antebrachial cutaneous nerves must be avoided. Frequently, the radial artery is intimately associated with the ganglion. When the ganglion arises from the scapho-trapezial-trapezoid joint or the carpometacarpal joint, the flexor carpi radialis tendon sheath must be opened and the ganglion dissected to its base.

Prognosis.   If the ganglion does not represent a significant arthritic process in the carpometacarpal joint, the scapho-trapezial-trapezoid joint, or wrist joint, the prognosis for full recovery should be good. However, other conditions if present will influence the final outcome.

LIGAMENTOUS AND JOINT DISORDERS

Trapeziometacarpal Joint

Clinical Findings

Two specific conditions involving the carpometacarpal (CMC) joint are seen in workers.[14] Symptomatic carpometacarpal joint degenerative arthritis is the most common and is a frequent complaint among middle-aged and older women whose work requires forceful and repetitive thumb motions. They complain to varying degrees of basal joint thumb pain that is attributed to activity. The primary symptom is arthritic pain that is improved with rest and exacerbated with activity. Physical examination localizes the pain to the carpometacarpal joint. The confirmatory sign is a painful grind test or subluxation. If there is no pain even when there is a positive grind, one should look for other causes.

The other type of carpometacarpal joint problem is painful instability. Some women have joint laxity, which can become symptomatic when associated with overuse. However, more frequently a patient falls or injures the thumb and sustains a tear of the deep volar ulnar ligaments. If the diagnosis is not established and the patient not treated acutely, a chronic symptomatic carpometacarpal joint laxity can develop. On physical examination, one can elicit a painful dorsal subluxation of the metacarpal from the base of the trapezium.

Confirmatory Tests

Routine radiographs of the carpometacarpal joint demonstrate osteoarthritis. Stress views can be obtained to confirm carpometacarpal joint laxity (Fig. 11-4).

Treatment

Patients who have symptomatic CMC joint instability after injury or even a congenital basis can often be restored to ex-

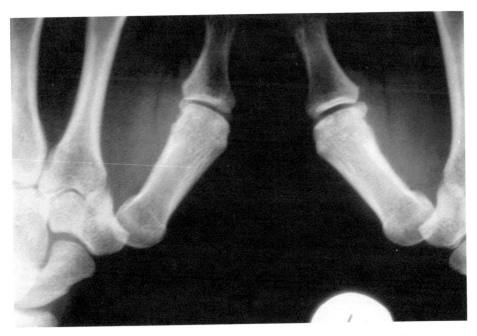

Fig. 11-4. Stress radiograph demonstrates bilateral thumb CMC laxity.

cellent function by CMC joint ligamentous reconstruction using a slip of the flexor carpi radialis tendon. When there are no degenerative changes within the joint, the procedure has a good record for restoring stability and strength to the CMC joint and alleviating pain.

Carpometacarpal joint arthritis in the worker should be treated conservatively with nonsteroidal anti-inflammatory drugs, splints, and job modifications. If these steps, especially job modification, are carried out, many patients can continue to work. Hand therapists who understand work issues are very helpful in these situations.

In general, trapezium arthroplasty with or without an implant or ligament reconstruction should not be recommended if the sole purpose is to allow the worker to return to work. If a stitcher or machine operator has symptomatic osteoarthritis that is controlled with conservative mea-sures so long as she is not doing that job, every attempt should be made to adjust the job. Trapezium arthroplasty is not without complications. Pinch strength averages 12 to 15 pounds in most studies (normal pinch strength is 17 to 20 pounds), and one cannot be certain that trapezium arthroplasty will restore enough function to allow the patient to return to those jobs.[16-19]

Prognosis

With job modification many patients with CMC degenerative joint arthritis can function well. Trapezium arthroplasty may not provide sufficient strength to allow patients to return to jobs requiring repetitive or forceful actions and is not recommended for manual or assembly line works.

Ligamentous reconstruction is an effective procedure for symptomatic ligamentous instability.

Scapho-Trapezial-Trapezoid Arthritis

Clinical Findings

The clinical findings are similar to those seen in carpometacarpal joint arthritis.[20,21] Pain is localized at the base of the thumb, is activity related, and may present abruptly or chronically. If the examiner is careful, the diagnosis can be suspected on physical examination. When the carpometacarpal joint is examined, the patient is pain free; however, pressure localized to the scapho-trapezial-trapezoid joint elicits the pain.

Confirmatory Tests

Radiographs confirm arthritis localized to the scapho-trapezial-trapezoid (STT) joint. Depending on the patient, the carpometacarpal joint may be normal or show degrees of arthritic involvement.

Treatment

Conservative treatment similar to that for carpometacarpal joint arthritis often eliminates the pain. For recurrent pain in workers who do repetitive forceful activities, job modification is preferable. The treatment for persistent symptomatic scapho-trapezial-trapezoid arthritis is fusion (Fig. 11-5). However, one should be cautious recommending this procedure to restore a worker to a manual job because a partial loss of wrist motion must be expected and the procedure is not without problems.

Prognosis

Conservative treatment including job modification is often effective in alleviating symptoms. Fusion should not be expected to uniformly allow patients to return to stressful manual jobs.

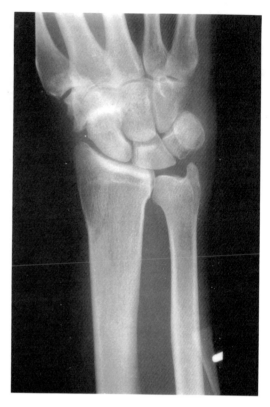

Fig. 11-5. Radiograph demonstrating an asymptomatic worker after a solid STT fusion for arthritis.

Scapholunate Dissociation

This condition can be seen in a variety of presentations, and the clinical picture, treatment, and prognosis will depend on the situation.[22,23]

Static Scapholunate Dissociation

Scapholunate dissociation results from a fall on the outstretched hand that tears the ligamentous support that stabilizes these bones. Patients have wrist pain, scaphoid tenderness, and instability to stress.[24]

Confirmatory Tests. Routine radiographs or stress views of the wrist demonstrate the scapholunate dissociation, which consists of gapping between the scaphoid and lunate on the PA projection and an increased scapholunate angle on the lateral x-ray (Fig.11-6).

Treatment. Depending on the chronicity, degree of instability, and needs of the patient, either acute repair, ligamentous reconstruction, or partial fusions are recommended. In acute situations (up to 3 to 6 weeks) open reduction of the scapholunate dissociation and ligamentous repair through the dorsal or volar approach are recommended.[25] In chronic situations, some authorities recommend ligamentous reconstruction by either the dorsal or volar[26] approach or a dorsal capsulodesis.[27] Other authorities recommend either scapho-trapezial-trapezoid fusion or scaphocapitate fusion.[28–30]

Prognosis. The most favorable prognosis follows reduction and ligamentous repair of acute scapholunate dissociation. When repaired acutely, the soft tissues heal, the reduction is maintained, and good range of motion and grip strength should be ex-

pected. Most workers should be able to return to full duty depending on the demands of their jobs.

The prognosis following reconstruction for chronic scapholunate dissociation is less predictable. It depends on the degree of displacement, the type of reconstruction possible, and the presence of any arthritis. Regardless of the procedures carried out, patients must expect to lose 30 to 60 percent of their normal range of motion.[30] In many cases grip strength and endurance can be restored to a satisfactory level to allow manual workers to return to full duty; however, normal function is not to be expected.

Dynamic Scapholunate Instability[23]

Clinical Findings. Patients present with varying degrees of wrist pain that is often associated with activity. They are usually women with generalized ligamentous laxity. The onset can follow one stressful

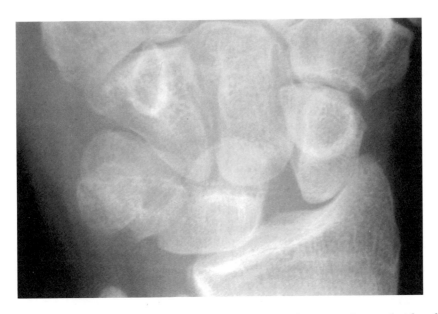

Fig. 11-6. Radiograph of an injured worker with a large gap between the scaphoid and lunate indicating a static scapholunate dissociation.

episode or be associated with repetitive and forceful motions. In addition to radial tenderness the diagnosis is suspected by eliciting a positive scaphoid instability test.[24] One feels a painful clunk when the fixed scaphoid is stressed.

Confirmatory Tests.   Routine radiographs including stress views are normal. Arthrography or magnetic resonance imaging may or may not demonstrate scapholunate ligament tear.

Treatment.   For dynamic instability, especially when it is associated with a negative arthrogram, prolonged conservative treatment is advised. Temporary job modification and joint protection instruction may be effective. Certainly, for persistent symptomatology, permanent job change is preferable to operation. For persistent disability various dorsal and volar ligamentous reconstructions or limited arthrodesis are recommended.[26,27]

Prognosis.   In many patients job modification, joint protection, and education about the condition are helpful in alleviating discomfort. Surgery is not without its problems and will certainly limit motion. However, when symptoms persist and patients have the proper expectations, surgery can be effective in restoring function.

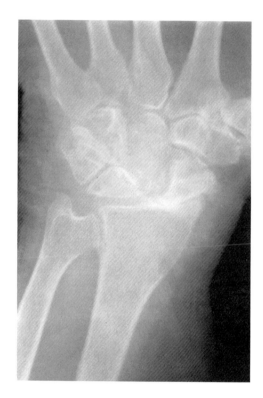

Fig. 11-7. Wrist radiograph demonstrating a SLAC deformity with proximal migration of the capitate with radio scaphoid and midcarpal arthritis.

Scapholunate Advanced Collapse

Clinical Findings
Scapholunate advanced collapse is a progressive degenerative arthritis following long-standing scapholunate dissociation.[31,32] The clinical picture depends on the severity of the arthritic changes, which begin with radioscaphoid arthritis and progress to capitolunate arthritis. Patients present with the onset of acute or progressive chronic wrist pain that is activity related. Physical examination dem-

onstrates various degrees of crepitation, synovitis, wrist instability, limited range of motion, and weakness of grip.

Confirmatory Tests
Routine radiographs confirm the degenerative changes and the severity of the arthritic process (Fig. 11-7).

Treatment
Treatment depends on the severity of the disability, the degree of arthritis, and the patient's needs. In some cases conservative therapy with splinting, nonsteroidal anti-inflammatory drugs, and job modification is effective in alleviating the pain. Many people with significant radiographic changes have surprisingly mild

symptoms and can be managed conservatively, especially if they can moderate their activities. When pain persists despite conservative treatment, options in surgical treatment include proximal row carpectomy, total wrist arthrodesis, or partial wrist arthrodesis with excision of the scaphoid with or without interpositional arthroplasty. Surgery can be expected to alleviate pain in most cases, but patients must expect a 40 to 60 percent loss of normal motion and a 20 to 50 percent loss of normal grip and strength. Most manual workers will need a modified job following any of these procedures.

Acute and Chronic Scaphoid Fracture

Clinical Findings
Clinical findings obviously depend on the situation. Acute scaphoid fractures cause moderate pain, and snuff box tenderness is the tell-tale sign.[33] Old non-

unions can become symptomatic after acute trauma or activity change

Confirmatory Tests
Most acute and chronic scaphoid fractures are evident by routine radiographs, including the scaphoid view (Fig. 11-8). Tomograms and CT scans are helpful in evaluating displacement or confirming a non-union. Bone scans are sometimes helpful in detecting undiagnosed and suspected scaphoid fracture.

Treatment
Treatment varies depending on the specific situation. Nondisplaced fractures should be treated in a cast. Usually the patient requires 6 weeks in a long thumb spica cast and then a short arm thumb spica cast until healed.[34] Certain displaced fractures require open reduction. Non-unions without arthritis require bone grafting,[35,36] whereas those with degenerative arthritis are treated similar to scapholunate advanced collapse (SLAC) wrists.

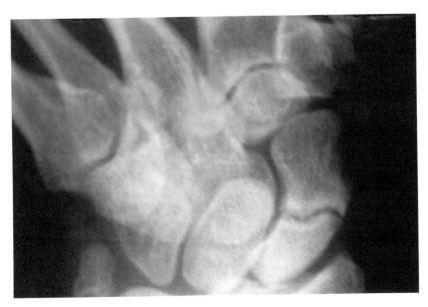

Fig. 11-8. Radiograph documenting a scaphoid non-union with sclerotic fracture margins.

Prognosis

Patients with acute and non-united scaphoid fractures that are treated and heal should be restored to excellent function. Their motion and grip strength may be limited somewhat, but they should be able to return to manual labor. The prognosis after wrist reconstruction procedures for non-union with degenerative arthritis are similar to those for SLAC wrist operations.

Kienböck's Disease

Clinical Findings

Kienböck's disease or avascular necrosis of the carpal lunate is generally felt to be caused by microfractures of the lunate associated with an abnormal blood supply[37-39] and usually of negative ulnar variance,[40] which result in the concentration of abnormal forces across the bone. The clinical findings vary and are related to the stage of the process and the severity of disease. Initially, patients complain of aching and mild pain that is usually activity related. As the process worsens the pain intensifies and eventually is constant. On examination one finds varying degrees of wrist stiffness, swelling, dorsal tenderness, crepitation, and weakness of grip strength. When dorsal tenderness is localized directly over the lunate, one should consider this diagnosis. The condition is not uncommon and is frequently seen in young men who do manual work.

Confirmatory Tests

Depending on the stage of the disease, routine radiographs may confirm the condition. In early stages, one sees increased density, sclerosis, and often a fracture line on the lateral radiograph. In more advanced stages there is collapse and fragmentation and eventually arthritis. In many cases one also sees a negative ulnar variance. It is now known that in the ear-

liest cases routine radiographs may be completely normal. Bone scans sometimes show a hot spot localized to the lunate, and magnetic resonance imaging[41] is sometimes helping in suggesting the diagnosis (Fig. 11-9).

Treatment

The treatment is controversial, but is somewhat related to the stages of the disease.[37,38] Because of the incidence of silicone synovitis, the previously recommended lunate prosthesis has fallen into disfavor.[42] Many authorities now recommend radial shortening for cases in early stages that have no collapse and have a ulnar negative variance.[43] This leveling operation redistributes the forces within the wrist, and patients often have relief of pain. There is some evidence that fractures sometimes heal. For advanced stages or in patients who have normal ulnar variance, intercarpal fusions are recommended to unload the lunate. Some recommend scapho-trapezial-trapezoid fusions,[44] and others recommend scapho-capitate fusions. These fusions are done either with or without lunate excision depending on the degree of lunate fragmentation or localized arthritis.

Prognosis

Most of the above procedures eliminate pain and improve grip strength. Radial shortening preserves motion, which is usually decreased by 50 percent after fusions. Grip strength is improved, but one should not expect the patient to have either normal strength or normal endurance after these procedures. Many workers should be able to return to manual jobs, but generally with some restrictions.

ULNAR-SIDED WRIST PAIN: VOLAR

Volar-sided ulnar hand and wrist pain is frequently seen among workers (Table 11-2). It can be caused by either acute or

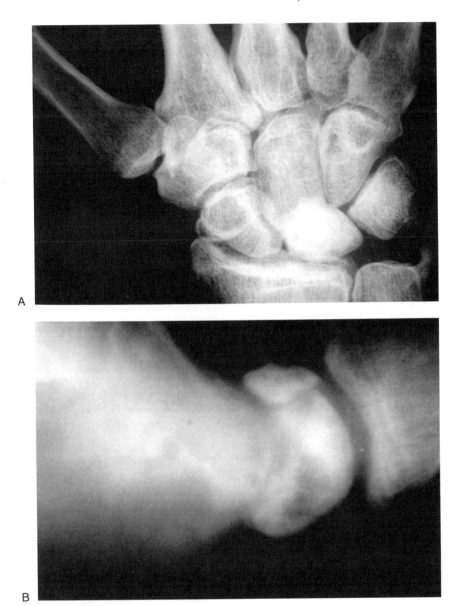

Fig. 11-9. A 53-year-old mechanic with advanced Kienböck's disease. (**A**) Radiograph demonstrating an increased density of the lunate and loss of carpal height. (**B**) Tomograms are often helpful to demonstrate a lunate fracture associated with Kienböck's disease. (*Figure continues.*)

chronic injuries. Acute injuries associated with direct trauma, twisting including hyperextension, and hyperpronation may result in any of the above conditions. Chronic trauma associated with repeated or unaccustomed activities can result in flexor carpi ulnaris (FCU) tendonitis, symptomatic pisotriquetrial arthritis, or hypothenar muscle strain (Fig. 11-10). Repeated blows to the base of the palm

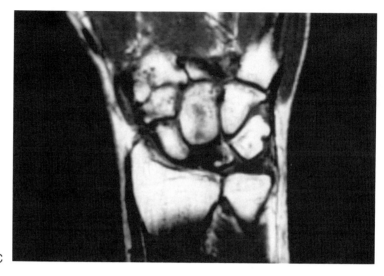

C

Fig. 11-9. (*Continued*). (**C**) Magnetic resonance imaging can confirm the diagnosis of Kienböck's disease with a loss of signal (*dark*) in the lunate.

is seen with hypothenar hammer syndrome can cause either thrombosis of the ulnar artery or ulnar nerve injury within Guyon's canal.

The diagnosis of these conditions is usually straightforward, is based on a careful history and physical examination, and is confirmed with radiographs. The treatment of these conditions is well established, and the prognosis for full recovery is good.

Table 11-2.   Ulnar-Sided
Wrist Pain: Volar

Flexor capri ulnaris tendonitis
Fracture pisiform
Pisotriquetrial arthritis
Ulnar nerve entrapment
Ulnar artery thrombosis
Hook of hamate fracture
Hypothenar muscle strain

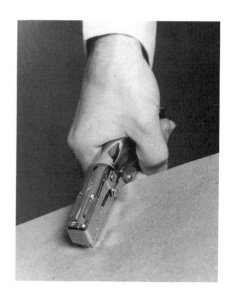

Fig. 11-10. Example of chronic repetitive trauma. (From Dawson et al.,[53] with permission.)

Flexor Carpi Ulnaris Tendonitis

Clinical Findings

Patients present with an acute or chronic onset of pain over the volar ulnar side of the wrist. This condition is sometimes seen when the patient begins a new job requiring excessive wrist flexion or after a brief episode of heavy lifting. It can also come on spontaneously. Examination shows tenderness over the FCU tendon, especially at the insertion. Pain is associated with resisted wrist flexion and passive wrist extension. In acute situations mild swelling or erythema may be noted.

Confirmatory Tests

A radiograph may show calcification within the FCU tendon (Fig. 11-11).

Treatment

In most cases conservative treatment using a wrist splint in slight ulnar deviation and neutral wrist flexion and NSAIDs alleviates the acute inflammation. Sometimes a steroid injection is indicated. However some patients develop a chronic FCU tendonitis and have recurrent bouts of pain. Occasionally, surgical excision of calcific deposits is necessary.

Prognosis

The prognosis is good for complete recovery. Most patients have one bout of FCU tendinitis, which never recurs. If the condition becomes chronic or if the patient has repeated bouts of acute FCU tendonitis associated with the job, modification to a less repetitive job might be curative. The prognosis for recovery after surgical excision of calcific deposits is usually good.

Pisiform Fracture

Clinical Findings

There is a history of a direct blow to the palm of the hand. The patient demonstrates direct tenderness over the pisi-

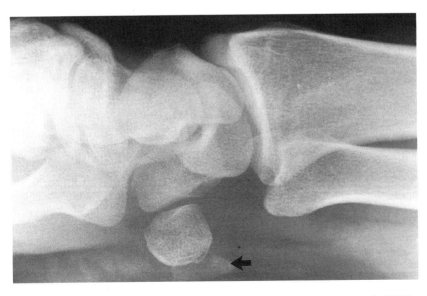

Fig. 11-11. Calcification (*arrow*) seen on a wrist radiograph in a patient with FCU tendonitis.

form. Evaluation of the ulnar nerve should be done.[45]

Confirmatory Tests

Routine radiographs may demonstrate the fracture. An oblique view 15 to 30 percent from the lateral and the carpal tunnel view may also be of some help in visualizing the fracture. The fracture may be linear, comminuted, or the avulsion type.[46]

Treatment

Casting or splinting for 3 to 4 weeks should result in fracture healing with alleviation of the pain. In rare cases where the fracture is displaced or the patient has persistent pain, pisiform bone excision is appropriate.[47]

Prognosis

The prognosis is good for full recovery following casting, and if excision is necessary patients should be able to return to normal jobs.

Pisotriquetrial Degenerative Arthritis

Clinical Findings

Patients may present after an injury or have a gradual or spontaneous onset of pain. The symptoms are similar to those of FCU tendonitis, but tenderness is located over the pisiform bone. The most specific sign is painful crepitus produced by grasping the pisiform and moving it from side to side over the triquetrum. Direct pressure over the bone may not elicit the pain.[49,50]

Confirmatory Tests

Radiographs of the pisotriquetrial joint demonstrate the arthritis. Lateral views in 30 to 40 percent of supination are nec-

essary to demonstrate the joint (Fig. 11-12).[48,49]

Treatment

Splinting, NSAIDs, steroid injections, rest, and altering activities often control the pain. However, for persistent or recurrent pain, pisiform excision is a successful operation that usually restores full use.[47,49,51,52]

Prognosis

Most patients do well and are able to resume normal activities after excision.

Ulnar Nerve Compression within Guyon's Canal

Clinical Findings

There are several presentations for ulnar nerve palsy within Guyon's canal depending on the anatomic site of entrapment.[53] A combined sensory and motor neuropathy, a complete or partial motor neuropathy, or an isolated sensory neuropathy may be seen. A spontaneous partial motor neuropathy is often associated with a ganglion arising from the triquetral-hamate joint and compressing the deep motor branch.[54] In these cases sensation and hypothenar muscle strength are normal since the compression is distal to these branches. After a direct blow or repeated blows to the palm both sensory and motor findings are usually noted. This can cause a syndrome known as hypothenar hammer syndrome, which is usually associated with ulnar artery thrombosis and is discussed later (Fig. 11-13).[55]

In addition to the neurologic findings tenderness is noted within Guyon's canal. Fractures, including the hook of hamate and pisiform, may be associated with this condition. Other masses including lipoma and aberrant muscles may also

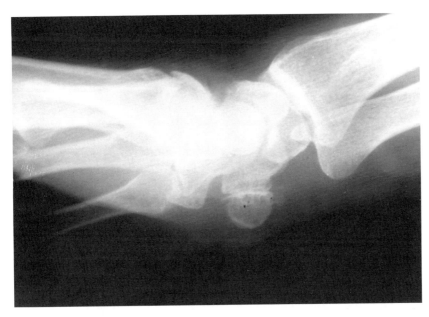

Fig. 11-12. Oblique radiograph demonstrating pisiform triquetrial joint arthritis.

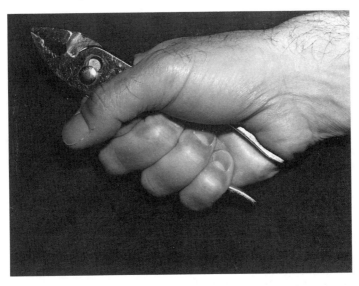

Fig. 11-13. Chronic repetitive forceful trauma to the wrist at Guyon's canal in a mechanic can cause pressure on the ulnar nerve. (From Dawson et al.,[53] with permission.)

be seen. The sensory branch of the ulnar nerve to the dorsum of the hand should be normal.

Confirmatory Tests

Electromyography and nerve velocity testing usually confirm the diagnosis and help localize the compression. More proximal entrapment is thereby excluded.

Treatment

Patients presenting with spontaneous paralysis should be explored because usually a mass is causing the paralysis. When there is an acute direct blow or a history of hypothenar hammer syndrome, one should allow time for spontaneous resolution of the paralysis. The amount of time required depends on the degree of sensory and motor loss. If resolution of the palsy does not occur, decompression and neurolysis are advised.

Prognosis

The prognosis is related to the cause and severity of the paralysis. Patients with spontaneous paralysis associated with a ganglion usually do well after exploration. Patients with blows to the palm with partial palsy also usually recover with conservative care.

Ulnar Artery Thrombosis

Clinical Findings

Patients usually present with either a painful or nonpainful mass within Guyon's canal, but they may present with pain alone.[55-57] There should be a history of acute or chronic trauma to the hypothenar region of the palm. Hypothenar hammer syndrome[55] is a condition seen in workers who use their hypothenar eminence for repeated blows as one would use a hammer. It has also been seen in cyclists.[58] A thrombosis of the ulnar artery develops.

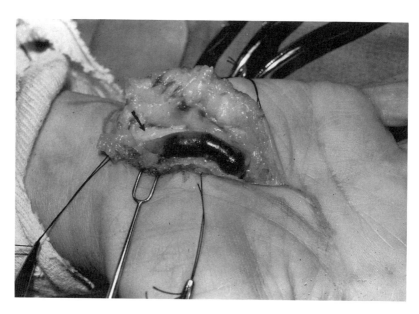

Fig. 11-14. Surgical exploration of Guyon's canal demonstrated a large thrombosed ulnar artery compressing the ulnar nerve (*arrow*). (From Dawson et al.,[53] with permission.)

Sometimes patients have evidence of the Raynaud's phenonema of cold intolerance or ischemia. The ulnar nerve may be compressed by the thrombosed vessel (Fig. 11-14). Examination usually demonstrates a tender mass. The Allen test is positive for ulnar artery thrombosis.

Confirmatory Tests
Ultrasound or arteriography diagnose the condition.

Treatment
Either resection of the thrombosed artery or reconstruction using a vein graph is appropriate.

Prognosis
The prognosis after surgery is usually good, and large percentage of patients can return to their previous job. Patients who work in cold environments may have some cold intolerance and have to change jobs.

Fracture of the Hook of Hamate

Clinical Findings
Most cases are associated with a fall on the outstretched hand or a direct blow.[59] However, the hook can also be fractured by indirect injury. Patients have sustained this injury when playing golf, racquet sports, and baseball and when hitting a solid object, i.e., the ground, or a wall. The patient develops pain and tenderness over the hypothenar area of the palm, although dorsal pain has also been reported. Routine radiographs are always negative, and usually the diagnosis is missed initially. When a patient complains of pain over the hypothenar aspect of the palm and there is tenderness over the hook of the hamate, one should have

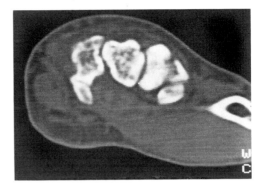

Fig. 11-15. CT scan demonstrating a fracture of the hook of the hamate. (From Dawson et al.,[53] with permission.)

a high suspicion for fracture. Sometimes direct pressure over the volar portion of the palm is not painful, but pressure over the ulnar side of the hook reproduces the symptoms. Again the pain and tenderness are not always severe, and patients can have the diagnosis delayed for months as it is missed by numerous physicians. Ulnar nerve symptoms or injury to the flexor tendons, especially to the small finger, may be seen.

Confirmatory Tests
Carpal tunnel views or oblique views of the hand with the forearm supinated 45 degrees and the wrist dorsiflexed sometimes demonstrate the fracture. However, a CT scan best delineates the fracture (Fig. 11-15). A bone scan obviously is positive over the hook of the hamate.

Treatment
If the diagnosis is made acutely, casting is often effective. The cast must include not only the fourth and fifth metacarpophalangeal joint but also the thumb in order to alleviate forces through the transverse carpal ligament. In cases of delayed diagnosis, most authors recommend excision of the hook. However, recent re-

ports have recommended reduction and screw fixation.[60]

Prognosis
In most cases excision of the hook should restore the hand to essentially normal function and allow the worker to return to most jobs.[59]

Hypothenar Muscle Contusion

Clinical Findings
Patients present with acute or chronic pain over the hypothenar region. A history of direct injury or chronic overuse is usually obtained. Tenderness over the muscles is demonstrated, and pain with resisted abduction of the fifth digit is noted. Other causes of pain are excluded. Discoloration or swelling may be noted when there is an acute injury.

Confirmatory Tests
This is a clinical diagnosis, and there are no tests to diagnose it.

Treatment
Conservative treatment, including rest, splinting, NSAIDS, and alteration of the activity is effective.

Prognosis
The prognosis is good especially when the condition is associated with an acute injury or with chronic overuse and the activity can be adjusted.

ULNAR-SIDED WRIST PAIN: DORSAL

In contrast to wrist disabilities of the volar-sided ulnar column, the diagnosis, treatment, and prognosis of problems of

Table 11-3.   Ulnar-Sided Wrist Pain: Dorsal

Extensor carpi ulnaris-tendonitis-subluxation
Distal radioulnar joint (DRUJ) disorders
Fractures into the DRUJ
Chondromalacia of DRUJ
DRUJ instability
Injuries of triangular fibrocartilage complex (TFCC)
Traumatic tears of TFCC
Degenerative tears of TFCC
Ulnar impaction syndrome
Disabilities of the ulnar carpus
Tears of lunotriquetrial ligament
Midcarpal instability

the dorsal column are much more difficult. In fact, the injuries to the dorsal column represent some of the most difficult reconstructive problems that hand surgeons are asked to correct (Table 11-3). Except for tendinitis of the extensor carpi ulnaris (ECU) or rupture of the ECU tendon sheath, manual workers with one of the joint problems usually cannot be expected to return to full manual duties that require heavy lifting, twisting, or forceful use of the hand and wrist.

The diagnosis of these conditions can also be difficult. When the patient presents with an acute injury and there is an obvious fracture or dislocation of the distal radioulnar joint, (DRUJ) the diagnosis is obvious and the treatment is more straightforward. However, in the majority of cases the patient is seen several weeks or months after a twisting injury to the wrist or a combination hyperextension and hyperpronation injury and has persistent pain. When the patient is initially seen in an emergency room, the condition is diagnosed as a sprain after negative radiographs are obtained. The wrist is splinted, and the patient may be treated with a NSAID. When the problem continues, the worker presents with a persistently painful wrist, with increasing pain associated with rotation and ulnar deviation, and with marked weakness of grip strength. On physical examination the physician should attempt to establish a diagnosis based upon the classification shown in Table 11-3.

Extensor Carpi Ulnaris Tendonitis

Clinical Findings

Patients present with acute or chronic pain over the ulnar side of the wrist that is exacerbated by active extension and ulnar deviation.[61] There may be a history of a recent change in activity or of a forceful twist or hyperflexion to the extended wrist. The diagnosis is often difficult to confirm on physical examination. Classically one finds tenderness along the course of the extensor carpi ulnaris tendon, and pain is associated with extension and ulnar deviation. The wrist should be examined in both pronation and supination as the ECU function and location differ in these positions. One should be able to palpate a tender tendon dorsally when the hand is supinated; when the hand is pronated, the tendon is felt over the ulnar side of the ulnar. Another finding is pain when the supinated wrist is stressed in flexion. In practice these physical findings are often subtle, and one should have a high level of suspicion for this condition. This condition can easily be misdiagnosed as an intra-articular problem, such as a tear of the triangular fibrocartilage complex.

Confirmatory Tests

Radiographs are negative. An arthrogram for possible triangular fibrocartilage complex tear is also negative.

Treatment

The treatment for this condition is usually conservative and consists or splinting and NSAIDs. Sometimes a steroid injection

may be needed. Rarely do patients have persistent problems; recurrent problems require tenosynovectomy and release of the ECU compartment.[61]

Prognosis

The prognosis is usually good for complete recovery after conservative treatment. Usually patients are able to return to their job regardless of the type of activity. However, when there is recurrence of tendonitis and it is associated with repetitive wrist rotation and ulnar deviation, some job modification may be necessary.

Subluxation of the Extensor Carpi Ulnaris Tendon

Clinical Findings

Patients present with a painful snapping of the ECU that is noted on ulnar deviation and rotation.[62,63] They might have experienced a traumatic event in which an actively supinated and extended wrist was forced into flexion and ulnar deviation, causing an acute rupture of the ECU retinaculum. In these cases the history suggests the diagnosis. Patients can also present with a chronic subluxation that becomes symptomatic. Some patients have a congenital subluxation of the ECU that becomes inflamed, especially when excessive wrist motions are carried out. On physical examination one should be able to see the ECU tendon sublux out of the ulnar grove as the patient rotates the wrist. In acute or inflamed cases pain may be associated with these motions.

Confirmatory Tests

There are no tests to confirm the diagnosis. It is a clinical diagnosis.

Treatment

For acute ruptures of the ECU subsheath, one might attempt casting in a pronated, dorsiflexed, and radial deviated position to see if the sheath will heal. If the subluxation persists in spite of the casting, then reconstruction of the ruptured tendon sheath is advised. It might require use of a strip of either the palmaris longus or ECU tendon, or the extensor retinaculum can be used. A similar type of reconstruction is required for patients who have a chronic ECU tendon subluxation and have repeated episodes of inflammation.[62,64,66]

Prognosis
Reconstruction of the ECU tendon sheath is usually quite successful, and in most cases patients are able to return to repetitive wrist activities. Obviously not all patients have this outcome, and job modification may be necessary for some. In patients with chronic subluxation who have recurrent bouts of inflammation associated with use, it is appropriate to recommend reconstruction of the sheath with the expectation that the patient will be able to return to work.

Distal Radioulnar Joint Disorders: Chronic Subluxation of the Distal Radial Ulnar Joint

Clinical Findings
The diagnosis of these acute injuries is usually relatively straightforward, although instability and chondromalicia of the distal radioulnar joint (DRUJ) can sometimes be difficult to confirm. In most cases there is a history of a remote injury, either a wrist fracture or dislocation of the DRUJ. The patient has pain on rotation, and there is tenderness over the DRUJ. Depending on the degree of arthritis and instability, one appreciates both grinding and subluxation when the DRUJ is manipulated. Comparison with the opposite wrist is necessary to confirm the instability.

Confirmatory Tests
Routine radiographs, tomograms, a CT scan, or an arthrogram may be needed to confirm the condition.

Treatment
For a chronic subluxation of the DRUJ that is not associated with arthritis, many soft tissue reconstructive procedures have been advocated. When there is arthritis of the DRUJ that is painful and not controlled conservatively, one of the reconstructive procedures is indicated. These include either complete or partial distal ulnar excision or the Sauve-Kapandji procedure, which consists of fusion of the distal radius and ulnar and resection of a 2 cm section of the ulnar proximally to allow rotation.

Prognosis
Although reconstructive procedures for instability of the DRUJ are difficult and require a detailed understanding of the complex anatomy and pathology of the DRUJ, good results can be seen after these procedures. One may expect a worker to be able to resume moderate activities after surgery and rehabilitation. However, the prognosis is not nearly as good after surgical procedures for arthritic conditions in the DRUJ. One should not expect most workers to return to heavy manual activities after these procedures. Grip strength is never normal, and stressful activities frequently cause pain.

Injuries, Traumatic Tears, and Degenerative Tears of The Triangular Fibrocartilage Complex: Ulnar Impaction Syndrome

Clinical Findings
These patients present a similar picture to the patients with above distal radioulnar joint disorders. They experience pain

over the ulnar side of the wrist associated with ulnar deviation and rotation. The patient may give a history of an injury that has not improved, or the pain may have appeared spontaneously. The physical findings are not obvious, and the diagnosis is more difficult to make than in the above group.

Patients have tenderness over the triangular fibrocartilage complex (TFCC)[68] with pain, but usually no instability when the distal radioulnar joint is stressed. If there is ulnar impaction, then forced ulnar deviation of the wrist is painful. Sometimes various clicks are elicited.

Confirmatory Tests
Routine radiographs are usually negative unless there is ulnar positive variance.[69] When the ulnar impaction syndrome is advanced, one might see cystic changes in the lunate or triquetrum, which are caused by degenerative changes associated with degenerative tear of the TFCC and long-standing impaction. The condition is best confirmed by an arthrogram (Fig. 11-16), but some authorities recommend arthroscopy for diagnosis.

Treatment
The treatment for these conditions is controversial and depends on the cause and magnitude of the problem. Patients generally do not improve conservatively and require surgery. The recommended procedures include arthroscopic debridement, open debridement, or repair of the TFCC; partial ulnar excision "wafer"; or formal ulnar shortening.[70]

Prognosis
The prognosis is guarded for any of these conditions. Although in many cases the pain can be either eliminated or relieved markedly and function can be improved, restoration to normal function, including

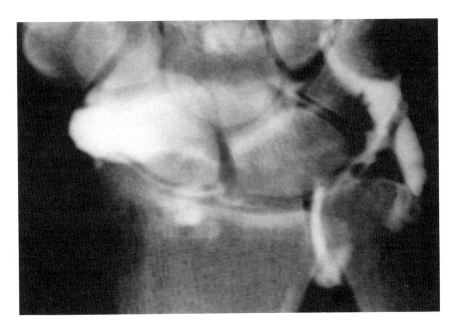

Fig. 11-16. Radiocarpal arthrogram in a patient with impaction syndrome with a positive ulnar variance and dye in the DRUJ and midcarpal joint. It demonstrates a TFCC and lunate triquetrial tear, which are often seen together in this condition.

grip strength or endurance, is unlikely. In most cases heavy manual workers should be advised that job modification might be needed. However, skilled workers, such as carpenters or electricians, should be able to return to these jobs in many cases.

Disabilities of the Ulnar Carpus, Tears of the Lunotriquetrial Joint, and Midcarpal Instability

Clinical Findings
The history is similar in these patients, who present with ulnar-sided wrist pain usually after an acute injury.[22,71,72] As with patients with triangular fibrocartilage complex tears, these patients may have negative routine radiographs and may have been diagnosed as having a sprain; yet, they have persistent wrist pain. The physical examination is positive for pain over the triquetrum or hamate. One can often elicit a painful click when the triquetrum is subluxed by applying pressure over the pisiform while the remainder of the carpus is stabilized. Radial and ulnar deviation also may cause a painful click. In cases of midcarpal instability where the instability is between the proximal and distal row, a loud clunking sound can be appreciated with radial and ulnar deviation of the wrist.

Confirmatory Tests
In most cases routine radiographs are negative. However, in some cases a volar intercalated segment instability (VISI) deformity may be seen. Arthrography or arthroscopy is indicated to confirm the diagnosis.

Treatment
The treatment for these conditions is controversial and not always successful. When patients have mild symptoms, con-

servative treatment, including splinting and avoiding activities that exacerbate the condition, is recommended. Surgical treatment includes various types of dorsal and volar ligament reconstructions or partial carpal fusions.[73,74]

Prognosis
The prognosis for returning to heavy work or work that requires stressful wrist motion is not good after these types of injuries. Obtaining adjusted work without surgery is often a wise choice because surgery is unlikely to allow the worker to return to unrestricted work.

REFERENCES

1. Froimson AI: Tenosynovitis and tennis elbow, 2117. In Green DP (ed): Operative Hand Surgery. 2nd Ed. Churchill Livingstone, New York, 1988
2. Finkelstein H: Stenosing tendovaginitis at the radial styloid process. J Bone Joint Surg 12:509, 1930
3. Grundberg AB, Reagan DS: Pathologic anatomy of the forearm: intersection syndrome. J Hand Surg 10A:299, 1985
4. Riddell DM: Spontaneous rupture of the extensor pollicis longus, J Bone Joint Surg 45B:506, 1963
5. Harvey FJ, Harvey PM, Horsley MW: de Quervain's disease: surgical or non surgical treatment. J Hand Surg 15A:83, 1990
6. Witt J, Pess G, Gelberman RH: Treatment of de Quervain's tenosynovitis. J Bone Joint Surg 73A:219, 1991
7. Arons MS: de Quervain's release in working women: a report of failures, complications and associated diagnoses. J Hand Surg 12A:540, 1987
8. Angelides AC: Ganglions of the hand and wrist, p. 2281. In Green DP (ed): Operative Hand Surgery. 2nd Ed. Churchill Livingstone, New York, 1988
9. Angelides AC, Wallace PF: The dorsal ganglion of the wrist: its pathogenesis,

gross and microscopic anatomy and surgical treatment. J Hand Surg 1:228, 1976

10. Gunther SF: Dorsal wrist pain and occult scapholunate ganglion. J Hand Surg 10A:697, 1985

11. Sanders WE: The occult dorsal carpal ganglion. J Hand Surg 10B:257, 1985

12. Fogel GR, Younge DA, Dobyns JM: Pitfalls in the diagnosis of the simple wrist ganglion. Orthopedics 6:990, 1983

13. Richman JA, Gelberman RH, Engber WD et al: Ganglions of the wrist and digits: results of treatment by aspiration and cyst wall puncture. J Hand Surg 12A:1041, 1987

14. Dray GJ, Eaton RG: Dislocations and ligament injuries in the digits, p. 800. In Green DP (ed): Operative Hand Surgery. 2nd Ed. Churchill Livingstone, New York, 1988

15. Eaton RG, Lane LB, Littler JW et al: Ligament reconstruction for the painful thumb carpometacarpal joint: a long term assessment. J Hand Surg 9A:692, 1984

16. Howard FM, Simpson LA Belsole RJ: Silastic condylar arthroplasty. Clin Orthop 195:144, 1985

17. Burton RJ: Basal joint arthritis; fusion; implant or soft tissue reconstruction. Orthop Clin North Am 17:493, 1986

18. Pellegrini VD, Burton RI: Surgical management of dorsal joint arthritis of the thumb. Part I: long term results of silicone arthoplasty. J Hand Surg 11A:309, 1986

19. Burton RI, Pellegrini VD: Surgical management of basal joint arthritis of the thumb. Part II: ligament reconstruction with tendon interposition arthroplasty. J Hand Surg 11A:324, 1986

20. Crosby EB, Linscheid RL, Dobyn JH: Scaphotrapezial-trapezoid arthrosis. J Hand Surg 3:223, 1978

21. Roger WD, Watson HK: Degenerative arthritis of the triscaphe joint. J Hand Surg 15A:232, 1990

22. Cooney WP, Garcia-Elias M, Dobyns JM et al: anatomy and mechanics of carpal instability. Surg Rounds Orthop Sept:15, 1989

23. Talesnik J: Current concept review: carpal instability. J Bone Joint Surg 70A: 1262, 1988

24. Watson HK, Ashmead D, Makhlouf MV: Examination of the scaphoid. J Hand Surg 13A: 657, 1988

25. Palmer AK, Dobyns JM, Lincheid RC: Management of post-traumatic instability of the wrist secondary to ligament rupture. J Hand Surg 3:501, 1978

26. Conyers DJ: Scapholunate interosseous reconstruction and imbrication of palmar ligament. J Hand Surg 15A:690, 1990

27. Blatt G: Capsulodesis in reconstructive hand surgery: dorsal capsulodesis for the unstable scaphoid and volar capsulodesis following excision of the distal ulnar. Hand Clin 3:81, 1987

28. Kleinman WB: Long term study of chronic scapho-lunate instability treated by scapho-trapezio-trapezoid arthrodesis. J Hand Surg 14A:429, 1989

29. Kleinman WB, Carroll C: Scapho-trapezio-trapezoid arthrodesis for treatment of amonic static and dynamic scapholunate instability: a 10-year perspective on pitfalls and complications. J Hand Surg 15A:408, 1990

30. Garcia-Elias M, Cooney WP, Linscheid RC et al: Wrist kinematic after limited intercarpal arthrodesis. J Hand Surg 14A:791, 1989

31. Watson HK, Ballet FL: The SLAC wrist: scapholunate advanced collapse pattern of degenerative arthritis. J Hand Surg 9A:358, 1984

32. Watson HK, Ryn J: Degenerative disorders of the carpus. Orthop Clin North Am 15:337, 1984

33. Gelberman RH, Wolock BS, Siegel DB: Current concepts review: fracture and non union of the carpal scaphoid. J Bone Joint Surg 71A:1560, 1989

34. Gellman H, Caputo RJ, Carter V et al: Comparison of short and long thumb spica casts for non-displaced fractures of the carpal scaphoid. J Bone Joint Surg 71A:354, 1989

35. Stark HH, Rickard TA, Zemel NP et al: Treatment of ununited fractures of the scapnoid by iliac crest bone grafts and Kinschner wire fixation. J Bone Joint Surg 70A:982, 1988

36. Amadio PC, Berquist TH, Smith DK et al: Scaphoid malunion. J Hand Surg 14A:679, 1989

37. Stahl F: On lunato malacia. Acta Chir Scand, suppl. 95:126, 1947
38. Almquist EE: Kienböck disease. Hand Clin 3:141, 1987
39. Gelberman RM, Bauman RD, Menon J et al: The vascularity of the lunate bone in Kienböck's disease. J Hand Surg 5:272, 1980
40. Gelberman RM, Salamon PB, Jurist JM et al: ulnar variance in Kienböck's disease. J Bone Joint Surg 57A:674, 1975
41. Trumble TE, Irving J: Histologic and magnetic resonance imaging correlations in Kienböck's disease. J Hand Surg 15A:879, 1990
42. Carter PR, Benton LJ, Dysert PA: Silicone rubber carpal implants: a study of the incidence of late osseous complications. J Hand Surg 11A:639, 1986
43. Almquist EE, Burns JC: Radial shortening for the treatment of Kienböck's disease—a 5–10 year follow up. J Hand Surg 7:348, 1982
44. Watson HK, Ryn J, DiBella A: An approach to Kienböck's disease: triscophe arthrodesis. J Hand Surg 10A:179, 1985
45. Howard F: Ulnar nerve palsy in wrist fracture. J Bone Joint Surg 43A:1197, 1961
46. Barton N: Fracture of Hand and Wrist. 1st ed. Churchill Livingstone, New York, 1988
47. Palmieri TJ: Pisiform area pain treatment by pisiform excision. J Hand Surg 17A:477, 1982
48. Vasilas A, Grieco RV, Barton NF: Roentgen aspects of injuries to the pisiform bone and pisotriquetral joint. J Bone Joint Surg 42A:1317, 1960
49. Green DP: Pisotriquetral arthritis: a case report. J Hand Surg 4:465, 1979
50. Jenkins SA: Osteoarthritis of the pisiform-triquetral joint: report of three cases. J Bone Joint Surg 33B:532, 1951
51. Johnson GH, Tonkin MA: Excision of pisiform in pisotriquetral arthritis. Clinical Orthopaed Rel Res 210:137, 1986
52. Carroll RE, Coyle MP: Dysfunction of the pisotriquetral joint: treatment by excision of the pisiform. J Hand Surg 10A:703, 1985
53. Dawson DM, Hallet M, Millender LH: Entrapment Neuropathies. 2nd Ed. Little Brown, Boston, 1990
54. Seddon HJ: Carpal ganglion—as a cause of paralysis of the deep branch of the ulnar nerve. J Bone Joint Surg 34B:386, 1952
55. Conn J Jr, Bergan JJ, Bell JL: Hypothenar hammer syndrome: post traumatic digital ischemia. Surgery 68:1122, 1970
56. Koman AL, Urbaniak JR: Ulnar artery thrombosis. Hand Clin 1:311, 1985
57. Newmeyer WL: Vascular disorders, p. 2404. In Green DP (ed): Operative Hand Surgery. 2nd Ed. Churchill Livingstone, New York, 1988
58. Eckman PB, Pearlstein G, Altrocchi PH: Ulnar neuropathy in bicycle rider. Arch Neurol 32:1304, 1975
59. Stark HH, Chao E, Zemel ND et al: Fracture of the hook of hamate. J Bone Joint Surg 71A:1201, 1981
60. Watson HK, Roger WB: Non union of the hook of the hamate: an argument for bone grafting the non union. J Hand Surg 14A:486, 1989
61. Hajj AA, Wood MB: Stenosing tenosynovitis of the extensor carpi ulnaris. J Hand Surg 11A:519, 1986
62. Bowers WH: The distal radioulnar joint, p. 985. In Green DP (ed): Operative Hand Surgery. 2nd Ed. Churchill Livingstone, New York, 1988
63. Doyle JR: Extensor tendons—acute injuries, p. 2050. In Green DP (ed): Operative Hand Surgery. 2nd Ed. Churchill Livingstone, New York, 1988
64. Burkhart SS, Wood MB, Linscheid RC: Post-traumatic recurrent subluxation of the extensor carpi ulnaris tendon. J Hand Surg 7:1, 1982
65. Eckhardt WA, Palmer AK: Recurrent dislocation of the extensor carpi ulnaris tendon. J Hand Surg 6:629, 1981
66. Spinner M, Kaplan EB: Extensor-carpi ulnaris: its relationship to stability of the distal radius ulnar joint. Clin Orthop 68:124, 1970
67. Bowers WH: The distal radioulnar joint, p. 939, In Green DP (ed) Operative Hand Surgery. 2nd Ed. Churchill Livingstone, New York, 1988
68. Palmer AK, Werner FW: The triangular

fibrocartilage complex of the wrist: anatomy and function. J Hand Surg 6:152, 1981

69. Palmer AK, Glisson RR, Werner FW: Ulnar variance determination. J Hand Surg 7:376, 1982

70. Darrow JC, Linscheid RL, Dobyns JH et al: Distal ulnar recession for disorders of the distal radioulnar joint. J Hand Surg 10:482, 1955

71. Alexander CE, Lichtman DM: Triquetrolunate and midcarpal instability, p. 274. In Lichtman DM (ed): The Wrist and Its

Disorders. WB Saunders, Philadelphia, 1988

72. Lichtman DM, Schneider JR, Swafford AR et al: Ulnar midcarpal instability—clinical and laboratory analysis. J Hand Surg 6:515, 1981

73. Pin PG, Young VL, Gilula LA et al: Management of chronic lunotriquetral ligament tears. J Hand Surg 14A:77, 1989

74. Viegas SF, Patterson RM, Peterson PD et al: Ulnar sided perilunate instability: an anatomic and biomechanic study. J Hand Surg 15A:268, 1990

12

The Carpal Tunnel Syndrome in the Work Place

Dean S. Louis, M.D.

The carpal tunnel syndrome has been the subject of increasing concern around the world. Its cause and its relationship to occupational tasks have evoked much controversy. This chapter discusses the history of the carpal tunnel syndrome with specific emphasis upon its epidemiology, pathology, and pathophysiology. Recommendations for treatment as it relates to the worker and the work place are suggested. It is assumed that the reader is concerned with an analysis of the problem as seen from the unique perspective of a hand surgeon. For this reason, there is little reference in this chapter to surgical specifics that are available elsewhere.

We are entering a time of change and a time of resolution regarding some of the issues relating to the occurrence of carpal tunnel syndrome in the work place. There is change in the circumstances which the carpal tunnel syndrome now occurs. There is resolution because more studies are being done to isolate the pathophysiology of the syndrome. Each worker that we deal with is different as an individual and as a person with a par-

ticular task. When we evaluate that worker we must know much about the person and much about the particular job. Whether the carpal tunnel syndrome in a particular worker is or is not caused by or aggravated by work can only be determined after careful analysis. Such an analysis must be based upon an understanding of the evolving literature and an evaluation of the worker and the job.

So much has been written about the carpal tunnel syndrome that it is possible that a reader unfamiliar with the problem may become confused. With this concern, the reference list for this chapter has been selected carefully and contains only those references that are considered pertinent to the subject.

HISTORICAL REVIEW

Although Paget[1] in 1857 is generally credited with the first reported case of median nerve compression at the wrist, Lipscomb[2] refers to an earlier case reported by Gensoul. Both of these patients had sustained distal radius fractures. There were a few scattered reports in the following years. Marie and Foix[3] in 1913 observed postmortem swelling of the median nerve proximal to the transverse carpal ligament in a patient with bilateral thenar atrophy. In subsequent decades increasing numbers of cases were reported. In 1946 Cannon and Love[4] reported a series of 38 cases of tardy median nerve palsy. Nine of their patients underwent median nerve decompression. Thus, recognition of the problem resulted in effective surgical management. Subsequently, in 1966 Phalen reported his personal experience with 439 patients. Only 40 percent of his patients underwent surgical release. He stated, "It is obvious that resting the hands or a change of occupation is indicated for the patient who has had a recent onset of symptoms after an unusual amount of manual labor." Although he did not consider carpal tunnel syndrome to be caused by occupational activities, Phalen did state that an occupation may aggravate it. Ten years later in 1976, Posch and Marcotte[6] reported on their experience with 1,201 cases.

Therefore, as the decades passed, there were increasing numbers of reports about the carpal tunnel syndrome and increasingly larger numbers of cases reported in individual series. In 1988, carpal tunnel release was the tenth most performed procedure in terms of dollars, spent under Medicare Part B.[7] The total cost in this older population group was over $15.5 million which, of course, does not include expenditures for the younger working population. Clearly, surgery for the carpal tunnel syndrome is one of the most frequently performed operations in adults in the United States. However, data on the frequency of this operation and the total dollar amounts expended in direct and indirect costs are not available.

EPIDEMIOLOGY

The personal experience of George Phalen perhaps reflects the increased awareness of this clinical problem. He made his first diagnosis of the syndrome in 1947. By 1949 he had treated three patients surgically. His subsequent report in 1966[5] involved 654 hands in 439 patients. Increased awareness of the clinical problem led to more frequent diagnosis of the condition and an increasing number of cases treated surgically. The majority of his patients were housekeepers or cooks, who were not thought to use their hands excessively. Excessive use of the hands in highly forceful and highly repetitive activities in the work place is now thought to be related to the genesis of the carpal tunnel syndrome in the industrial environment.[8-10]

One can only speculate about the changes that have occurred in the work place in the past 30 years and their relationship to the increasing reports of carpal tunnel syndrome.[11-18] Many tasks have been made more intensive (constantly repetitive) rather than intermittent in nature. A few obvious examples are the increasing use of computers for data entry, optical scanners at grocery check-out counters, and word processors. When the automotive industry is in high gear, shifts may lengthen to 10 hours per day, 6 days per week, increasing the workers' exposure to repetitive acts. Most notable among the occupations that have been reported as related to the carpal tunnel syndrome are butchers,[14] poultry workers,[15] assembly line workers,[16] cash register operators,[17] telegraphers,[18] and garment workers.[19]

After an extensive review of the literature and a carefully designed study, Silverstein[10] proposed that repetitiveness, force, awkward posture, and vibrating and nonvibrating hand tools were risk factors for the development of cumulative trauma disorders, including the carpal tunnel syndrome.

These investigators found the literature on cumulative trauma disorders wanting in several aspects, including lack of controls, observer bias, and survivor bias in studied populations. They then designed a careful study involving 574 workers in six plants. The jobs were categorized according to the forcefulness and repetitiveness of the tasks performed. Low repetitive jobs were those in which the fundamental cycle time was more than 30 seconds, or less than 50 percent of the cycle time was involved in performing the same kind of fundamental cycle. Highly repetitive jobs were defined as those having a cycle time of less than 30 seconds or in which more than 50 percent of the cycle time involved performing the same kind of fundamental cycle. Force determinations were made by observation of the tasks and the size and weight of the objects handled. Electromyographic observations were also made to determine the forearm flexor force used for each of the tasks. Each specific job studied was then classified into high force or low force and high repetition or low repetition. Thus, there were four categories of jobs: (1) low force and low repetition, (2) high force and low repetition, (3) low force and high repetition, and (4) high force and high repetition. Thirty-three percent of the study population had cumulative trauma disorders on interview, and 19.5 percent had cumulative trauma disorders on physical examination and interview. The high force and high repetition groups consistently exhibited an increased risk for all hand-wrist cumulative trauma disorders, tendonitis, and carpal tunnel syndrome. Force seemed to be a more important risk factor than repetitiveness for most hand-wrist cumulative trauma disorders. Repetitiveness appeared to be more important than

force as a risk factor for carpal tunnel syndrome. The prevalence of cumulative trauma disorders in women was twice that of men. However, there was no significant association between sex and the carpal tunnel syndrome. Neither was there an observed association between exposure and health history or recreational activities. Age and years on the job were associated with most cumulative trauma disorders, but this association was not statistically significant.

This study was extensive, exhausting, and unlike any other in its effort to control variables and confounders. It is quoted frequently and is now key to our understanding of the relationship between the nature of work and the development of cumulative trauma disorders, in particular the carpal tunnel syndrome. Conducting such a study is very difficult. In order to do such an analysis, the workers involved must be away from their assigned tasks for a considerable time to participate in interviews and other evaluations, resulting in a net loss of productivity for the business involved. This is one of the reasons why similar comprehensive studies are not available.

Yet, it is evident that more controlled studies are needed to assess accurately the relationship of work to cumulative trauma disorders and the carpal tunnel syndrome. The development of the Agency for Health Care Policy and Research, and funding for outcome studies should be helpful in this regard. This newly developed agency is in the Department of Health Services.

PATHOLOGY AND PATHOPHYSIOLOGY

What changes occur within the carpal tunnel to precipitate the clinical symptom complex that we call the carpal tunnel syndrome? It is easy to understand how a fracture or dislocation can cause an attenuation in its dimensions, thereby placing increased pressure on the median nerve. Yet, what happens when the anatomy of the carpal canal is unaltered?

Gelberman et al[20] in 1981 reported their results of wick catheter carpal tunnel pressure measurements in 15 patients with the carpal tunnel syndrome and in 12 normal controls. In the controls, with the wrist in neutral position, the average pressure was 2.5 mmHg. In full flexion the average pressure was 32 mmHg, and in extension it was 30 mmHg. In patients with the carpal tunnel syndrome, the corresponding pressures were 32, 90, and 110 mmHg, respectively. Szabo and Chidgey in 1989[21] reported similar findings with the slit catheter technique and then carried their study one step further. The pressure measurements that they obtained were recorded after cyclic passive exercises at a rate of 30 cycles per minute. They then measured pressures at 30-second intervals over the next 10 minutes. Patients with carpal tunnel syndrome had a slower rate of return to pretest values than normal subjects. Gellman and associates[22] using the wick catheter technique studied a group of paraplegic patients who relied upon the extended wrist position exclusively for activities of daily living, including propelling a wheelchair and transferring to and from a wheelchair. They found the pressures in the carpal tunnel in the neutral wrist position in the paraplegic patients were higher than in the nonparaplegic patients without the carpal tunnel syndrome, but were lower than nonparaplegic patients with the carpal tunnel syndrome. The pressures in the carpal tunnel in paraplegic patients in the extended position were higher than those in nonparaplegic patients with or without the carpal tunnel syndrome. They argue that the forced extension of the wrist and the repetitive trauma to the volar aspect of the wrist were related to the high frequency of the carpal tunnel syndrome in paraplegic patients. The use of the extreme extended posture of the wrist in a repetitive fashion while performing other activities can presumably result in the same problem.

Thomas and Fullerton[23] noted a diminished fiber size of the median nerve in a postmortem study of a patient with the carpal tunnel syndrome. In addition there was an increase in the perineural connective tissue. Phalen[5] in 1966 obtained biopsy specimens of the tenosynovium and noted fibrosis in 91 of 181 specimens. In a more recent study by Schwind and colleagues[24] specimens of the tenosynovium were obtained from 21 patients with idiopathic carpal tunnel syndrome. Their inclusion and exclusion criteria were sufficiently rigorous to eliminate any other possible confounders. Electrodiagnostic recovery was one of the major inclusion criteria. They observed three types of histologic change in the tenosynovium: grade I—isolated tenosynovial hypertrophy; grade II—fibrous hypertrophy with localized necrotic areas; and grade III—fibrous hypertrophy with localized necrotic areas and empty spaces similar to serous bursae. In the more advanced lesions there was an absence of fibroblasts, and in some areas there were accumulations of rounded cells that had the appearance of chondroid metaplasia. In no instance was there evidence of any inflammatory cellular reactions. They believed that these changes were typical of connective tissue undergoing degeneration as a result of repeated mechanical stress.

It is unfortunate that such terms as tenosynovitis, and tendonitis, and synovitis are used so loosely when referring to the response within the carpal tunnel to repetitive trauma. This putative cause of the carpal tunnel syndrome (inflammation) does not appear to be appropriate when we are considering repetitive mechanical stress within the carpal tunnel as is seen in the work place.

DIAGNOSTIC STUDIES

The median nerve is the least rigid and therefore the most easily compressible structure within the carpal tunnel. Its response to increased pressure has been measured by several methods.

The carpal tunnel syndrome is primarily a clinical syndrome; that is, the diagnosis can be suspected with a high degree of accuracy based upon the history and physical examination alone. A clinical history of numbness and tingling in the median nerve distribution associated with pain in the hand or wrist, nocturnal paresthesias, and proximal radiation to the elbow or shoulder is strongly suggestive of carpal tunnel syndrome. Subsequent evaluations, including electrodiagnostic tests, radiographs, and chemical profiles where indicated may be helpful. Electrodiagnostic tests should now be considered to be a standard part of the work-up of a patient suspected of having carpal tunnel syndrome. It is now necessary to do these tests—perhaps defensively for legal reasons—although they are not always cost effective when the clinical symptomatology is specific. It should be recognized, however, that a small percentage of patients will have all of the usual symptoms and signs of the carpal tunnel syndrome and yet have normal electrodiagnostic studies. In such patients, Grundberg[25] achieved symptomatic relief with carpal tunnel release in 30 of 32 hands, Green[26] and Gelberman[27] obtained excellent relief with steroid injections. They also felt this response had prognostic significance; a good response from the injection usually meant a good response to surgery.

Gelberman and associates[28] in a study of 12 volunteers applied external compression to the median nerve with varying pressures from 40 to 70 mmHg for periods from 30 to 240 minutes and then measured the response to four sensory tests. Two-point discrimination, both moving and static; Semmes-Weinstein pressure monofilaments; and vibration were measured. The threshold tests (Semmes-Weinstein monofilaments and vibration tests) showed gradual decreases in nerve function both subjectively and with electrical testing. The innervation density tests (static and moving two-point discrimination) remained normal until almost all sensory conduction had ceased. These studies may provide an explanation as to why in some instances the electrodiagnostic tests are normal in the face of clinical symptoms consistent with the carpal tunnel syndrome. There appears to be a sensitive threshold where symptoms may occur even though the currently available tests fail to reveal any abnormalities.

Electrodiagnostic studies may be helpful in confirming the diagnosis. They may also help exclude other diagnoses, especially generalized peripheral neuropathies, no matter what the cause.

EVALUATION

When a worker is seen with symptoms suggestive of the carpal tunnel syndrome, a detailed history is imperative. The usual general medical history is, of course, appropriate. It should ask specifically about past or present illnesses, especially previous trauma and systemic diseases, such as diabetes, rheumatoid arthritis, and thyroid disease.

A past employment history is also very important. Has the worker changed from a less hand-intensive activity to one that puts more functional demands upon the upper extremity? Has the worker been employed only in the household and then embarked upon a highly repetitive task? Is the worker resuming employment after many years away from the work place? What social factors are involved in the worker's current situation? Is the worker being forced by a family situation to return to the work force, without great enthusiasm and even reluctance because of personal circumstances? What about the job? Are the demands always the same? How many tasks are performed? How frequently are the tasks performed (cycle time)? Have there been any recent change in the way the job is performed or the rate at which it is performed? Such a question relates to the work station and the tools or machines involved. It is important to ascertain the worker's attitude about the current job and previous jobs and the level of satisfaction with the current work. Is there any evidence of depression? Home life and leisure activities should also be evaluated. Hand-intensive leisure activities, such as racquet sports, computer use, knitting, and similar activities, may contribute to the worker's overall symptom production.

It is important to know when symptoms occur and when they subside. Are the symptoms intensified as the work day progresses? Are they relieved or diminished during periods away from work, such as nights, weekends, or vacation periods?

The results of these inquiries will be subject to a great deal of interpretation by the physician. Motivation is dealt with elsewhere in Chapter 16. Paul Brown has also discussed motivation from the unique perspective of a hand surgeon.[29] The recent Kappa Delta Award paper by Bigos et al.[30] emphasizes how nonphysical factors affect the worker's response to medical treatment.

The desire of the worker to get well and return to work will have a major influence upon progress toward this goal. If the carpal tunnel syndrome in a given individual is deemed compensable, then there may be no motivation to return to work, especially when there is collateral insurance to cover car and house payments. Subjective pain and discomfort are largely unmeasurable and confound the situation. Symptoms may thus persist even when objective evaluation after surgery shows that electrophysiologic parameters have reverted to normal. All of this is to say that patient management should proceed cautiously. The recent reports by Jones and Scott[31] and by Nancollas, Peimer, and Wheeler[32] support this approach.

MANAGEMENT

Each patient with the carpal tunnel syndrome must be managed individually. No standard formula applies to their care. If no confounding problems, such as previous trauma or underlying disease processes, complicate the occupationally related carpal tunnel syndrome, then a conservative approach is clearly indicated. My own experience has firmly convinced me that an aggressive surgical approach to the management of the carpal tunnel syndrome when it is related to hand-intensive activities at work frequently does not restore the worker to an asymptomatic state. This observation has also been made by others.[33]

Conservative management may involve time away from work, light duty assignments, splinting, steroid injections, nonsteroidal anti-inflammatory drugs, or various combinations of the above. Because there is no good prospective study that measures the effectiveness of any of these measures in relationship to specific job tasks, their use is empiric. The progress through several conservative programs also gives the physician an opportunity to get to know the patient better and to assess motivation.

The following commonly observed scenario supports the usefulness of this empiric approach. After a challenging exposure to a hand-intensive job, the worker develops symptoms and signs compatible with the carpal tunnel syndrome. He is taken away from that task either completely, is placed on light duty, or is given a medical leave of absence. While away from the hand-intensive work, his symptoms subside. He then returns to the original task and the symptoms return. This exposure response cycle is the occupational equivalent of Koch's postulates. The relationship to the task under these circumstances should not be a matter of dispute when there is objective evidence to confirm the diagnosis and its resolution, i.e., electrodiagnostic tests. The problem becomes more difficult when there is a manifest psychological component to the symptoms and little objective evidence for them. This aspect of the problem is discussed elsewhere in this volume (see Chapter 7). Ireland[34] and Hadler[35-37] have strongly disputed a causal relationship between job activities and the carpal tunnel syndrome. The issue of work relatedness is not at all clear-cut.

If a worker has been removed from the specific hand-intensive job and fails to respond symptomatically to conservative means, and with the coincident failure of improvement in electrodiagnostic studies, then surgery may be indicated. Under these circumstances, however, it must be agreed that the worker will return to less hand-intensive work. How long to continue with new operative measures before acknowledging their failure is a matter of individual discretion and is usually somewhere between 3 to 6 months.

If the worker has no other related problems, such as degenerative arthritis of the wrist or of the carpometacarpal joint of the thumb, then symptomatic relief should be the expected outcome in the short term. After a course of conservative treatment, then resumption of the hand-intensive work becomes the issue. Job modifications or change, work hardening, and ergonomic assessment may be appropriate measures under these circumstances. The success of these measures will depend to a large extent upon the original task that provoked the problem. If the task is one of intermittent intensity in terms of hand usage, such as a teacher, clerk typist, dental hygienist, then the likelihood that the individual will have long-lasting relief is great in my experience. The converse is true for typical assembly line and production employees. Most workers who are employed in these continuously repetitive jobs will experience a recurrence when returned to their original jobs.

Some people will never return to employment either because they do not want to, some of their symptoms were due to other causes, (i.e., degenerative arthritis at one level or another), or because of real but undiagnosed vague symptoms that have eluded our individual diagnostic snares. Others will not return to work because of specific recognizable complications relating to the surgery.[38,39]

SUMMARY

The management of a patient with the carpal tunnel syndrome that occurs in relationship to the work environment is a complex process. The equation—symptoms + physical findings + abnormal electroneuromyographic studies = surgery = relief = return to former job—is not tenable. The process is much more prolonged and requires patience and understanding of the worker; it must emphasize a conservative approach and surgical restraint.

REFERENCES

1. Paget J: Lectures on Surgical Pathology, 1st ed. Lindsay and Blakiston, Philadelphia, 1854
2. Lipscomb PR: Historical perspective on nerve compression syndromes. In Szabo RM (ed): *Nerve Compression Syndromes Diagnosis and Treatment.* Slack, Inc., Thorofare, NJ, 1989
3. Marie P, Foix C: Atrophie isole de l'eminence thenar d'origine nevritique: role du ligament annulaire anterieur du carpe dans la pathogenie de la lesion. Rev Neurol 26:647, 1913
4. Cannon BW, Love JG: Tardy median palsy: median neuritis and median thenar neuritis amenable to surgery. Surgery 20:210, 1946
5. Phalen GS: The carpal tunnel syndrome: seventeen years' experience in diagnosis and treatment of six hundred fifty-four hands. J. Bone Joint Surg 48A:211, 1966
6. Posch JL, Marcotte, DR: Carpal tunnel syndrome: an analysis of 1201 cases. Orthop Rev 5:25, 1976
7. Data on Volume and Changes for Medicare Services by Orthopaedic Surgeons, 1986-1988. American Academy of Orthopaedic Surgeons, Center for Research, Park Ridge, IL, 1990
8. Occupational disease surveillance: carpal tunnel syndrome. Morb Mort Wkly Rep 38:485, 1989
9. Occupational disease surveillance: carpal tunnel syndrome. Centers for Disease Control. JAMA 262:88, 1989
10. Silverstein B: The prevalence of upper extremity cumulative trauma disorders in industry. Ph.D. dissertation, University of Michigan, Ann Arbor MI, 1985
11. Birkbeck MQ, Beer TC: Occupation in relation to the carpal tunnel syndrome. Rheumatol Rehab: 14:218, 1975
12. Cannon LJ, Bernacki EJ, Walter SD: Personal and occupational factors associated with carpal tunnel syndrome. J Occup Med 23:225, 1981
13. Dimberg L, Olafsson A, Stefansson E et al: The correlation between work environment and the occurrence of cervicobrachial symptoms. J Occup Med 31:447, 1989
14. Finkel ML: The effects of repeated mechanical trauma in the meat industry. Am J Indust Med 8:375, 1985
15. Armstrong TJ, Foulkes J, Joseph BS, Goldstein S: An investigation of cumulative trauma disorders in a poultry processing plant. Am Indust Hyg Assoc J 43:103, 1982
16. Morse LH: Repetitive motions: musculoskeletal problems in the microelectronics industry. State Art Rev. Occup Med 1:167, 1986
17. Margolis W, Kraus JF: The prevalance of carpal tunnel syndrome symptoms in female supermarket checkers. J Occup Med 29:953, 1987
18. Hocking B: Epidemiologic aspects of repetition strain injury in Telecom Australia. Med J Aust 147:218, 1987
19. Punnet L, Robins JM, Wegman DH, Keyserling WM: Soft tissue disorders in the upper limbs of female garment workers. Scand J Work Environ Health 11:417, 1985
20. Gelberman RH, Hergenmoeder PT, Hargens AR et al: The carpal tunnel syndrome: a study of carpal canal pressures. J Bone Joint Surg 63A:380, 1981
21. Szabo RM, Chidgey LK: Stress carpal tunnel pressures in patients with carpal tunnel syndrome and normal patients. J Hand Surg 14A:624, 1989
22. Gellman H, Chandler DR, Perasek J et al: Carpal tunnel symdrome in paraplegic patients. J Bone Joint Surg 70A:517, 1988
23. Thomas PK, Fullerton PM: Nerve fiber size in the carpal tunnel syndrome. J Neurol Neurosurg Psychiatr 26:520, 1963
24. Schwind F, Ventura M, Posteek JL: Idiopathic carpal tunnel syndrome: histologic study of flexor tendor synovium. J Hand Surg 15A:497, 1990
25. Grundberg AB: Carpal tunnel decompression in spite of a normal electromyography. J Hand Surg 8:348, 1983

26. Green DP: Diagnostic and therapeutic value of carpal tunnel injection. J Hand Surg 9:850, 1989

27. Gelberman RH, Aronson D, Weissman MH: Results of a prospective trial of steroid injection and splinting. J Bone Joint Surg 62A:1181, 1980

28. Gelberman RH, Szabo RM, Williamson RV, et al: Sensibility testing in peripheral nerve compression syndromes: an experimental study in humans. J Bone Joint Surg 65A:632, 1983

29. Brown P: The role of motivation in the recovery of the hand, p.1 In Kasdan M (ed): Occupation Hand and Upper Extremity Injuries and Diseases. Hanley & Belfus, Philadelphia, 1991

30. Bigos SJ, Bottie MC, Spengler DC et al: A longitudinal prospective study of industrial back injury reporting. Paper presented at American Academy of Orthopaedic Surgeons, 58th Annual Meeting, Anaheim, CA, March 1991

31. Jones BF, Scott FA: Carpal tunnel release. The effect of workers' compensation on clinical outcome. Paper presented at American Academy of Orthopaedic Surgeons 58th Annual Meeting, Anaheim, CA, March 1991

32. Nancollas MP, Peimer CA, Wheeler DR: Long term results of carpal tunnel release. Paper presented at American Academy of Orthopaedic Surgeons 58th Annual Meeting, Anaheim, CA, March 1991

33. Masear VR, Hayes JM, Hyde AG: An industrial cause of carpal tunnel syndrome. J Hand Surg 11A:222, 1986

34. Ireland D: Psychological and physical aspects of occupational arm pain. J Hand Surg 13B:5, 1988

35. Hadler NM: Occupational illness: the issure of causality. J Occup Med 26:587, 1984

36. Hadler NM: Work related disorders of the upper extremity: Part I. Cumulative trauma disorders: a critical review. Occup Probl Med Pract 4:1, 1989

37. Hadler NM: Cumulative trauma disorders: an iatrogenic concept. J Occup Med 32:38, 1990

38. MacDonald RI, Lichtman DM, Hanlon JJ et al: Complications of surgical release for carpal tunnel syndrome. J Hand Surg 3:70, 1978

39. Louis DS, Greene TL, Noellert RC: Complications of carpal tunnel syndrome. J Neurosurg 62:352, 1985

13

Occupational Injuries of the Elbow

Barry P. Simmons, M.D.
Edwin T. Wyman, Jr., M.D.

Although work-related elbow injuries represent a small percentage of total work injuries, their incidence is significantly increased when rapid and repetitive arm motion, particularly in the wrist and fingers, is involved. Increased strength requirements, poor tool design, machine pacing, strained work positions, and cold temperatures tend to increase the incidence of these cumulative trauma disorders. In the elbow, pathology includes several tendonitis patterns, milder forms of arthritis, nerve entrapment syndromes, un-united or malunited fractures, and olecranon bursitis. In the management of cumulative trauma disorders it is important for the treating physician to realize that regardless of treatment, whether surgical or nonsurgical, it is unlikely that the patient will be able to return to the same job unless it is modified to remove the harmful effects that caused or aggravated this disorder.

LATERAL ELBOW PROBLEMS

Lateral Epicondylitis (Tennis Elbow)

Clinical Picture

Lateral epicondylitis is the commonest form of cumulative trauma disorder at the elbow. In industry it is usually associated with repeated gripping activities, particularly if the elbow is extended and the wrist flexed. Repeated forced supination and the presence of vibration also seem to be instigating or aggravating factors. Pathology is said by some to be secondary or tearing of the common extensor tendon,[1] whereas others believe that the point of inflammation is at the attachment of the common extensor tendon to periosteum.[2] Still others indict the synovium over the radial head as the key to the problem.[3]

In any case, symptoms involve pain over the lateral aspect of the elbow that is sharply localized to the area of the lateral epicondyle and joint line in the area of the radial head (Fig. 13-1). Occasionally there is radiation of pain into the lateral forearm, which can cause confusion with the radial tunnel syndrome. Grip strength is often weakened because of pain. True radicular pain radiated into the forearm should not occur. Physical examination should elicit tenderness directly over the lateral epicondyle, common extensor tendon, or radial head. Discomfort is increased with elbow extension and wrist flexion, by stretching the extensor musculature, and by resisted extension of the wrist and finger extensors. There is commonly a permanent flexion contracture if these symptoms have lasted for some time.

Confirmatory Tests

The diagnosis is made by physical examination. Routine x-rays are indicated, and the presence of calcific deposits in the area of the common extensor tendon confirms the diagnosis. EMG and nerve conduction studies may be carried out to rule out the radial entrapment syndromes.

Treatment

Rest by means of sling or splint, hot or cold applications, nonsteroidal anti-inflammatory agents, and physical therapy modalities, such as ultrasound, are commonly used in the conservative treatment of the acute phase of this condition. Stretching exercises to eliminate elbow permanent flexion contracture, as well as muscle strengthening exercises for the wrist and finger extensors, are important later.[4] Steroid injections in the the painful areas are commonly used. It is important not to inject a steroid into the elbow joint itself, but rather into the tendon and periosteal area of the epicondyle. Injections of this sort can be used several times over a few months, but should not be used for a longer period. Surgery is reserved for the most resistant cases and involves releasing the common extensor tendon at the lateral epicondyle with or without exploration of the lateral compartment of the elbow joint (Fig. 13-2).[5] Many feel that the major benefit of these procedures is the elimination of an inflammatory reaction by scar production.

Prognosis

Regardless of treatment, the symptoms will probably recur if the patient returns to the same job that produced or aggra-

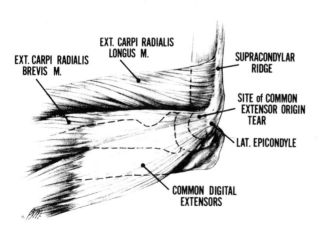

EXT. CARPI RADIALIS BREVIS M.

EXT. CARPI RADIALIS LONGUS M.

SUPRACONDYLAR RIDGE

SITE of COMMON EXTENSOR ORIGIN TEAR

LAT. EPICONDYLE

COMMON DIGITAL EXTENSORS

Fig. 13-1. Anatomic features of the lateral side of the elbow showing the site of the common extensor origin tear found in cases of tennis elbow. (From Green,[21] with permission.)

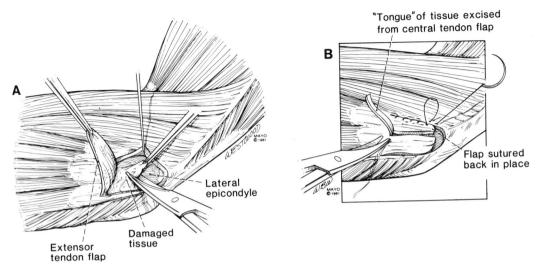

Fig. 13-2. Surgery of extensor origin problems. (**A**) Lateral view of the lateral epicondyle showing the underside of the central tendon and removal of damaged tissue in that area. (**B**) Reinsertion of the tendon remnants into the remainder of the extensor origin mass. (From Evarts,[22] with permission.)

vated the condition. Thus, the treating physicians should emphasize either job modification or job retraining. Job modification may include changing the work environment, the tools used, or the rapidity of work demands.[6]

In the chronic condition, a large element of operant conditioning may be involved in the patient's total symptoms. This effect can be elicited by inconsistent physical findings, which may help the treating physician both in diagnosis and treatment, in particular the avoidance of surgery. Such inconsistent physical findings are patterned along the lines of those outlined by Waddell for evaluation of industrial chronic low back pain and include tenderness above rather than at the lateral epicondyle, increased pain with resisted finger and wrist *flexion*, pain being the same with the elbow flexed or extended when the wrist is held in flexion, and tenderness over the olecranon.

Although work place ergonomic changes are most important in the prevention of this condition, medical preventive techniques include work hard-

ening activities to prevent permanent flexion contractures and to increase finger and wrist extensor muscle strength. Occasionally, it is helpful to use a pressure splint that places pressure over the lateral extensor muscle mass just distal to the common extensor tendon and radial head during work activities.

Radial Nerve Entrapments: Resistant Tennis Elbow, Posterior Interosseous Nerve Syndrome, Radial Tunnel Syndrome

Clinical Picture

Radial nerve entrapments around the elbow are rare. Anatomically, the radial nerve courses anterior to the elbow and then laterally beneath the brachioradialis. There it divides into a sensory nerve that terminates as the superficial branch in the first web space and the posterior interosseous nerve that supplies the extensor muscles of the ulnar side of the wrist (ECU) and the fingers (EDC, EIP, EDQ, APL, APB) and thumb (EPL). The division in the forearm occurs at the supinator. At that site the nerve can be entrapped by a leash of vessels or the origin of the supinator that constitutes the arcade of Frohse[8] (Fig. 13-3). Distally it can also be trapped at the edge of the supinator.

If the entrapment mainly involves the posterior interosseous branch the patient may present with pain at the site of entrapment and/or weakness in the digital extensors. Appropriately, this condition is known as *posterior interosseous nerve syndrome* (PIN).[9] If the entrapment involves the sensory branch, known as the *radial tunnel syndrome*, there is no weakness and rarely any sensory loss, but both pain and tenderness occur at the site of entrapment.[10,11] Note that there is no difference in the site of entrapment; the only

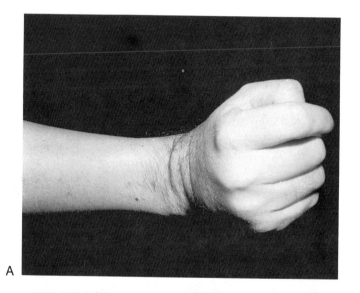

A

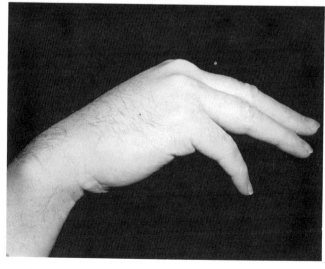

B

Fig. 13-3. (**A & B**) Patient with posterior interosseous nerve palsy. Note radial deviation with wrist extension and wrist flexion to produce MCP extension. (*Figure continues.*)

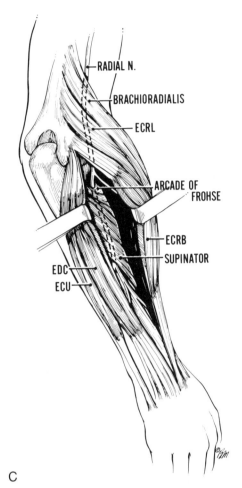

RADIAL N.

BRACHIORADIALIS

ECRL

ARCADE OF
FROHSE

ECRB
SUPINATOR

EDC
ECU

C

Fig. 13-3 (*Continued*). (**C**) The posterior muscle splitting approach to the radial tunnel and the arcade of Frohse. (Figs. A & B from Dawson et al.,[23] Fig. C from Green,[21] with permission.)

difference is which branch is more compromised. PIN is primarily a motor lesion, which may even present without pain, and radial tunnel syndrome is a pain syndrome.

Radial tunnel syndrome is also known as *resistant tennis elbow*. Classically this disorder is seen in workers who have to perform multiple repetitive motions, especially if they involve significant wrist dorsiflexion (extension), with or without force. Its onset may be gradual or acute

and, in the latter case, can be severe enough for patients to seek emergency treatment because of the pain. On rare occasion patients present because of inability to extend their wrist or digits, rather than because of pain. On examination patients have tenderness over the nerve at the site of entrapment; that is, beneath the brachioradialis (Fig. 13-3). This site is approximately 4 to 6 cm distal to the lateral epicondyle or over the radiocapitellar joint. Frequently the patient is symptomatic at both areas and can have both disorders. There may be no further findings, but a patient may have increased pain at the site of entrapment with wrist flexion, antagonism of wrist extension, or a positive "middle finger test." This test is performed by having the wrist in neutral and the middle finger fully extended; the examiner tries to passively flex the middle finger. However, probably the most reliable of these relatively nonlocalizing tests is direct tenderness of the nerve at the site of entrapment, especially if a positive Tinel's sign is present.

If there is motor involvement, it can be partial or complete. In complete posterior interosseous nerve palsy, the patient has radial wrist extension, but absent finger and thumb extension (Fig. 13-3). The examiner must be sure to have the wrist extended to test properly for digital extension. If patients cannot extend their digits, they will tend to flex the wrist, which produces digital extension by a tenodesis effect. Flexing the interphalangeal joints to isolate metacarpophalangeal joint extension also demonstrates the palsy.

Confirmatory Tests

In addition to the studies for lateral epicondylitis, an EMG and nerve conduction study (NCS) should be ordered.[12] In posterior interosseous nerve palsy these studies can be confirmatory. Unfortunately, in a pure pain picture, these studies are negative in 80 percent of cases; the development of dynamic EMG/NCSs and/or near nerve studies may increase the accuracy. However, it is still of value to obtain these studies not only because of the small percentage that are positive but also to rule out other sites of entrapment, such as the cervical spine, in these difficult-to-treat patients.

Treatment

In posterior interosseous nerve syndrome, rest is the initial treatment. A cock-up wrist splint and sling may be sufficient; NSAIDs may also help. The patient should not return to work. If spontaneous resolution of the palsy occurs, then a rehabilitation program can be initiated. However, if the weakness recurs, this program should be stopped. If, after a period of 6 to 8 weeks of rest, there is no resolution of the palsy, surgical decompression is indicated. If there is a question as to whether improvement is occurring, a repeat EMG may be of help.

In radial tunnel syndrome, as in lateral epicondylitis, rest is the initial treatment. If symptoms have improved, then rehabilitation emphasizing stretching of the wrist and digital extensors and subsequent strengthening is indicated (Mill's exercises). With resolution of symptoms, work simulation and work hardening can begin. However, recurrence of symptoms is an indication that a new job will be necessary.

If symptoms fail to resolve with nonoperative treatment and the patient is unable to perform daily activities, then surgery is indicated.[11] It is extremely unlikely that such a patient will return to the original employment.

Prognosis

The prognosis is guarded. In posterior interosseous nerve palsy, there is a possibility that the worker may return to the original job. However, as in lateral epicondylitis, this is unlikely. The same is true for radial tunnel syndrome. Certainly, in the older, unskilled worker whose job involves repetitive motion, the prognosis is poor.

Radiocapitellar Arthritis

Clinical Picture

Posttraumatic arthritis of the radiocapitellar joint may occur after fracture or may simply be part of a generalized degenerative arthritis of the elbow that becomes symptomatic in the radiocapitellar area because of repeated pronation and supination work activities. There is usually a permanent flexion contracture, and pronation and supination are limited. Crepitation may be found, and there may be a history of locking if loose bodies are present secondary to the arthritis.

Mild arthritic changes consisting of early cartilaginous fraying, roughening, and splitting may also occur. These changes may be caused by heavy work activities, such as handling heavy vibrating tools, e.g., jackhammers. Discomfort is noted over the lateral aspect of the elbow, which is differentiated from lateral epicondylitis and the radial tunnel syndrome by its accentuation by pronation and supination and crepitation.

Confirmatory Tests

All but the earliest stages of radiocapitellar arthritis are seen on plain x-rays. Loose bodies may also be visible on these studies, if they are not cartilaginous. Early chondral changes are not seen. Arthroscopy may help both with diagnosis and treatment by means of a minimally invasive debridement.

Treatment

Rest by slings and splints and the use of nonsteroidal anti-inflammatory agents often help. Occasional débridement by arthroscopy is beneficial. However, open surgery for debridement rarely proves beneficial, except to remove loose bodies. In late arthritis with limited and painful pronation and supination resistant to less invasive treatment, excision of the radial head may be considered, but only in conjunction with major job modification.

Muscle strengthening through work hardening has relatively limited application in the treatment of work-aggravated arthritis unless the pathology is very early in its course.

Prognosis

Return to a job similar to one that caused or aggravated the elbow arthritis is very doubtful, even with job and work environment modifications as noted above. Regardless of treatment and recedence of symptoms, return to such a job often causes a recurrence of symptoms. The best alternative is job retraining, but since the diagnosis usually occurs in the older worker, this option is often resisted by the employer and insurance company. Although the diagnosis is usually not difficult in these cases, at times x-rays may be negative and yet symptoms may persist for many months, allowing the chronic pain syndrome to be superimposed. In that case, inconsistencies of physical findings may be helpful in making this latter diagnosis. Pain on elbow *flexion*, tenderness of the soft tissues of the upper forearm, and abnormal sensory changes in the absence of a nerve entrapment syndrome may help diagnostically.

Non-Union/Malunion Fracture Lateral Epicondyle

Clinical Picture

This is a rare condition that does not usually pose a diagnostic problem as there is a history of trauma to the elbow, often when the worker was a child. The onset of discomfort is usually more gradual than in the case of lateral epicondylitis, although the symptoms are quite similar. Often there is asymmetric swelling of the lateral epicondyle. Tenderness occurs directly over the lateral epicondyle and radiocapitellar joint. Motion may be limited in pronation and supination, and there is often a permanent flexion contracture of the elbow. On occasion, cubitus valgus occurs, which may be associated with a tardy ulnar nerve palsy.

Confirmatory Tests

In this instance there is no problem in diagnosis, as plain x-rays reveal either a fracture that has healed only by fibrous tissue or a malunion of the lateral epicondyle. Comparison x-rays with the normal elbow often are necessary to reveal minor changes. At times the lateral epicondyle may be separated from the humeral metaphysis by several millimeters.

Treatment

In cases with mild symptoms, nonspecific conservative measures, which as rest, temporary splinting, nonsteroidal anti-inflammatory medication, and later gradual work hardening and muscular strengthening exercises, may be helpful. Steroid injections in these cases are usually not beneficial and should not be used.

In rare instances, surgery to excise the area of non-union and insert bone graft may be carried out. However, usually the epicondylar bone fragment is small and is therefore excised on the rare occasions that surgery is performed for this condition.

Prognosis

In cases that are aggravated by light repetitive activity, tool and work environment changes may allow the patient to return to this type of job. More often, a job change is indicated. Most cases are not diagnostic problems, and treatment is successful in alleviating symptoms associated with activities of daily living. Return to a job requiring heavy and repetitive use of the arm is not uncommon, but certainly is not assured.[6]

POSTERIOR ELBOW PROBLEMS

Triceps Tendinitis

Clinical Picture

Pain over the posterior aspects of the elbow is the hallmark of this diagnosis, which is associated with work activities involving frequent pushing with the arms or lifting over the head. Occasionally it is a secondary condition superimposed over other elbow joint pathology. Physical findings include point tenderness over part of the attachment of the triceps tendon into the olecranon. There may be localized swelling in this area. Pathology usually includes either minor tearing of the triceps tendon or a traumatic inflammatory reaction secondary to irritation at the point of maximal tenderness. Permanent flexion contracture may occur when the symptoms have been present for some period of time, either by an impinging spur formation at the tip of the olecranon or from protective muscular spasm.

Confirmatory Tests

Routine x-rays, particularly the lateral view, often confirm the diagnosis by showing the presence of calcium at the area of maximal tenderness. Without such evidence, however, there are only the physical findings noted above to make the diagnosis.

Treatment

Conservative management by rest with a sling or splint and nonsteroidal anti-inflammatory drugs may be helpful. As symptoms abate, gradual resumption of motion and muscle strengthening exercises are instituted, but must progress slowly in order not to re-exacerbate symptoms. Steroid injections have been used, but may cause further degeneration in the tendon if they are injected directly. Repeated injections are not indicated. Surgery is occasionally used to remove calcium deposits or debridé part of the olecranon if it is blocking full extension, but these procedures are rarely needed and if carried out will probably ensure that the patient cannot return to the former occupation, even with major work environment modifications.

In patient whose x-rays are negative and who have no classical physical findings, the elicitation of inconsistent physical findings again may warn the treating physician of the presence of operant conditioning. Tenderness over other parts of the olecranon or humerus and increased posterior discomfort on full extension of the elbow without any mechanical block to full extension are examples of these inconsistencies.

Prognosis

In general, this diagnosis is usually readily apparent, treatment is successful, and return to work activities of the sort that aggravated the condition is usually possible, probably because alternative methods of pushing are available. However, small, symptomatic, unrecognized partial tears of the triceps tendon may lead, with further unmodified work, to complete rupture.

Triceps Tendon Rupture

Clinical Picture

As noted above, at times complete rupture follows one or more episodes of "tendinitis," which actually were small partial tears in the triceps tendon. The rupture occurs as an acute injury, located at the attachment of the triceps tendon to the olecranon or just proximal to it. It also can occur as an avulsion fracture with the tendon taking a piece of the olecranon with it. The rupture may be undisplaced, in which case the medial and lateral triceps expansions are intact, or it may be displaced, in which case these expansions are torn.

Physical examination reveals weak or absent extension of the elbow against gravity and tenderness, ecchymosis, and swelling occur over the tip of the olecranon and distal triceps. Often a palpable gap in the continuity between the triceps muscle and olecranon is noted.

Confirmatory Tests
Although one would think that the diagnosis would be simple in a complete tendon rupture, the patient often is relatively comfortable with the elbow in extension or even in 60° of flexion and may not seek immediate medical attention. When the patient does seek care, one must remember the possibility of this diagnosis, with careful examination of the back of the elbow for the above physical findings.

X-rays are only valuable if there is an avulsion fracture of the olecranon. Rarely an MRI may reveal the defect, but in most cases it should be apparent by careful physical examination.

Treatment
Partial tears may be misdiagnosed as tendinitis, but little is lost since treatment is the same. Complete but undisplaced triceps tendon ruptures are treated with splint immobilization for a period of 4 to 6 weeks, followed by gradual development of range of motion and muscle strengthening exercises, with an expected total recovery time of 3 months. Complete and displaced triceps tendon ruptures requires surgical intervention that repairs both the medial and lateral

triceps expansions, as well as the major tendon rupture itself (Fig. 13-4).

Prognosis
Full recovery may be expected, although it may take several months and there is commonly a mild decrease in flexion of the elbow, as well as a permanent flexion contracture. Triceps tendon ruptures usually are not difficult to diagnose if one does a careful physical examination; the treatment is usually successful. One can expect a return to similar work activities unless there is an unusually continuous need for full forceful triceps function or completely full elbow range of motion.

Olecranon-Trochlear Arthritis

Clinical Picture
Symptoms related to this compartment of the elbow are seldom isolated and are commonly combined with those of radiocapitellar arthritis. An exception is post-traumatic arthritis secondary to malunions of olecranon fractures. There is usually a permanent flexion contracture and, in later cases, a decrease also in flexion. There may be some chondromalacia, swelling of the joint, and locking in the presence of loose bodies. If the changes are early, only thinning, fraying, and splitting of the articular cartilage are present, and x-rays are negative. Symptoms include pain in the posterior and medial aspect of the elbow that is accentuated by motion. Crepitation is present only after arthritic changes are fairly well developed.

Confirmatory Tests
Plain x-rays usually show joint space narrowing and periarticular lipping, but earlier cartilaginous changes are not visible by x-ray. Arthroscopy can be considered

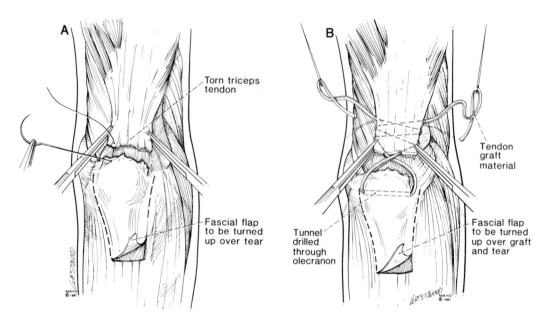

Fig. 13-4. Surgery of triceps avulsion repair. **(A)** The ruptured triceps is shown being reattached to the olecranon. In addition, a flap of fascia and periosteum hinged proximally is being developed from the posterior olecranon. **(B)** A bone tunnel through the olecranon with a plantaris tendon graft passed through the tunnel. The triceps tendon has been augmented by the criss-cross plantaris tendon graft, and over this graft the periosteal flap will be turned and sutured. (From Evarts,[22] with permission.)

as a diagnostic tool, but is more effective in visualizing loose bodies than articular damage in this compartment because of anatomic constrictions.

Treatment

Nonspecific measures, such as rest and nonsteroidal anti-inflammatory medications, are usually helpful. After symptoms abate, general exercises to redevelop motion and muscle strength, as well as specific work hardening routines, often are quite successful in improving function.

Rarely arthroscopy can be used to debride the joint and remove loose bodies. In some cases where the posttraumatic arthritis is secondary to an olecranon fracture malunion, excision of the olecranon may be considered. Surgery in these cases is not done until the process is advanced, and it is extremely unlikely that after surgery the patient will be able to return to any work activity that requires full use of the elbow even if the work environment does not include heavy or repeated flexion and extension activities.

Prognosis

For the most part, this diagnosis is not difficult, and treatment methods are well established and usually successful. Return to full work activities requiring normal function of the elbow, however, is unlikely, and if work activities require maximum elbow function, then vocational rehabilitation and job modification will be necessary regardless of the type or success of treatment.

Non-union/Malunion Fracture of Olecranon

Clinical Picture

Both non-union and malunion affect the narrow space tolerances of the trochlear-olecranon relationship, and thus early symptomatic posttraumatic arthritis is common. Range of motion tends to be diminished, and in cases of nonunion, there may be tenderness over the subcutaneous surface of the olecranon. A permanent flexion contracture is commonly present, with flexion somewhat limited, but pronation and supination are usually unaffected. Normal function of the elbow is unusual so symptoms are increased with work activities that require only moderate activity stresses.

Confirmatory Tests

Plain x-rays always give the diagnosis of a non- or malunion and, in conjunction with the physical examination, should enable a clear diagnosis.

Treatment

Since there is pathology in the elbow before the onset of work-related symptoms, the usual conservative measures may improve those acute or subacute symptoms, but do not restore the elbow to normal. If these measures relieve work symptomatology, then only job modification will be needed. If they do not, however, then surgical intervention is possible through either (1) a bone grafting procedure for the non-union or (2) excision of the olecranon with reattachment of the triceps tendon to the remaining olecranon in cases of malunions or nonunions.

Prognosis

These patients usually do not present difficulty in diagnosis, and therapy almost always improves symptoms. However, since a normal joint cannot be achieved, a job change is usually indicated. Modifying the work environment but keeping the same job is less successful.

Olecranon Bursitis

Clinical Picture

The olecranon bursa that is most commonly inflamed lies between the subcutaneous tissue and the olecranon. Although inflammation can occur spontaneously, it is usually associated with single or multiple direct trauma. It is usually related to a job injury, rather than an activity, unless the job requires constant leaning on the elbows against a hard surface. The diagnosis is simple, as the condition creates a large swelling over the subcutaneous surface of the olecranon; the swelling is usually only mildly discomforting. If the injury involves a break in the skin, the bursitis may possibly become septic, in which case there is considerably more pain and inflammatory reaction. Olecranon bursitis does not affect the triceps mechanisms or the elbow joint itself, so examination of these structures is negative.

Confirmatory Tests

No confirmatory tests are necessary to make the diagnosis as it is obvious on physical examination, and the history will inform the examiner whether the changes are acute or chronic. The only diagnostic question is whether there is sepsis. Aspiration of bursal fluid for culture establishes the presence of sepsis.

Treatment

Aspiration as a treatment maneuver, has limited success as there is a considerable incidence of recurrence. Often, aspiration is carried out once, with application of a pressure dressing and immobilization of the elbow in acute flexion to decrease the dead space. The major indication for this procedure is discomfort.

If the condition persists or recurs frequently, surgical excision may be carried out. This is usually successful, although there is some discomfort over the area for many months when leaning that elbow on a hard surface.

Prognosis

Prognosis for return to work is good, since the only work environment modification needed is to prevent chronic trauma to this area caused by leaning on hard surfaces. Padded surfaces or wearing pads over the elbows at work can prevent chronic trauma may be facilitated by the use of doughnut-shaped pads over the area to minimize pressure on the area of the bursa even when leaning on hard surfaces.

This condition does not pose a diagnostic problem, and therapy is successful although the recovery time is somewhat longer than one would expect for a condition that is apparently so minor. Return to full function with minimal if any work environment modification is typical.

MEDIAL ELBOW PROBLEMS

Medial Epicondylitis

Clinical Picture

Medial humeral epicondylitis has many of the same features as lateral epicondylitis, but is less common. Anatomically the joint-ligament-tendon relationship is less complicated than on the lateral side because of the absence of the radial head. Physical examination reveals tenderness directly over the medial epicondyle or medial collateral ligament. Pain may be accentuated by resisted flexion of fingers and wrist, although this is not as predictable a physical sign as on the lateral side. Because the ulnar nerve lies immediately posterior as it courses the cubital canal, there can be some confusion between medial epicondylitis and the cubital canal syndrome (Fig. 13-5). Point tenderness over the medial epicondyle or ulnar collateral ligament of the joint line and not distally, lack of tenderness over the ulnar nerve or soft tissues distal to the medial epicondyle, and absence of any subluxation of the ulnar nerve on flexion and

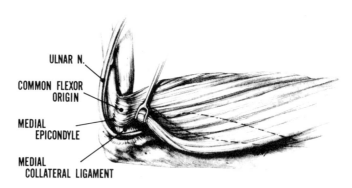

ULNAR N.

COMMON FLEXOR ORIGIN

MEDIAL EPICONDYLE

MEDIAL COLLATERAL LIGAMENT

Fig. 13-5. Note the close proximity of the anatomic features of the medial aspect of the elbow and the diagnostic importance of differentiating tenderness over the medial epicondyle from the cubital canal. (From Green,[21] with permission.)

extension of the elbow should establish the diagnosis.

Confirmatory Tests
As on the lateral side, x-rays may reveal calcification within the ulnar collateral ligament or at its attachment to the medial condyle, in which case the diagnosis of medial epicondylitis is greatly supported. As there is no other confirmatory test for medial epicondylitis, one must depend on testing for the cubital canal syndrome being negative to support further the diagnosis of medial epicondylitis.

Treatment
Conservative measures are the same as for lateral epicondylitis: rest with a sling or splint, nonsteroidal anti-inflammatory medication, physical therapy modalities, such as ultrasound, and occasional steroid injections into the area of maximal tenderness but not into the joint. As symptoms abate, range of motion exercises with stretching to decrease any permanent flexion contracture and work hardening exercises to strengthen the finger and wrist flexors are of help.

Surgical intervention to release muscular attachments or remove calcium is done very rarely, much less frequently than on the lateral side. When x-rays are negative, the physical findings not definite, and the symptoms chronic, testing for inconsistency in physical findings may help the examiner establish whether operant conditioning is increasing symptoms. These findings include tenderness over the olecranon or the medial humeral ridge proximal to the medial condyle, increased discomfort caused by forced *extension* of fingers and wrist, and sensory changes without any indications of a nerve entrapment syndrome.

Prognosis
The diagnosis may be difficult to establish and treatment may be less than successful, since this diagnosis commonly occurs with cumulative trauma. It is unlikely that the patient will be able to return to the job that caused or aggravated this condition, even if symptoms have abated, without either job or work place modifications.

Ulnar Nerve Entrapment: Cubital Canal Syndrome

Clinical Picture
Ulnar nerve entrapments at the medial epicondyle are the second most common nerve entrapment in the upper extremity. The ulnar nerve can be entrapped at the intermuscular septum proximal to the elbow or at the cubital canal directly or as it passes between the two heads of the flexor carpi ulnaris just distal to the elbow. The presentation can vary from complaints of weakness in the hand, numbness and/or dysesthesia in the ulnar nerve distribution, or just pain along the medial aspect of the elbow. The onset is usually gradual and spontaneous. As in so many other work-related disorders, its cause may be repetitive motions or heavy lifting. However, because the canal narrows in flexion, the disorder may be seen only when prolonged elbow flexion is necessary even in workers who do not do repetitive motions.

Findings on examination can vary. There may be tenderness along the course of the nerve at the elbow, which is often associated with a positive Tinel's sign radiating into the ulnar nerve distribution; decreased sensibility to light touch or two-point discrimination; and weakness in the small muscles of the hand and the flexor digitorum profundus to the small and ring fingers. On occasion, as the elbow is flexed, the nerve subluxes anteriorly. Ulnar palsy findings, such as wasting in the hypothenar muscles, inability to cross the index and middle fingers, and a positive Froment's and Jeaune sign, may be present (Fig. 13-6). A provocative test may be used to elicit symptoms by keeping the elbow at maximum flexion; the wrist must be kept in neutral to avoid a false positive result if there is also ulnar nerve entrapment at the wrist (Guyon's canal syndrome).

Confirmatory Tests
EMG is often, although not always, positive; positive results can be increased with near nerve conduction studies. Semmes-Weinstein monofilament testing may define ulnar nerve hypesthesias.

Treatment
Unfortunately, there is limited nonoperative treatment for cubital canal syndrome. Often, if the symptoms are mild and pain is not a large part of the picture, behavioral modification is sufficient. The worker who works with the elbows flexed at 90° or more for a prolonged period of time should either be given a workbreak to extend the elbows or modification of the job so the elbows do not have to be as flexed. If patients are symptomatic at night, again behavioral modification is of help. The cubital canal syndrome is often seen in people who sleep prone and flex their arm to support their chest; sleeping with a pillow under their chest helps prevent this condition. A splint in 30° of flexion can also be used intermittently, but is tolerated poorly. Injections and/or NSAIDs are of little help.

If symptoms persist, surgery may be indicated. However, although approximately 80 percent of patients obtain relief from surgery, they may not return to their original job. With mild symptoms and no significant weakness, especially in the older worker, a period of rest and then work hardening is preferable to surgery. If patients fail to improve, then job modification is probably best. If there is significant weakness or pain, surgery is indicated.

Prognosis
The prognosis is variable and unpredictable. Using the guidelines mentioned under treatment, it is reasonable to expect the worker to return to the original job if symptoms are mild. If, however, a return to work exacerbates old symptoms, whether surgery was performed or not, job modification is the best choice.

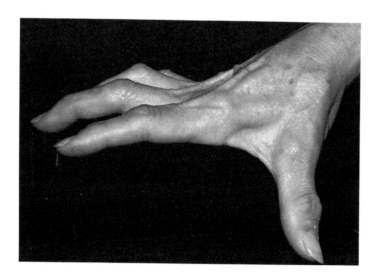

Fig. 13-6. Ulnar palsy findings in cubital canal syndrome. (from Dawson et al.,[23] with permission.)

Medial Compartment Arthritis

Since arthritis of the medial compartment is identical to olecranon-trochlear arthritis, the clinical picture, confirmatory tests, treatment, and prognosis are the same as those described above under that section.

Non-Union/Malunion Fracture of Medial Epicondyle

The clinical picture, confirmatory tests, treatment, and prognosis for these complications of pre-existing fractures of the medial epicondyle are the same as for those on the lateral side of the elbow except for the location (Fig. 13-7). Because of the proximity of the ulnar nerve, there is more likelihood of an associated chronic ulnar nerve entrapment syndrome.[13] The treatment of the ulnar nerve entrapment takes precedence over treatment of the epicondylar non-union or malunion, at least initially. After the entrapment is treated, if symptoms persist, then therapeutic measures noted for non-union and malunion in the lateral epicondyle can be adopted.

ANTERIOR ELBOW PROBLEMS

Distal Biceps Tendon Ruptures

Clinical Picture

Ruptures of the distal end of the biceps occur as a sudden injury with maximum contraction of the biceps. There is discomfort in the anterior elbow, nonspecific physical findings, and negative x-rays, so the acute diagnosis is often missed. Elbow flexion strength remains because of brachialis function but supination is significantly weaker. There is loss of prominence of the biceps tendon and tenderness over the anterior elbow to deep pressure.

Because of the unusual anatomic prominence of the bicipital tuberosity, there may be fraying of the biceps tendon on pronation and supination, with rupture occurring with less than a maximal flexion/supination effort. This condition may be confused with median nerve entrapment syndromes, but there should be no positive Tinel sign nor any sensory or motor changes.

Confirmatory Tests

There are no good confirmatory tests, although an MRI occasionally may be helpful in localizing pathology to the area of the biceps tendon and bicipital tuberosity. Rarely there may be an avulsion of the bicipital tuberosity with this injury that, of course, is visible on plain x-rays.

Treatment

Conservative treatment consisting of immobilization of the elbow in flexion for a period of 4 to 6 weeks allows healing, although flexion and supination strength is permanently weakened and the muscle will have an abnormal shape. In the younger worker, operative repair has also yielded good results. Even late repairs requiring a tendon graft have been worthwhile. The surgery is extensive and the rehabilitation lengthy, up to 6 to 12 months, but one can expect the worker to return to the original employment, including heavy work.

Prognosis

In this condition the diagnosis can be somewhat elusive, and careful physical examination is important. Treatment is also difficult and not uniformly success-

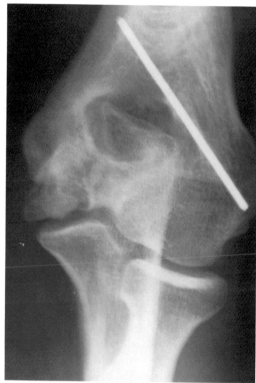

Fig. 13-7. Ulnar nerve entrapment after remote elbow fracture. Epicondylectomy and cubital tunnel release are planned since it is unlikely with prior trauma that cubital tunnel release alone will be sufficient. **(A)** Note the deformity of the medial condyle of humerus after remote fracture. Retained Kirschner wire from original surgical intervention. **(B)** Cubital tunnel is released, demonstrating compressed ulnar nerve (*arrow*). (*Figure continues.*)

A

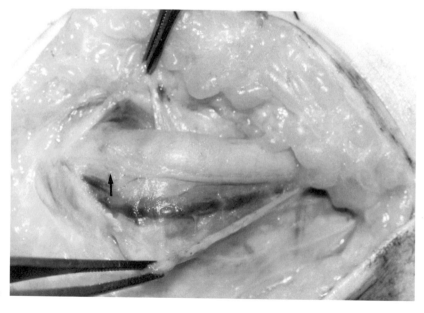

B

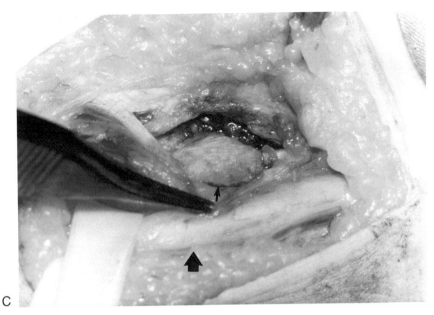

C

Fig. 13-7 (*Continued*). (**C**) Medial epicondyle exposed before epicondylectomy. Note the small medial epicondyle (*arrow*) similar to that seen on x-ray. Ulnar nerve is retracted (*large arrow*). (From Dawson et al.,[23] with permission.)

ful. Since the injury occurs after extremely heavy lifting, either work environment changes to negate the need for this activity will be needed for the patient to return to the original job or the worker will need to change jobs to avoid intensive flexion-supination elbow function.

Pronator Syndrome: Anterior Interosseous Nerve Syndrome, Pronator Teres Syndrome

Clinical Picture

As with radial nerve entrapments, median nerve entrapments in the forearm are rare. The median nerve courses under the ligament of Struthers at the distal humerus and then anteriorly and distally. The nerve passes under the lacertus fi-brosis and the arcade constituting the origin of the flexor digitorum superficialis to the middle finger and then divides into the main branch and anterior interosseous branch, which passes under the pronator teres. Entrapment can occur at any one of those areas, although the pronator teres is the most common site. Entrapment proximal to the elbow by the ligament of Struthers is least common and usually occurs only if a supracondylar process is present; this can be defined on x-ray.[14,15] Distally, as with the radial nerve, the findings depend upon which portion of the nerve is compromised most significantly. If the entrapment involves the anterior interosseous nerve predominantly, the patient may complain of pain in the anteromedial forearm, usually about 7 cm distal to the elbow, but most often complains of weakness in the hand.[12,16–18] This disorder is seen more

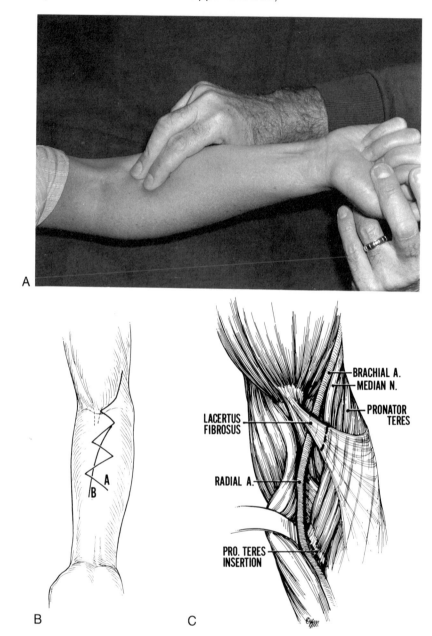

Fig. 13-8. (**A**) In patients with a pronator teres or anterior interosseous nerve syndrome, there is tenderness of the median nerve at the site of entrapment. This is beneath the tendon of the pronator or origin of the middle finger superficialis. A positive Tinel's sign may also be present. (**B**) Surgical approach to the median nerve in the forearm. (**C**) The lacertus fibrosus and/or deep head of the pronator teres can be the site of entrapment. (*Figure continues.*)

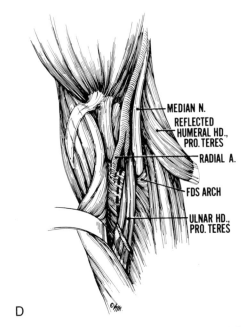

D

Fig. 13-8 *(Continued)*. **(D)** The origin of the flexor digitorum superficialis to the middle finger can also be the site of entrapment. Here it is shown after the other two structures have been released. (From Green,[21] with permission.)

commonly in the younger, more muscular patient, especially if the job involves heavy lifting. Examination may disclose tenderness in the forearm, a positive Tinel's sign at the site of entrapment, and weakness of the pronator quadratus, the flexor pollicis longus, and/or flexor digitorum profundus to the index finger (Fig. 13-8). On occasion there is total paralysis of all of these muscles; the patient is unable to make an "O" by pinching the thumb and index as the interphalangeal joint of the thumb and the distal interphalangeal joint of the index collapse into hyperextension (Fig. 13-9). Pronator quadratus function can be tested by resisting attempted forearm pronation, starting from a position of full supination, with the elbow in about 100° of flexion to eliminate the pronator teres. Although

there can be sensory changes, the anterior interosseous nerve syndrome is classically a motor disorder. Interestingly, clinical studies have disclosed that the nerve is usually entrapped at the pronator teres.[18]

The pronator teres syndrome, like the radial tunnel, is mostly a syndrome of pain.[19,20] However, it is seen in older patients with less muscular activity. Patients complain of pain in the forearm in the area noted in the anterior interosseous nerve syndrome above. Clinically, the picture is very similar, except there are minimal motor changes in the hand and more sensory changes. Patients may complain of numbness and tingling in their hand, and there may be demonstrable decreases in sensibility not only in the median nerve distribution of the hand but also in the palmar cutaneous nerve distribution over the thenar eminence. Provocative tests may help make the diagnosis. In addition to the positive Tinel's sign from percussion over the nerve, which is probably the most reliable test, there may be a positive Tinel's sign and increased pain with antagonism of either pronator teres function or middle finger flexor digitorum superficialis (FDS) function. Pronator teres function is assessed by having the elbow in extension and forearm in supination and then asking the patient to pronate while the examiner resists the maneuver. Middle finger FDS function is assessed by asking the patient to flex the middle finger proximal interphalangeal joint while the examiner resists. At surgery, any of the three sites distal to the elbow lacertus fibrosus, origin of FDS, or the deep head of pronator teres—may cause the entrapment. Both of these clinical pictures may be seen in patients who do multiple repetitive motions and/or heavy lifting. Anterior interosseous nerve syndrome may be seen in weight lifters, suggesting that heavy muscular exercise may be a causative factor.

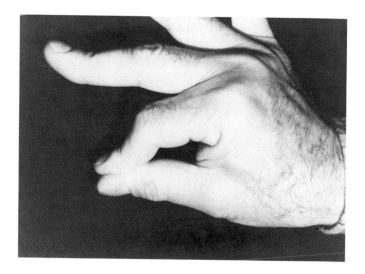

Fig. 13-9. With paralysis caused by the anterior interosseous nerve syndrome, the flexor pollicis longus and index flexor digitorum profundus are weak. As a result, patients are unable to make an "O" by pinching the index finger to the thumb tip. (From Dawson et al.,[21] with permission.)

Confirmatory Tests

X-rays of the elbow may disclose a supracondylar process, implying thickening of the ligament of Struthers. An EMG/NCS should always be obtained. There is a high percentage of accuracy in making the diagnoses of an anterior interosseous nerve syndrome because of the muscular weakness. However, in the pronator teres syndrome, the electrical studies are negative about 80 percent of the time. Still, they should be obtained, not only to confirm the clinical impression but also to rule out a carpal tunnel syndrome, which may sometimes present with a similar picture.

Treatment

Again, as with radial nerve entrapments at the elbow, the prognosis in pronator teres syndrome is guarded, especially in the older unskilled worker whose job involves multiple repetitive motions. If the usual nonoperative treatment of rest, NSAIDs and/or rehabilitation is unsuccessful, then surgery is indicated. This consists of decompression of the nerve from the lacertus fibrosis to the pronator

teres; only if there is a supracondylar process or evidence of proximal entrapment on electrical studies is decompression proximal to the elbow indicated.

In anterior interosseous nerve syndrome, which may recover spontaneously, a period of rest and/or splinting is the first approach. If recovery is not apparent at about 3 months, then surgical decompression is indicated. A repeat EMG/NCS at 6 to 8 weeks helps document clinically subtle recovery. The operative approach is the same as for pronator teres syndrome.

Prognosis

The prognosis is guarded. In the pronator teres syndrome, especially in older unskilled workers, a new job will probably be necessary even if they respond positively to surgery. Work hardening and work stimulation can be tried. In the anterior interosseous nerve syndrome, the prognosis is somewhat better. These patients, whether they respond to nonsurgical or surgical treatment, may well be returned to their old jobs.

REFERENCES

1. Conrad RW, Hooper WR: Tennis elbow: its course, natural history, conservative and surgical management. J Bone Joint Surg 55A:1177, 1973
2. Nirschl RP, Pettrone FA: Tennis elbow: the treatment of lateral epicondylitis. J Bone Joint Surg 61A:832, 1979
3. Friedlander HL, Reid RL, Cape RF: Tennis elbow. Clin Orthop 51:109, 1967
4. Mills GP: The treatment of "tennis elbow." Br Med J 12, January 7 1928
5. Boyd HB, McLeod AC: Tennis elbow. J Bone Joint Surg 55a:1183, 1973
6. Schultz-Johnson K: Assessment of upper extremity—injured person's return to work potential. J Hand Surg 12A:950, 1987
7. Waddell G, et al: Nonorganic physical signs in low back pain. Spine 5:117, 1980
8. Spinner M: The arcade of Frohse and its relationship to posterior interosseous nerve paralysis. J Bone Joint Surg 50B:809, 1968
9. Capener N: Posterior interosseous nerve lesions. Proceedings of the Second Hand Club. J Bone Joint Surg 46B:770, 1966
10. Roles NC, Maudsley RH: Radial tunnel syndrome. Resistant tennis elbow as a nerve entrapment. J Bone Joint Surg 54B:499, 1972
11. Lister GD, Belsole RB, Kleinert HE: The radial tunnel syndrome. J Hand Surg 4:52, 1979
12. Rosen I, Werner CO: Neurophysiological investigation of posterior interosseous nerve entrapment causing lateral elbow pain. EEG Clin Neurophysiol 50:125, 1980
13. Bernstein SM et al: Fractures of the medial epicondyle of the humerus. Contemp Orthop 3:637, 1981
14. Terry RJ: A study of the supracondyloid process in the lining. Am J Phys Antropol 4:129, 1921
15. Laha RK, Diyovny M, DeCastro C: Entrapment of median nerve by supracondylar process of the humerus. J Neurosurg 46:252, 1977
16. Kiloh LG, Nevin S: Isolated neuritis of the anterior interosseous nerve. Br Med J 1:850, 1952
17. Spinner M: The anterior interosseous nerve syndrome. J Bone Joint Surg 52A:84, 1970
18. Hartz CR, Linscheid RL, Gromse RR, Daube JR: The pronator teres syndrome: compressive neuropathy of the median nerve. J Bone Joint Surg 63a:885, 1981
19. Johnson RK, Spinner M, Shrewsbury MM: Median nerve entrapment syndrome in the proximal forearm. J Hand Surg 4:48, 1979
20. Seyffarth H: Primary myoses in the M. Pronator teres as cause of lesion of the N. medianus (the pronator syndrome). Acta Psychiatr Scand, suppl. 74:251, 1951
21. Green DP (ed): Operative Hand Surgery. 2nd Ed. Churchill Livingstone, New York, 1982
22. Evarts CM (ed): Surgery of the Musculoskeletal System. 2nd Ed. Churchill Livingstone, New York, 1989
23. Dawson D, Hallett M, Millender LH: Entrapment Neuropathies. 2nd Ed. Little, Brown, Boston, 1991

14

Disorders of the Neck and Shoulder in Workers

Robert D. Leffert, M.D.

The problem of defining the complex entity of work-related disorders of the neck and shoulders can be likened to the folk-tale of the group of blind men given the task of describing an elephant. Four of them declare the beast to resemble a broad and leathery tree-trunk, one claim it to be the spitting image of a vacuum cleaner hose, and one, reaching up, proclaim that the creature has all the earmarks of a large sail. So it is that groups of physicians, therapists, researchers, lawyers, and insurance companies have tried to come to grips with the common problem of the worker disabled by complaints of pain in the neck and shoulder. Because of their differing orientations and, in some cases, diverse agendas, each group has tended to focus on one or only a few of the facets of the problem. On the contrary, in an attempt at uniform nomenclature, the excessively comprehensive terms "occupational cervicobrachial disorder" and "repetitive strain injury" have become firmly established in the literature. Although these names are applicable to some cases, they should be understood clearly as not being pertinent and appropriate for all workers with similar symptoms. The neck and shoulder are interrelated in a complex manner such that a disorder of either one can significantly influence the other, and each area has its own unique set of pathologic entities, all of which must be considered in the diagnosis of each worker's symptoms and signs. The fact that the shoulder is the most mobile joint in the body and that it serves as a way station for the nerves and vessels of the upper extremity makes it impossible to group the various diagnostic entities into a neat format wherein complaints are limited to only one anatomic locus. For example, patients with anterior instability of the shoulder may complain of posterior discomfort because of stretch of the ligaments in back of the joint, and rotator cuff tear pain is often felt anterolaterally in the midarm despite the fact that the lesion is actually within the confines of the subacromial space.

Clearly, there are many disorders in this area that can and do occur independently of any industrial exposure or causation, whereas some can be confidently attributed to the work place. Some represent combinations of both causes in varying proportions. From the standpoint of accurate diagnosis and treatment, as well as the fair and equitable disposition of the administrative aspects of these cases, it is the responsibility of the examining physician to obtain as accurate a history as possible so that these issues can be resolved. The history-taking process is discussed further in the next section.

GENERIC DIAGNOSTIC APPROACH TO THE WORKER WITH NECK/SHOULDER PAIN

In an ideal world, the doctor-patient relationship in a compensation case would be conducted on the same unbiased, courteous, and understanding basis as with any other patient. From a practical standpoint, however, the encounter can conceivably be influenced by the fact that the physician's fee is being paid by the employer or insurance company, or the patient has been referred by a plaintiff's lawyer. Nevertheless, every effort must be made to exclude these factors from the deliberations and the ultimate opinion that is rendered.

The History

The onset of symptoms may involve a single traumatic incident, in which case a detailed description of its circumstances is needed to fully understand the mechanism of injury. This detailed description is particularly important with shoulder problems, where the position of the arm at the time of application of the force may greatly clarify the type of injury to be expected. For example, a worker whose arm is twisted in abduction and lat-

eral rotation is likely to have an injury to the anterior capsule and ligaments, whereas one who has a weight fall on an abducted arm and suddenly has it forced to the side is more likely to have sustained an acute injury to the rotator cuff. The height of a fall and the type of surface to which the worker fell are important, as are details of any additional injuries sustained. The initial symptoms and whether there was a delay between the accident and their onset should be noted carefully. In all cases, it is vital to inquire about a history of prior injury or symptoms and if they have changed with the passage of time. All treatments and their result should be assessed both from the patient's history and the available medical records. Occasionally, there is a significant divergence between the two, and this should be noted if present.

In situations in which there is no single episode of trauma but the presumption is that of chronic stress with repeated motions of the upper extremity or neck or perhaps the maintenance of a static or uncomfortable position, the chronic stress should be described. As part of the examination, the worker should be asked to duplicate the position of the body, and particularly the neck and shoulder, assumed during the work activity. Measurements should be made of the degree of elevation and rotation of the arm with reference to the body during this demonstration, and the amount of weight that would be lifted during the maneuver should be ascertained.[1]

If a number of patients are seen from the same plant with the same complaint and the physician is retained by the company, it may be necessary to make an on-site inspection of the work place so that its ergonomics may be determined accurately. Videotapes or movies of the process may be extremely useful in documentation[2,3] so that preventive measures may be instituted.

It is important to know whether the patient works on an assembly line. If so, does the product come from the right or left, does it have to be lifted or handed to the next station or worker, and if so, how much does each unit weigh? How many units or pieces are handled in the course of an hour? If tools are used repeatedly, how much do they weigh, how is the arm positioned during their use, and is significant effort required to complete the required task? All of these questions should be answered when substantiating the relationship between the injury and the work environment.[3]

For workers who do not produce a tangible product of significant size or weight, such as keypunch operators or cashiers, the number of keystrokes per hour and the height of the keyboard or machine with reference to their sitting height are important parts of the history.[4] The hours of work and whether there are breaks in the routine should also be recorded.

Finally, and especially when the worker has been seen by multiple physicians who have produced complex diagnostic evaluations, it is most important to review all of the prior records. This can be a very tedious, but most important part of the evaluation, which can be made considerably easier by having a secretary arrange the material chronologically and eliminate any duplications.

The Physical Examination

Important information relevant to the physical examination may be obtained even before the introduction to the patient if the physician has the opportunity to observe the worker in the waiting-room interacting with office personnel, or other patients. Station and gait, as well as whether the head, neck, and upper limbs are moved normally in conversation or in the course of gesticulating, can be noted for future reference and compared with their status during the course of the formal examination. Within the boundaries of decorum and appropriate modesty, observing how the patient disrobes or adjusts the clothing may clarify further the veracity of some findings that may be difficult to interpret during the course of the examination.

The way in which the patient is dressed for the physical examination of the neck and shoulders is important. The room must be maintained at a comfortable temperature and the patient put at ease, but it is also necessary to be able to observe and palpate all areas under examination directly. A simple gown with ties, open to the back, is used for female patients. They are instructed to disrobe completely above the waist with the exception of the brassiere. The gown may be alternately tied beneath each axillae so that each shoulder girdle may be examined in turn (Fig. 14-1A and 1B).

The examination of the head and neck is included in every evaluation of a patient with a shoulder problem, and specific note is made of the range of motion in the cervical spine, as well as the presence or absence of spasm or tenderness of the paravertebral musculature. The condition of the trapezius muscles is particularly important, and one can obtain valuable information by palpation and assessment of the bulk of these important suspensors of the shoulder girdle.

The foraminal closure test is helpful in the identification of cervical radiculopathies. It is done by laterally flexing and extending the neck so as to narrow the intervertebral foramina on the affected side. If positive, it causes pain or paresthesias in the shoulder or upper extremity. The supraclavicular fossae are palpated for the presence of masses or tenderness, and if there is a question of thoracic outlet compression, the area over

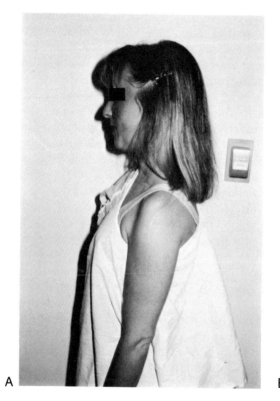
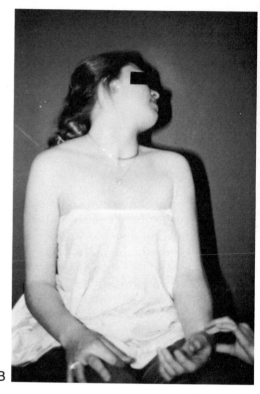

A   B

Fig. 14-1. This gown allows all pertinent areas to be examined. **(A)** This patient has an osteosynthesis of an non-united clavicle and a shoulder fusion for brachial plexus injury. **(B)** Both sides may be examined simultaneously in the Adson's test for thoracic outlet compression.

the subclavian vessels is auscultated with a stethoscope as the arm is placed in the various provocative positions. The presence of a bruit is usually determined just before the radial pulse is extinguished.

In the examination of the shoulder girdle, it is vitally important to remember that this complex is actually composed of three true joints, one functional "joint," and one "space," which is often the site of pathology. The three joints are the acromioclavicular, sternoclavicular, and glenohumeral, each of which must be evaluated separately for range of motion, as well as the presence or absence of instability, inflammation, or tenderness. It is helpful to palpate the overlying and adjacent musculature during this part of the

examination so that the tone of the muscles, particularly the occurrence of spasm concurrently with the subjective complaint of discomfort, can be noted.

The scapulothoracic interval must be assessed in terms of its motion and whether it is painful or accompanied by crepitus. In addition, the position of the scapula with reference to the rib cage and the contralateral scapula is noted both at rest and in bilateral elevation of the arms. By watching as the arms are lowered from an overhead position, this relationship, called scapular rhythm, can be assessed. An asymmetric relationship is usually an indication of pathology.

The subacromial space is the origin of much of the shoulder pain that is observed in patients with industrially re-lated complaints, and although the temp-tation is to ascribe all shoulder pains to "bursitis," in reality, primary subacro-mial bursitis is an unusual entity. If this anatomic locus has been identified cor-rectly, the pathology is usually a result of rotator cuff derangement.[5] Therefore, it is most important to be able to correctly di-agnose the various disorders that origi-nate in this small but important area. Fur-ther discussion of this subject is found in the section devoted to the rotator cuff.

One should not neglect to carefully ex-amine the distal portions of the upper limb and the contralateral one as well, since if they are normal or asymptomatic, they serve as a control with which to in-terpret abnormalities found in the limb under scrutiny. A neurologic examination is an indispensable part of the evaluation. Finally, it must be remembered that the shoulder may be the site of referral of pain that originates elsewhere. The cervical spine and thoracic outlet are two of the more common loci, but cardiac disease, as well as pathology within the abdomen or chest, may also be initially expressed in this manner, much to the consternation of both patient and physician.

Radiographic Studies

The available radiographic techniques for the evaluation of the shoulder are dis-cussed in the context of the various patho-logic entities seen in the industrial set-ting. In addition to the routine studies that can and should be obtained when-ever there is a question whether the cer-vical spine is the origin of pain in this area, the additional techniques of mye-lography and MRI are available.

The chest x-ray is an important part of the evaluation of a patient with pain in the shoulder (Fig. 14-C2).

Electrodiagnostic Studies

Although most patients with cervico-brachial or shoulder pain can be diag-nosed correctly on the basis of a carefully done history and physical examination, there are several situations wherein the diagnosis requires further clarification, which can then be provided by electro-diagnostic techniques. These tests in-clude electromyography, the determina-tion of the velocity of conduction of the peripheral nerves, as well as F responses, and somatosensory evoked potentials. The most obvious application is electro-myographic examination of the muscles to detect evidence of denervation that re-sults from cervical radiculopathy. In ad-dition, proper differentiation of the atro-phy of disuse from that caused by nerve deficit is easily accomplished by these means. Although this examination is an objective one that cannot be influenced by the patient, it must be appreciated that it is subject to the interpretation of the examiner.

Atrophy of the muscles of the rotator cuff is not rare in massive and long-stand-ing tears of the tendon, in which case it represents the atrophy of disuse. How-ever, similar atrophy may result from le-sions of the suprascapular nerve that may occur either independently or occasion-ally with rotator cuff tears. Herein, elec-tromyography is done, and the latency of the suprascapular nerve from Erb's point to the involved muscle is compared with the other side and with normative data. This combination of tests will clarify a dif-ficult diagnostic problem.

It would be very convenient if the di-agnosis of thoracic outlet syndrome could be absolutely confirmed by electrodi-agnostic techniques. Unfortunately, this is not the case, as has been suggested by Wilbourn and Lederman[6] and personally confirmed by other workers, including the author.

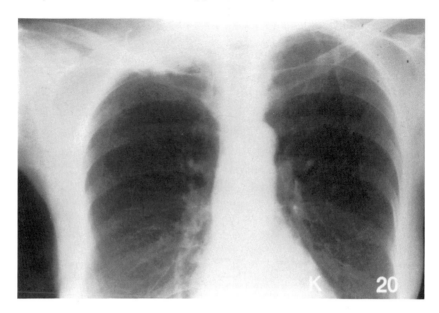

Fig. 14-2. This 41-year-old woman who smoked 20 cigarettes per day had severe pain in the right shoulder and was referred for consideration of decompression of her thoracic outlet. After this chest radiograph, her diagnosis of apical lung cancer required resection of the upper lobe of the lung and four ribs.

OCCUPATIONAL CERVICOBRACHIAL DISORDER

All patients should be subjected to the identical evaluation process in order to assess their complaints fully and to avoid missing important diagnostic information. The specific conditions that are most commonly seen in the industrially related situation are detailed in this section. Some of them are more common than others, and they are discussed in the order of frequency in which, in my experience, they are observed. However, depending on the locale and nature of a physician's practice, there may be wide variations in the types of patients seen. For example, a practice in proximity to a shipyard where many welders are employed will have a high percentage of patients with rotator cuff derangements,[7,8] whereas one located in an area with a large population of office workers, cashiers, and keypunchers, will see complaints of neck discomfort more often.[4]

The term "occupational cervicobrachial disorder" is used to describe symptoms of pain in the neck, paracervical musculature, and shoulders in workers who are doing either repetitive motions of the shoulders and arms or who must maintain a constant position of the neck and shoulders while performing stereotyped tasks with the wrists and hands. It is a most unfortunate and imprecise term that will survive on the basis of a large amount of literature that has mostly come from Japan (where the term originated)[9] and Australia, where it is known as repetitive strain injury (RSI).[10] The problem with the use of these terms is significant, since there are no specific anatomic or pathologic criteria for diagnosis other than symptoms of discomfort in the general location of the neck and shoulders, with occasional radiation of the pain into the upper extremities. Because of this lack of diagnostic precision, it is virtually impossible to compare various affected groups of workers described in the literature with any confidence, although attempts have been made to relate them according to type of work[11] or morphologic characteristics.[12] In addition, the organic nature of the diagnosis is called into serious question by the epidemic growth of RSI in Australia where it increased 30-fold within the span of 2 to 3 years.[13] Although some studies have attempted to establish the possible pathophysiologic mechanism of mechanical stress on the neck and shoulders,[14,15] this is difficult to accomplish; it is more easily documented for the shoulders.[7,8]

The question that one must ask then is whether there is any value at all in the use of the term "occupational cervicobrachial disorder." If not, how does one classify those patients with pain in the neck and shoulders associated with sitting at a computer terminal or typewriter, or workers, such as cashiers, who have a high incidence of these complaints? I believe that there is a genuine need to be able to diagnose and treat these patients, since their symptoms constitute a significant problem for industry and for themselves, so this would be a useful term if sufficiently restricted in its application. It has been established that habitual use of the arms above shoulder height, even for the performance of light repetitive tasks, can produce chronic neck and shoulder pain that can be relieved by lowering the arms[15] and by the institution of periodic rest periods.[16] For the worker typing at a desk, the simple measure of adjusting the height of the seat with reference to the keyboard can be beneficial (Fig. 14-3). At the same time, information gained from ergonomic studies should be applied to refine diagnosis, prevention, and treatment.[3]

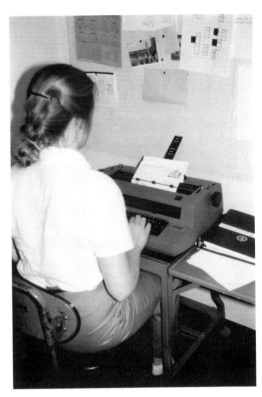

Fig. 14-3. This typist is positioned so there is minimal strain on the shoulder musculature. Work stations should be designed to minimize such strain.

Confirmatory Tests

Because of the sometimes vague nature of the complaints voiced by workers suffering from the effects of chronic strain of the suspensory muscles of the shoulder girdles and the neck musculature, it would be extremely desirable to have an objective test that would confirm what for the moment is a clinical diagnosis. Unfortunately, such a test does not exist. However, the clinical picture of muscle spasm and "trigger points," atrophy and weakness in the trapezius muscle, and tenderness at the insertion of the levator scapulae should be considered good presumptive evidence of the disorder. In addition to these findings, it has also been noted that symptomatic workers tend to have weaker shoulder and neck musculature than workers without these problems.[3]

Treatment

The symptoms of chronic muscle strain about the neck and shoulders are easier to prevent than to treat for many workers. Notwithstanding the psychosocial epidemics of this problem,[10] the physician who treats workers from assembly lines, shops, and offices must deal with patients suffering from the effects of chronic contraction of their neck and shoulder muscles due to maintaining postures at their work stations. In addition to altering the ergonomics of the job, which may or may not be practical or possible, some simple measures can be helpful. Periodic work breaks, during which the worker gets up, moves about, exercises, and stretches, can reduce the tonic contractions. General bodily conditioning and recreational exercise are also useful, particularly for those who are sedentary by nature. Strengthening and postural exercises can be done as a home program after proper instruction by a knowledgeable physical therapist. Oral nonsteroidal, anti-inflammatory agents, local heat and massage, and occasional injections of trigger points with local anesthetics and steroids are useful. The commitment of the patient to long courses of formal physical therapy with repeated application of various types of superficial and deep heat should be avoided. Occasionally, in very severe cases, a worker may have to be off work for weeks or months, but I have seen patients who had been away from the job for as long as a year with no reduction in the level of subjective complaints. These patients have invariably had minimal physical findings.

Prognosis

The prognosis for recovery from occupational cervicobrachial disorder is extremely difficult to predict, although, as one could expect, the more severe the degree of impairment, the longer it is likely to persist.[4]

In my opinion, it is important to restrict the use of the term "occupational cervicobrachial disorder" to these conditions of muscular stress as described above and to eliminate from this designation other such entities as thoracic outlet syndrome[11] and pathologic conditions of the glenohumeral joint and subacromial space for which specific medical or surgical modes of therapy exist. These are discussed below.

ROTATOR CUFF DERANGEMENTS

In 1934 E. A. Codman wrote, "Complete rupture of the supraspinatus is the most common cause of prolonged disability from industrial accidents to the shoulder. . . . The incomplete form accounts for the majority of shoulder disabilities."[15] It was Codman who first brought the pathology of the rotator cuff of the worker to the attention of both the medical profession and the workers' compensation authorities. His statement came as a result of 30 years of careful observations on hundreds of shoulders and was the groundwork upon which our understanding of this most important problem is based. His analyses have been reiterated and reproduced by others, but the basic problem of the effect of strain on the rotator cuff of the worker who must maintain the arms in an abducted or flexed position or must repeatedly raise and lower them remains. Much work has been done in this area.[1,3,7,8,14,17]

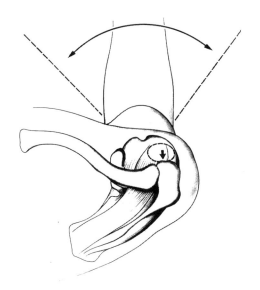

Fig. 14-4. Functional range of the shoulder and how it can cause wear of the supraspinatus by impingement of the anterior acromion or acromioclavicular joint. (From Neer,[19] with permission.)

Despite considerable attention to the problem, controversy still exists over the etiology of the derangements of the rotator cuff. Neer[19] has written extensively on the phenomenon of the impingement syndrome, a mechanical explanation of the interaction of the anterior acromion and the underlying cuff that glides beneath it as the arm is raised. Neer makes the point that most activities of daily living are done with the arms forward flexed, which can bring the supraspinatus area of cuff insertion into contact with the anterior edge of the acromion (Fig. 14-4). If there is excessive overhead use of the arms, edema and hemorrhage in the cuff (Stage I) will result in even further impingement. As this sequence is repeated, the cuff and the subacromial bursa become thickened and scarred (Stage II). Finally, due to continued impingement, the cuff tears (Stage III). Neer raises the questions of why many heavy laborers do not get cuff tears and why many tears occur in people who do not do heavy work. He suggests that the shape of the anterior acromion is a determinant of the susceptibility to cuff tear and uses this as the rationale for anterior acromioplasty. The reader is reminded that the type of cuff tear under consideration here is a wholly different entity from the one that occurs in young athletes as a result of severe trauma. In those situations, the tissues of the cuff are essentially normal before the application of forces greater than they can resist.

The vascular anatomy of the rotator cuff has also been proposed as a reason for the pathology of cuff tear and the poor healing once rupture has occurred.[5,20,21] This concept has also been considered by Herberts and his co-workers,[7,8] within the context of the dynamic use of the arms in industry. They studied shipyard workers for rotator cuff tears and found an 18.3 percent incidence in welders and a 16.2 percent incidence in steelplate workers. Their biomechanical studies confirmed the fact that the shoulder muscles, particularly the supra- and infraspinatus, are heavily loaded when the arms are elevated. Since welding often requires that the arms be maintained in this position for long periods of time, this tonic contraction would result in high intramuscular pressures that, in turn, accentuate the hypovascularity of the supraspinatus tendon and contribute to its fibrosis and ultimate failure (Fig. 14-5).

In my opinion, the two explanations for cuff tears are mutually complimentary, rather than being contradictory. In addition, one must not consider the subacromial space as being independent of the scapula and its position with reference to the ribcage as determined by the suspensory musculature. If, for example, the trapezius is fatigued or otherwise weakened, then the normal mechanics are disturbed so that the scapula tends to be displaced laterally and anteriorly. This

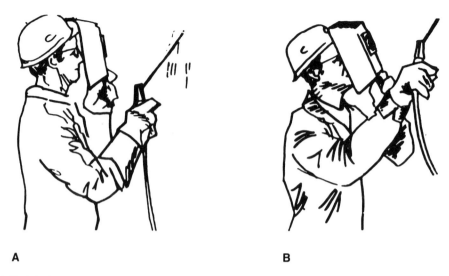

A   B

Fig. 14-5. Working postures investigated in a muscle fatigue study. (**A**) In shoulder level work there was no evidence of fatigue. (**B**) In overhead work there was significant fatigue in the deltoid, supraspinatus, and trapezius muscles of inexperienced welders and in the supraspinatus muscle of both experienced and elderly welders with shoulder pain. (From Herberts,[8] with permission.)

brings the anterior edge of the acromion closer to the underlying cuff where impingement can occur.

Clinical Picture

The clinical presentation of the worker with a rotator cuff problem depends on the stage of the pathology, although in all cases there is pain as the arm is elevated or abducted. Pain may be in the subacromial area or is often felt as a vague ache in the upper lateral arm at the level of the deltoid tuberosity. The discomfort on examination is usually present in only part of the arc of range of motion. With the arm at the side, there is little pain, but as the arm is brought to the horizontal and then medially rotated, pain occurs. As the horizontal plane is passed, the pain dimin-

ishes. Neer's "impingement sign" is elicited by forced upward elevation of the humerus against the acromion and is confirmed by injection of local anesthetic beneath the acromion, which abolishes the pain if it is due to impingement.[19]

There is a variable amount of crepitus, and again, depending on whether there is a complete tear, there is weakness. It tends to be "mid-range" in character as well, but in some patients it is not only present in attempted abduction and forward flexion, but if the infraspinatus is torn, also in attempted lateral rotation (Fig. 14-6). In a massive tear, the patient may not be able to raise the arm at all.

Most patients with rotator cuff tears do not have significant stiffness, although some do, and particularly in long-standing, large tears, there is atrophy of the muscles in the supraspinous and infraspinous fossae. This can raise the diagnostic possibility of a suprascapular nerve lesion, which admittedly is much less

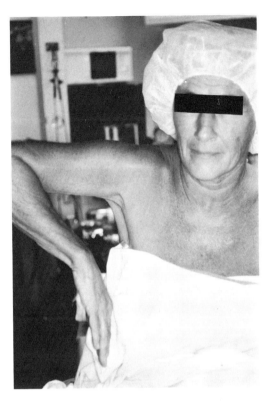

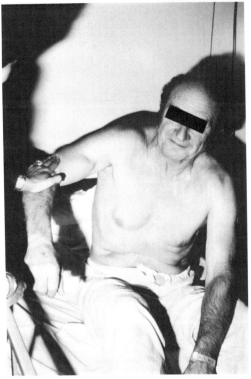

Fig. 14-6. This patient with a rotator cuff tear could not prevent her arm from medially rotating when she abducted it because of weakness of the infraspinatus muscle.

Fig. 14-7. This patient presented with a rupture of the long head of the biceps. He also has mid-range weakness of abduction and an arthrogram that demonstrates a rotator cuff tear.

common but can occur, either separately or in combination with a tear.

Finally, in some patients with a rotator cuff tear, the first indication of pathology is the spontaneous rupture of the long head of the biceps.[22] This rupture should not be viewed as an isolated phenomenon, but is usually a result of impingement (Fig. 14-7). Further discussion of this problem is found in the next section.

Confirmatory Tests

Standard radiographs of the shoulder are obtained in the anteroposterior view, both in internal and external rotation; an axillary view is obtained as well. The findings obviously depend on the extent and duration of the lesion of the cuff. Some patients have normal radiographs. As the degree of pathology increases, one observes cyst formation at the level of the greater tuberosity or flattening and sclerosis of that structure. With larger, complete tears, there is cephalic migration of the humeral head with reference to the glenoid and acromion. The humeroacromial distance is then usually less than 7 mm.[23] As the process continues, there is demonstrable articulation of the head with the underside of the acromion, resulting in the development of a "pseudojoint." This situation represents a very large and chronic tear (Fig. 14-8).

The most reliable means of demonstrating a complete tear of the rotator cuff is contrast arthrography (Fig. 14-9), although it is an invasive and occasionally painful procedure. It may also be combined with CT scanning for additional information. Although arthrography has been considered the "gold standard" for diagnosis of rotator cuff tears,[19] there has been considerable interest recently in the use of noninvasive techniques, particularly ultrasound and MRI.[24–27] Correct interpretation of an ultrasonographic examination of the shoulder requires a dedicated and experienced radiologist who is especially interested in the procedure;

such clinicians are not generally available. However, in some institutions, such radiologists have made it possible to rely on the test primarily.[25]

MRI has the appeal of being noninvasive, and experience is being gained with it, which improves its accuracy, but for the differentiation of tendinitis from a partial tear, it is still not sufficiently reliable.[24] It has the further problem of being considerably more expensive than either ultrasound or arthrography. The use of arthroscopy in the routine diagnostic evaluation of a rotator cuff tear is to be condemned as unnecessarily invasive, expensive, and unproven in its efficacy.

For those occasional patients who present with the differential diagnosis of atro-

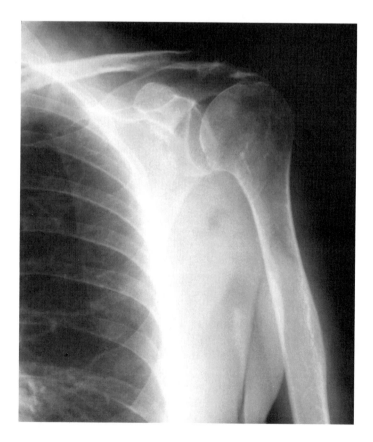

Fig. 14-8. Plane radiographs of a patient with a large rotator cuff tear. The space normally occupied by the rotator cuff is virtually gone.

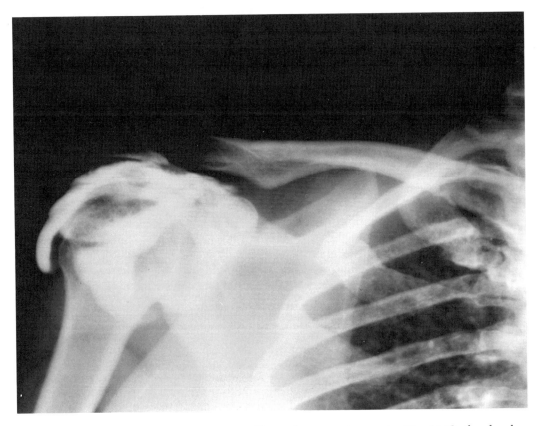

Fig. 14-9. In this patient with a rotator cuff tear (same patient as in Fig. 14-7), the dye has leaked through the rent in the cuff and filled the subacromial bursa.

phy of the supra- and infraspinatus muscles, the possibility of suprascapular nerve lesion can be eliminated by means of electromyography.

Treatment

The treatment of Stage I impingement is conservative. If it is possible to modify any job-related shoulder motions that might be contributing to the continuing impingement and irritation of the rotator cuff, this should be done; if not, it may be necessary to take the worker off the job altogether until the lesion heals. The judicious use of nonsteroidal anti-inflammatory agents can be of benefit, but to prescribe them on a long-term basis is unjustified, as is the use of multiple intrabursal injections of cortisone and local anesthetic.

The differentiation of Stage II impingement from a tear of the cuff is clarified by the above diagnostic maneuvers, but some patients do not appear to have complete tears and yet continue to be disabled by their symptoms of pain whenever they do anything but light activities or use their arms overhead. These workers sometimes have partial tears that can be very symptomatic, and ultimately they are not able to function. If they have had 6 months of conservative therapy and are still disabled, they should be considered for surgical decompression.

At this juncture it is necessary to comment on the role of physical therapy in these patients, because there is a tendency to keep them in therapy indefinitely, often to the demoralization of all concerned. The modalities of therapy for delivering heat to the shoulder are useful for symptomatic relief, but in established lesions, they do not promote healing. They can be useful as an adjunct to active range of motion and strengthening exercises, but even these exercises are not to be continued if they cause persistent pain or are not followed by significant improvement within a month or so. At that point, maintenance of gentle range of motion is done until surgery can be scheduled.

The worker with documented failure of a conservative program of therapy as outlined above or one who presents with an acute inability to elevate the arm after a trauma should be studied radiographically for the possibility of rotator cuff tear and considered for surgery.

Surgery of the rotator cuff is tailored to the pathology that is found at surgery. For the patient with an intact cuff, a significant bursitis, and evidence of impingement, treatment should be an anterior acromioplasty with resection of the coracoacromial ligament. It is important to avoid acromionectomy, removal of the bony attachment of the deltoid muscle, since this results in considerable disability and weakness of the deltoid (Fig. 14-10).

The patient with a documented rotator cuff tear should, whenever possible, have the tear repaired if the shoulder is weak and painful. Arthroscopic debridement of such tears does not in any way restore the integrity or function of these cuffs, although in the absence of a complete tear, arthroscopic decompression of the subacromial arch (acromioplasty) may be accomplished by those skilled and experienced in these techniques.[29–23] For those

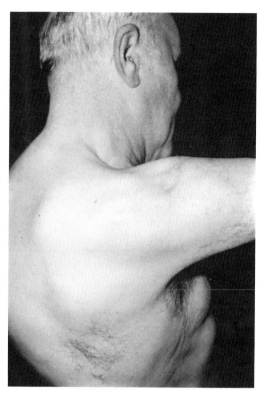

Fig. 14-10. This patient underwent a resection of the anterior and lateral acromion because the surgeon believed that this procedure would decompress his rotator cuff. Postoperatively, his deltoid muscle detached and retracted down the arm, leaving him with a permanently weak and painful shoulder.

patients whose cuffs have been massively avulsed and in whom repair is not technically possible, the decompression of the coracoacromial arch by removal of the anteroinferior acromion and coracoacromial ligament can bring significant pain relief, but it does not improve the active control or strength of the shoulder.

Prognosis

The prognosis for recovery of the patient with a derangement of the rotator cuff depends on the degree and duration of the pathology and the occupational demands that are to be placed upon the shoulder, either during or after treatment has been completed. For those workers with a relatively benign Stage I impingement, the prognosis is good as long as those factors that have brought about the condition are alleviated. In some inexperienced workers, this impingement will be temporary until they develop more experience in the job and learn to do it without hurting themselves. For workers with a significant tendinitis or a frank tear, the outlook is more problematic. If there is no tear, then with decompression one can expect that the rehabilitation process will be relatively rapid and successful. With jobs requiring heavy use of the arm, this process will require about 3 to 4 months off work. The patient with a significant tear cannot expect to return to light work for at least 6 months after repair. Welders or electricians with a large tear may never be able to go back to their original job even though they will be capable of lifting or use of the arms at table height without difficulty.

The patient with a large tear who chooses not to undergo surgery has a significant risk of developing a particularly painful type of arthritis called cuff arthropathy.[34]

BICIPITAL TENDINITIS

Of all the structures in and about the shoulder, none has been the subject of greater controversy than the long head of the biceps. Because it has an intra-articular portion, enjoys an intimate relationship with the rotator cuff, and then passes through a rigid tunnel between the greater and lesser tuberosities of the humerus, it has been an object of intense interest and scrutiny since Cowper described a case of tendinitis nearly 300 years ago.[35] In addition, it has been

falsely accused of being the cause of shoulder pain in countless shoulders, which have then been subjected to numerous operative procedures. A historical review of the anatomic studies, theories of pathogenesis, and surgery is beyond the scope of this chapter. Suffice it to say that Codman[5] believed that the tendon was rarely if ever the primary cause of symptoms, which were usually caused by one of the adjacent structures. After multiple swings of the pendulum of opinion, that is the prevalent opinion of most shoulder surgeons today.

The pain thought to be due to bicipital tendinitis is usually associated with anterior glenohumeral instability, lesions of the glenoidal labrum in the absence of instability, and impingement or tear of the rotator cuff. Even when the presenting complaint is an acute rupture of the long head of the biceps, with the acute onset of pain in the anterior aspect of the shoulder and the sudden retraction of the muscle to give the "Popeye" appearance of the arm, it is usually caused by an associated rotator cuff tear that has resulted from attrition. These patients should all be studied with either shoulder arthrograms or MRI to rule out a cuff tear. Primary rupture of the biceps tendon in the absence of rotator cuff tear is an unusual lesion in my experience. The "clunk" that may be found on examination and is thought to be a dislocating biceps tendon usually results from either a cuff tear or anterior instability.

Yet, one occasionally encounters the unusual patient who does have anterior shoulder pain in the absence of any of the conditions listed above. I can remember a particularly perplexing case of a man of 50 years of age with exactly that situation who was vice president of a major pharmaceutical company. The etiology of his pain defied discovery until he casually mentioned that his major hobby was "sawing up a few cords of wood every weekend"!

If one has ruled out instability, other labral lesions, and rotator cuff derangements, a biceps rupture in most cases can be treated conservatively, without resorting to operative tenodesis in the bicipital groove. Usually the pain subsides spontaneously, and the worker may resume the use of the shoulder as comfort determines, depending on occupational demands.

THE STIFF AND PAINFUL SHOULDER: FROZEN SHOULDER AND ADHESIVE CAPSULITIS

The worker who presents with a stiff and painful shoulder should not be immediately labeled as having a "frozen shoulder" or adhesive capsulitis. Not only may several different entities present in this way[36] but the term may also convey an inappropriate sense of negativism to the treatment plan that will prove costly to all concerned. Many painful conditions, even at hand level, that result in immobilization of the limb over a protracted period of time, can cause painful stiffness of the shoulder. What is indicated is to work through the differential diagnosis to determine the cause of the pain and then to correct the primary problem so that the shoulder may be mobilized appropriately. It is important to be able to recognize the entity of adhesive capsulitis. The diagnosis, treatment, and prognosis of the other varieties of the stiff and painful shoulder are dealt with in their respective sections.

Clinical Presentation

Adhesive capsulitis[37] is a distinct entity that occurs uncommonly in manual workers and far more commonly in persons who are sedentary in their habits. The eti-ology is unknown, although there have been many theories.[38] Usually the patients are in the 40 to 60-year age group, and it is more common to see the nondominant limb affected. Although the presentation is variable, there is usually no history of significant antecedent trauma, either acute or chronic. Pain in the shoulder is the presenting complaint, and it is often very severe. Usually, pain diminishes within a few weeks, being replaced by gradually increasing stiffness over the span of weeks to months. With the passage of time, however, the shoulder gradually "unfreezes," and motion is restored. This entire process may take as long as 12 to 18 months.

Confirmatory Tests

In addition to the general examination as detailed above, routine radiographs of the shoulder demonstrate the absence of calcific deposits or arthritis. It is mandatory to obtain a contrast arthrogram in all cases where the diagnosis of adhesive capsulitis or frozen shoulder is suspected. In this way, rotator cuff tears, which usually do not cause severe restriction of motion but which do cause significant pain, can be ruled out. Diagnostic signs of adhesive capsulitis are the characteristic arthrographic picture of the severely diminished capacity of the joint capsule and the diminished axillary recess (Fig. 14-11).[39–41] MRI may be substituted for the contrast arthrogram, which may be technically difficult to accomplish in the patient with a small capsule.

Treatment

The treatment of adhesive capsulitis, as is the etiology, is controversial.[38,40,42,43] Patients are best treated with analgesics and nonsteroidal anti-inflammatory agents in the initial "freezing" phase and are advised to use their shoulders within

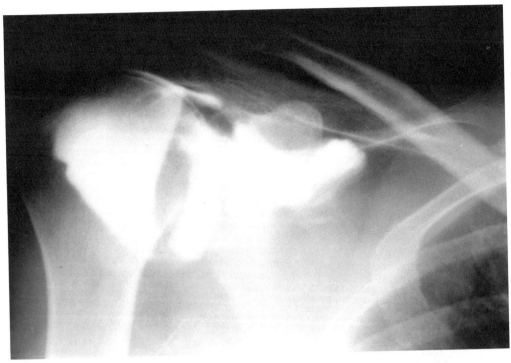

Fig. 14-11. Contrast arthrogram of a patient with adhesive capsulitis or "frozen shoulder." Note the tight appearance of the joint due to its diminished capacity and the medial extravasation as more dye is pushed into the joint.

their limits of comfort. When pain abates, the shoulder can be gradually mobilized with gentle range of motion and strengthening exercises. In my opinion, manipulation under anesthesia is seldom indicated, and surgery is reserved for those unusual cases that fail to regain useful range of motion.[44]

Prognosis

Most of the patients that I have observed over the years have regained their full range of motion. This is the general experience,[45] although an occasional patient does not recover completely. Recurrence in the same shoulder is extremely rare, although the contralateral shoulder may be involved at a later date.

CALCIFIC TENDONITIS AND BURSITIS

The presence of a calcific deposit in a radiograph of the shoulder— usually in the supraspinatus tendon adjacent to the greater tuberosity of the humerus— may give rise to spurious conclusions regarding the relationship of that finding to the patient's symptoms or their etiology. Although it would be tempting to ascribe the lesion to a worker's job, it is generally agreed that such is not the case.[46] According to Uhtthoff,[46] Ruttimann in 1959 found calcifications in the shoulder radiographs of 20 percent of asymptomatic individuals. Welfling et al[47] found an incidence of asymptomatic calcifications in 7.5 percent of 200 individuals. The over-

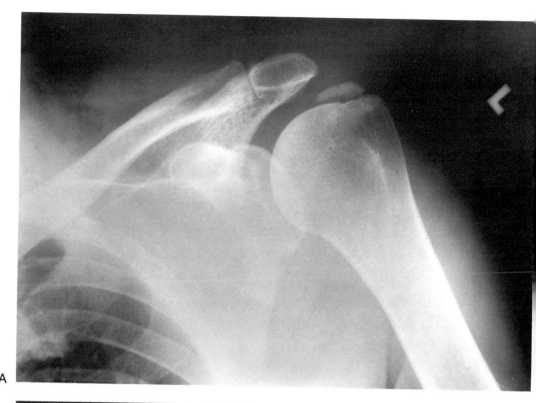

A

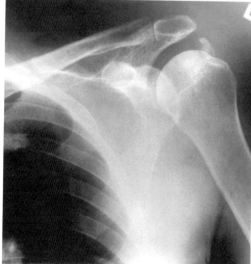

B

Fig. 14-12. The calcific deposit in the supraspinatus tendon as seen in (**A**) lateral rotation, (**B**) medial rotation, and (**C**) axillary view. (*Figure continues.*)

all incidence of shoulder calcifications has varied considerably in different series.[48,49]

The symptoms that are associated with the presence of a calcium deposit depend on the location of that deposit. In the majority of cases, it is located within the substance of the supraspinatus tendon, and since it constitutes a space-occupying lesion under the subacromial arch, it can produce symptoms of impingement. It is conceivable that, in this situation, if the worker was engaged in an activity involving continued overhead work that would ordinarily predispose to the development of the symptoms of impingement, then the presence of the calcification could enhance the effect of the overhead work on the rotator cuff, but the work per se does not cause the deposit to form. The second expression of the calcific deposit is a reflection of the natural history of the lesion, which is that the deposit may work its way out of the tendon and ultimately rupture into the subacromial bursa, where it is very irritating and produces severe, but time-limited pain in the shoulder.[5]

Confirmatory Tests

It is important to obtain radiographs of the shoulder both in the anteroposterior plane with the arm medially and laterally rotated and in an axillary view so as to be able to locate the calcific deposit accurately (Fig. 14-12A-C). As previously stated, the supraspinatus tendon is predilected, but deposits can occur in other tendons. One must differentiate the scattered, small radiopacities adjacent to the greater tuberosity that are associated with chronic rotator cuff tear from calcific deposits, for these are different entities that require different treatment.

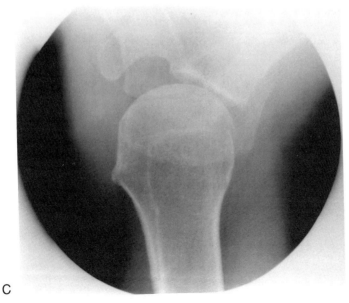

C

Fig. 14-12 (*Continued*).

Treatment

The treatment of the calcific deposit depends on the stage in its natural history. Because many calcific deposits about the shoulder are totally asymptomatic, they do not require treatment. If they are seen because of impingement on the subacromial arch, the pain occurs only during a specific arc in the range of motion, which is usually when the arm is forward flexed and then medially rotated. In these situations, the treatment is that of impingement, which includes rest and avoidance of the position that provokes pain. This treatment may require that the worker's job be changed temporarily, or if that is not possible, the employee may have to simply stop work for a week or two. One or two subacromial injections of steroids and local anesthetic may be very beneficial at this stage, as is the use of oral nonsteroidal anti-inflammatory agents. Repeated injections into the shoulder are to be avoided, however.

The worker who presents with an acute calcific bursitis has very severe pain. The use of a sling and local applications of ice rather than heat are indicated. The pain is often severe enough to warrant oral narcotic analgesics. Occasionally, it is possible to aspirate a fluid deposit from the subacromial bursa, but in most cases, the severe pain disappears spontaneously over a few days as the deposit is absorbed.

Prognosis

The prognosis for most patients with symptoms due to either impingement or acute calcific bursitis is good. The symptoms subside within a few weeks with adequate rest and supportive treatment. For those who have either multiple recurrences or in whom the impingement continues to be a problem, then surgery is indicated to remove the deposit and decompress the subacromial arch.

THORACIC OUTLET SYNDROME

This entity results from compression of the nerves and vessels that supply the upper limb within the area of the thoracic outlet. This space extends from the axilla to the neck and encompasses the area between the clavicle and the first rib. Because it is adjacent to and so intimately associated with the shoulder complex, it is not unexpected that the two areas are mutually influential.[50] Unfortunately, thoracic outlet syndrome (TOS) is the subject of great controversy regarding pathogenesis and treatment, and it tends to be included in the general topic of cervicobrachial syndromes. In my opinion, it should be considered separately in an attempt to improve the care rendered to individuals with TOS.

The symptoms are those of pain in the neck, shoulder, and upper limb, which is often accompanied by paraesthesias and numbness that may have a predilection for the medial aspect of the arm, forearm, and hand; alternatively, the entire limb may be affected. There is often a complaint of nocturnal paraesthesias, and activities that involve lifting or use of the limb at shoulder level or above may also produce symptoms. Sometimes, holding the arms out in front of the body as one might in steering an automobile causes pain as well. There may be complaints of weakness in the hand. All of the above symptoms are manifestations of compression of the lower trunk of the brachial plexus at the level of the first rib. Intermittent swelling of the arm may result from compression of the subclavian vein. Rarely, there may be symptoms stemming from thrombosis of the vein or the subclavian artery,[51-54] but fortunately, these are rare.

The diagnosis is made by history and physical examination. The position of the scapula is an important part of the pathology of this entity,[55,56] despite the fact that early interest was focused on the scalene muscles. Anatomic variations within the thoracic outlet continue to be of interest and importance.[57-60] However, in my clinical practice more patients have postural abnormalities as the major cause than have definable cervical ribs or bands.[61] It is this postural abnormality that serves as both the common denominator and the explanation for the occurrence of TOS in the industrial population. It may result from a wrenching injury that alters the supporting structures of the shoulder girdle, or it may be caused by repetitive weight-bearing motions performed many times per day in the course of factory work. Sometimes it can develop because of a relatively trivial injury distally in the hand, which then, over a protracted period of time, causes disuse atrophy of the shoulder girdle. The actual incidence of TOS in the industrial population is difficult to establish, but has been noted to be as high as 18 percent of a varied group of workers.[11]

The ability to reproduce the symptoms by positioning the arm in abduction and external rotation with the shoulder braced has been the most consistently useful test in my experience. The pulse is usually occluded at the wrist with this maneuver, but pulse obliteration by itself should not be taken as a positive test. There are often subtle findings of neurologic loss in the hand, which are usually limited to the muscles supplied by T1 and C8, as well as the sensory territory of the ulnar aspect of the forearm and hand. In long-standing compression, particularly when there is a congenital band compressing the nerves, the atrophy of the hand muscles may be severe.[68]

Additional Testing

In all cases of suspected TOS, the patient should have a radiograph of the cervical spine and chest. Note should be made of the presence of long transverse processes at C7 or the cervical ribs. The chest film is important in ruling out the possibility of a Pancoast tumor of the lung. MRI and CT scanning have not contributed materially to the diagnosis of TOS. Comment has already been made above regarding the lack of reliability of electrodiagnostic studies in confirming the diagnosis of TOS.[6] These studies are most applicable in cases where a double crush syndrome is suspected[63] or in the differential diagnosis with a more peripheral lesion of the median or ulnar nerves. The use of both noninvasive and invasive studies of the vascular system to establish the diagnosis of TOS is a difficult problem, since one would assume that, because the pulse may be obliterated during the provocative maneuvers, they would be helpful in confirming the diagnosis. Unfortunately, the symptoms of TOS are usually the result of neural compression and not vascular compression. Furthermore, since it is possible to occlude the pulse in many totally asymptomatic and normal young women, it would seem inadvisable to perform invasive vascular testing on those suspected of having TOS unless there is evidence of an aneursym of the subclavian artery. Noninvasive testing in the form of digital plethysmography has been described,[64] but in my personal experience has produced a high percentage of both false negative and false positive results. In fact, 50 percent of the asymptomatic contralateral arms in my patients with TOS who underwent surgery had false positive digital plethysmographic studies. In my opinion, the diagnosis remains a clinical one.

Treatment

In most cases of TOS the initial treatment is nonoperative unless there is significant and objective neural loss, impending vascular catastrophe, or documented failure of a carefully supervised program of exercise therapy. All other patients are treated with a routine of exercises to strengthen the shoulder girdle suspensory muscles and to correct any postural malalignments. If the patients are overweight, they are advised to lose weight. Wherever possible, some adjustment in the working conditions is tried as an alternative to surgery, particularly with overhead work or that involving heavy lifting. If the conservative routine has failed after 4 to 6 months and the patient is still symptomatic, then surgery in the form of a resection of the first rib[65] is considered. The results of this surgery in well-motivated workers are generally quite good, but because of the possibility of secondary gain in continued postoperative complaints of pain, they may be difficult to interpret. Assuming all goes well, however, most clerical workers should be able to resume full duties within 2 to 3 months. The return to work of heavy manual laborers is somewhat problematic. There have been fewer cases of TOS in such workers, as it is considerably more common in women than men. As the composition of the work force continues to change with time, this group of manual laborers with TOS will be interesting to follow.

GLENOHUMERAL INSTABILITIES

Glenohumeral instability is not usually seen as a problem related to chronic industrial use of the shoulder. It should, however, be considered in the differential diagnosis of shoulder pain from an acute injury or in situations wherein the worker has failed to recover with treatment for what was thought to be an impingement syndrome. In the case of the acute injury, the history of having sustained a wrenching of the arm into abduction and external rotation should alert the examiner to the possibility of a tear of the anterior glenohumeral ligaments. Although these patients may not describe dramatic episodes of dislocation of the shoulder, they may experience pain in the anterior aspect of the shoulder and feelings of instability along with crepitus. These symptoms may be misinterpreted as resulting from impingement, and I have seen a number of patients who have failed to respond to technically satisfactory surgery for impingement because they were actually unstable and required correction of that defect. For workers who fall on the flexed and internally rotated shoulder, the possibility of posterior instability should be considered.

The physical examination may be supplemented by examination under anesthesia, at which time the shoulder is stressed and compared to the other side. In some situations, arthroscopic examination is valuable in defining the problem further, but it should not be needed for the routine patient in whom glenohumeral instability is suspected. Before these more invasive tests are done, MRI and CT arthrogram may be used, although they too must be interpreted with caution. Sometimes, several of these measures may be needed to make the precise diagnosis, since the physical findings may be quite subtle.

DEGENERATIVE ARTHRITIS

I have been unable to find documentation of the association of osteoarthritis of the shoulder with industrial use, either in my own practice or the literature. There is, however, an intriguing paper by Waldron[66] in 1989 in which he describes having examined the skeletons of 367 English workers who died between 1729 and 1869 and for whom detailed occupational histories were available. His analysis failed to show a relation between occupation and osteoarthritis of the shoulder.

PERIPHERAL NERVE COMPRESSION LESIONS

Industrially related lesions of the peripheral nerves have been well documented at the elbow and distally in the forearm and hand.[67] They are, however, rare in the region of the shoulder. Although one might expect that the mechanisms that have been described for nerve entrapments of the peripheral nerves about the shoulder girdle would result in a significant number of them being recognized as a result of repetitive motion and lifting, this has not proved to be so in my experience. In addition, Post[68] reported seeing 2,520 patients over a 3-year period for painful shoulder problems; of these he was only able to identify ten patients with suprascapular nerve entrapments, and only one of these cases was occupationally related.

Serratus palsy has been reported in slaughterhouse workers from carrying heavy weights on their shoulders,[69] but I have not seen the lesion in a worker who had not sustained a significant single trauma or had some other non-work-related cause. In a review of my own office practice for the 2-year period of October, 1988 to October 1990, there were 22 patients seen for the diagnosis of serratus palsy, but none from carrying heavy weights on the shoulder or making repetitive movements with the upper extremity.

Compression of the axillary nerve and the posterior circumflex humeral artery resulting in pain and paraesthesias in the upper extremity and pain in the shoulder, yet not associated with trauma, has been described by the term "quadrilateral space syndrome."[70] It is said to be difficult to diagnose. Flexion or abduction of the humerus is claimed to aggravate the symptoms, and neurologic examination and electrodiagnostic studies are normal. Cahill[7] recommends an arteriogram as an aid to diagnosis. I have never recognized a case of quadrilateral space syndrome in 25 years and would not advise that patients with vague tenderness about the shoulder be subjected to arteriography even if their symptoms are made worse by abduction and external rotation. Some of these patients will have unstable shoulders, and others TOS, and I do not recommend arteriography in either case unless there is a real question of an aneurysm of the subclavian artery.

Confirmatory Tests

Clearly, although entrapment lesions of the peripheral nerves of the shoulder beyond the intervertebral foramina and the thoracic outlet are uncommon, they are even more so in industrial circumstances, and the diagnosis should be made with great caution. Although I would be willing to accept a clinical diagnosis of TOS in the absence of positive electrodiagnostic findings, this has come from the knowledge that the technical aspects of measurement of conduction velocity through the thoracic outlet and the intermittent and complex nature of the disorder make accuracy extremely difficult. Nevertheless, one must be extremely rigorous in the clinical assessment of these disorders. For entrapment lesions of the peripheral nerves in this area, the threshold for acceptance of the lesions as industrially related should be extremely high.

REFERENCES

1. Garg A: An evaluation of the NIOSH guidelines for manual lifting, with special reference to horizontal distance. Am Indust Hyg Assoc J 50:157, 1989
2. Amano M, Umeda G, Nakajima H, Yatsuki K: Characteristics of work actions of shoe manufacturing assembly line workers and a cross-sectional factor-control study on occupational cervicobrachial disorders. Sangyo Igaku 30:3, 1988
3. Bjelle A, Hagberg M, Michaelson G: Work-related shoulder-neck complaints in industry: a pilot study. Br J Rheumatol 26:365, 1987
4. Ohara H, Mimura K, Oze Y, Itani T et al: Studies on the cervico operators. Part 2. A review on clinical findings and working conditions of patients. Sangyo Igaku 24:65, 1982
5. Codman EA: The Shoulder. Thomas Todd Co, Boston, 1934
6. Wilbourn AJ, Lederman RJ: Evidence for conduction delay in thoracic-outlet syndrome is challenged. N Engl J Med 310:1052, 1984
7. Herberts P, Kadefors R: A study of painful shoulder in welders. Acta Orthop Scand 47:381, 1976
8. Herberts, P, Kadefors R, Hogfors C, Sigholm G: Shoulder pain and heavy manual labor. Clin Orthop 191:166, 1984
9. Keikenwan SI: Report of the committee on occupational cervicobrachial disorder of the Japan Association of Industrial Health, 1973
10. Browne CD, Nolan B, Faithful D: Occupational repetition strain injuries. Med J Aust 140:329, 1984
11. Sallstrom J, Schmidt H: Cervicobrachial disorders in certain occupations with special reference to compression in the thoracic outlet. Am J Indust Med 6:45, 1984

12. Onishi N, Nomura H, Sakai K, Yamamoto T et al: Shoulder muscle tenderness and physical features of female industrial workers. J Hum Ergol (Tokyo) 5:87, 1976
13. Hocking B: Epidemiological aspects of "repetition strain injury" in Telecom Australia. Med J Aust 147:218, 1987
14. Hagberg M: Occupational musculoskeletal stress and disorders of the neck and shoulder: a review of possible pathophysiology. Int Arch Occup Environ Health 53:269, 1984
15. Wiker SF, Chaffin DB, Langolf GD: Shoulder posture and localized muscle fatigue and discomfort. Ergonomics 32:211, 1989
16. Tarumi K, Nagami M, Kadowaki I: An inquiry into the factors affecting the complaints of subjective symptoms in VDT operators. Sangyo Igaku 32:77, 1990
17. Christensen H: Muscle activity and fatigue in the shoulder muscles during repetitive work. An electromyographic study. Eur J Appl Physiol 54: 596, 1986
18. Neer CS II: Anterior acromioplasty for the chronic impingement syndrome in the shoulder. J Bone Joint Surg 54A:41, 1972
19. Neer CS II: Impingement lesions. Clin Orthop 173:70, 1983
20. Rathbun JB, Macnab I: The microvascular pattern of the rotator cuff. J Bone Joint Surg 52B:540, 1970
21. Rothman RH, Parke WW: The vascular anatomy of the rotator cuff. Clin Orthop 41:176, 1965
22. Neer CS II, Bigliani LU, Hawkins RJ: Rupture of the long head of the biceps related to subacromial impingement. Orthop Trans 1:111, 1977
23. Cotton RE, Rideout DF: Tears of the humeral rotator cuff. A radiological and pathological necrosy survey. J Bone Joint Surg 46B:314, 1964
24. Buirski G: Magnetic resonance imaging in acute and chronic rotator cuff tears. Skeletal Radiol 19:109, 1990
25. Crass JR, Craig EV, Feinberg SB: Ultrasonography of rotator cuff tears: a review of 500 diagnostic studies. J Clin Ultrasound 16:313, 1988
26. Hodler J, Fretz CJ, Terrier F, Gerber C: Rotator cuff tears: correlation of sono-

graphic and surgical findings. Radiology 169:791, 1988

27. Tsai JC, Zlatkin MB: Magnetic resonance imaging of the shoulder. Radiol Clin North Am 28:279, 1990

28. Neer CS II, Marberry TA: On the disadvantages of radical acromionectomy. J Bone Joint Surg 63A:1981, 1981

29. Biedert R, Kentsch A: Arthroscopic revision of the subacromial space in impingement syndrome. Unfallchirurg 92:500, 1989

30. Esch JC: Arthroscopy update #4. Arthroscopic subacromial decompression. Surgical technique. Orthop Rev 18:733, 1989

31. Esch JC, Ozerkis LR, Helgager JA, Kane N et al: Arthroscopic subacromial decompression: results according to the degree of rotator cuff tear. Arthroscopy 4:241, 1988

32. Gartsman GM: Arthroscopic acromioplasty for lesions of the rotator cuff. J Bone Joint Surg 72A:169, 1990

33. Ogilvie HDJ, D'Angelo G: Arthroscopic surgery of the shoulder. Sports Med 9:120, 1990

34. Neer CS II, Craig EV, Fukuda H: Cuff arthropathy. Orthop Trans 5:447, 1981

35. Cowper W: Myotomia Reformata. London, 1694

36. Neviaser RJ: Painful conditions affecting the shoulder. Clin Orthop 173:63, 1983

37. Neviaser JS: Adhesive capsulitis of the shoulder: study of pathological findings in periarthritis in the shoulder. J Bone Joint Surg 27:211, 1945

38. Leffert RD: The frozen shoulder. p. 199. Instructional Course Lectures, American Academy of Orthopaedic Surgeons, XXIV, 1985

39. Neviaser JS: Adhesive capsulitis and the stiff and painful shoulder. Orthop Clin North Am 11:327, 1980

40. Neviaser RJ, Neviaser TJ: The frozen shoulder diagnosis and management. Clin Orthop 223:59, 1987

41. Reeves B: Arthrographic changes in frozen and post-traumatic and stiff shoulders. Proc Roy Soc Med 59:827, 1966

42. Haines JE, Hargadon EJ: Manipulation as the primary treatment of the frozen shoulder. J Roy Coll Surg Edinburgh 27:5, 1982

43. Quigley TB: Indications for manipulation and corticosteroids in the treatment of stiff shoulders. Surg Clin North Am 43:1715, 308, 1963

44. Rowe CR, Leffert RD: Idiopathic chronic adhesive capsulitis ("frozen shoulder"), p. 155. In Rowe CR (ed): The Shoulder. Churchill Livingstone, New York, 1988

45. Grey RG: The natural history of idiopathic frozen shoulder. J Bone Joint Surg 60:564, 1978

46. Uhthoff HK, Sarkar K: Calcifying tendinitis, p. 774. In Rockwood CA Jr., Matsen FA III (ed): The Shoulder. WB Saunders, Philadelphia, 1990

47. Welfling J, Kahn MF, Desroy M et al: Les calcifications de lepaule. IILa. maladie des calcifications tendineuses multiples. Rev Rheum 32:325, 1965

48. Bosworth DM: Calcium deposits in the shoulder and subacromial bursitis: a survey of 12, 122 shoulders. JAMA 116:2477, 1941

49. DePalma AF, Kruper JS: Long term study of shoulder joints afflicted with and treated for calcific tendinitis. Clin Orthop 20:61, 1961

50. Leffert RD, Gumley G: The relationship between dead arm syndrome and thoracic outlet syndrome. Clin Orthop 223:20, 1987.

51. Cormier JM, Amrane M, Ward A, Laurian C et al: Arterial complications of the thoracic outlet syndrome: fifty-five operative cases. J Vasc Surg 9:778, 1989

52. Gloviczki P, Kazmier FJ, Hollier, LH: Axillary-subclavian venous occlusion: the morbidity of a nonlethal disease. J Vasc Surg 4:333, 1986

53. Hassen KR, Batt M, Gagliardi JM, Duane B et al: Venous involvement in the thoracic outlet syndrome (apropos of 30 cases). Phlebologie 41:818, 1988

54. Shuttleworth, RD, van der Merwe DM, Mitchell WL: Subclavian vein stenosis and axillary vein 'effort thrombosis.' Age and the first rib bypass collateral, thrombolytic therapy and first rib resection. S Afr Med J 71:564, 1987.

55. Swift TR, Nichols FT: The droopy shoulder syndrome. Neurology 34:212, 1984

56. Todd TW: The descent of the shoulder

after birth. Anatomischer Anzeiger Centralbatt fur die gesamte wissenschaftlichje Anatomie 14:385, 1912

57. Adson AW: Surgical treatment for symptoms produced by cervical ribs and scalenus anticus muscle. Surg Gynecol Obstet 85:687, 1947

58. Adson AW: Thoracic outlet syndrome——symposium: the classic surgical treatment for symptoms produced by cervical ribs and the scalenus anticus muscle. Clin Orthop 207:3, 1986

59. Adson AW, Coffey JR: Cervical rib: method of anterior approach for relief of symptoms by division of scalenus anticus. Ann Surg 85:839, 1927

60. Roos DB: Congenital anomalies associated with thoracic outlet syndrome. Anatomy, symptoms, diagnosis and treatment. Am J Surg 132:771, 1976

61. Leffert RD: Surgery of the thoracic outlet, p. 1427. In Chapman MW (ed): Operative Orthopaedics. JB Lippincott Co, Philadelphia, 1988

62. Bonney G: The scalenus medium band: a contribution to the study of thoracic outlet syndrome. J Bone Joint Surg 47:268, 1965

63. Wood VE, Biondi J: Double crush nerve compression in thoracic outlet syndrome. J Bone Joint Surg 72:85, 1990

64. Roos DB: Plethysmography: a simple method of studying and following peripheral vascular disorders. Surg Clin North Am 49:1333, 1969

65. Roos DB: Transaxillary approach to the first rib to relieve thoracic outlet syndrome. Ann Surg 163:354, 1966

66. Waldron HA, Cox M: Occupational arthropathy: evidence from the past. Br J Indust Med 46:420, 1989

67. Harris W: Occupational pressure neuritis of the deep palmar branch of the ulnar nerve. Br Med J 1:98, 1929

68. Post M, Mayer J: Suprascapular nerve entrapment. Clin Orthop 223:126, 1987

69. Porsman O: Serratus anterior paresis as an occupational disease in slaughterhouse workers. An occupational medicine analysis. Ugeskr Laeger 139:291, 1977

70. Cahill BR: Quadrilateral space syndrome, p. 602. In Omer GE, Jr, Spinner M (eds): Management of Peripheral Nerve Problems. WB Saunders, Philadelphia, 1980

15

Rheumatologic Problems in the Worker

Don L. Goldenberg, M.D.

Every systemic and localized rheumatic condition may have an impact on one's occupation. Rather than attempting to cover all such possible rheumatic disorders, this chapter focuses on two rheumatic conditions: rheumatoid arthritis (RA) and fibromyalgia (also known as fibrositis). These two disorders are superb models by which to evaluate the role of any rheumatic condition in the work place. They are both common, primarily affect individuals during their peak work-production years, and are chronic, painful disorders. However, although the disability in RA is generally considered to be related to obvious anatomic joint changes, the etiology of disability in fibromyalgia is controversial and speculative. Nevertheless, recent studies have described the similar adverse effects of both conditions on the worker. Furthermore, the work disability in both conditions may be related more to social and demographic factors than to specific disease factors.

To set the stage for this discussion, it is necessary to review the clinical characteristics of RA and fibromyalgia. RA may affect 1 percent of the population, is two to three times more common in women, and peaks between ages 30 to 40.[1] Although RA is extremely variable in its clinical features and natural history, a substantial number of patients develop progressive pain, deformities, and dysfunction. These manifestations are especially problematic in the upper extremities. Diagnostic criteria for RA[1] have been revised recently (Table 15-1). The cardinal clinical feature is a symmetric, chronic polyarthritis involving the small joints of the hands and feet. Rheumatoid nodules and the presence of rheumatoid factor in the blood are helpful but not essential diagnostic features. Most patients feel systemically ill, with prominent fatigue and often some weight loss. Such patients also are anemic, and blood tests reveal elevated acute-phase reactants, such as the erythrocyte sedimentation rate (ESR), but these are nonspecific. Therapy initially consists of salicylates or other nonsteroidal anti-inflammatory medications (NSAIDs), physical therapy, joint protection when appropriate, and patient education. When these measures

203

Table 15-1. 1988 Revised ARA Criteria for Classification of Rheumatoid Arthritis*

Criteria	Definition
Morning stiffness	Morning stiffness in and around the joints lasting at least 1 hour before maximal improvement
Arthritis of three or more joint areas	At least three joint areas have simultaneous soft tissue swelling or fluid (not bony overgrowth alone) observed by a physician. The 14 possible joint areas are (right or left): PIP, MCP, wrist, elbow, knee, ankle, and MTP joints
Arthritis of hand joints	At least one joint area swollen as above in wrist, MCP, or PIP joint
Symmetric arthritis	Simultaneous involvement of the same joint areas (as in 2) on both sides of the body (bilateral involvement of PIP, MCP, or MTP joints is acceptable without absolute symmetry)
Rheumatoid nodules	Subcutaneous nodules over bony prominences, or extensor surfaces, or in juxta-articular regions, observed by a physician
Serum rheumatoid factor	Demonstration of abnormal amounts of serum "rheumatoid factor" by any method that has been positive in less than 5 percent of normal control subjects
Radiographic changes	Radiographic changes typical of RA on PA hand and wrist x-rays, which must include erosions or unequivocal bony decalcification localized to or most marked adjacent to the involved joints (osteoarthritis changes alone do not qualify)

* For classification purposes, patients are said to have RA if they have satisfied at least four of the above seven criteria. Criteria 1 through 4 must be present for at least 6 weeks. Patients with two clinical diagnoses are not excluded. Designation as classic, definite, or probable rheumatoid arthritis is *not* to be made.[1]

are not sufficient to control the illness, more powerful medications, which may include antimalarials, gold, methotrexate, and the judicious use of corticosteroids, and surgical management are added to the baseline regimen.

Fibromyalgia is a form of soft tissue, rather than joint, rheumatism. Therefore, it is more analogous to chronic idiopathic low back pain or chronic neck and shoulder pain problems. Although patients often present with a more localized pain condition initially, eventually most patients report that they "hurt all over." Yet, they appear to have no structural anatomic problems to account for their pain. Fibromyalgia may affect 2 to 5 percent of the population, is ten times more common in women, peaks between ages 30 to 50, and, like RA, is associated with fa-

tigue, sleep disturbances, and stiffness.[2] However, unlike RA, there is no joint inflammation and no laboratory or radiologic abnormalities. Most patients report months or years of generalized pain, almost always involving the neck, shoulders, and back. They may feel that their joints are swollen or that their muscles are weak, but synovitis or myositis is not present at the time of examination. Most patients are exhausted, never feel refreshed in the morning, and are often depressed. The patients also report numbness and tingling in their muscles and extremities, skin sensitivity, and frequent headaches. They often describe symptoms of irritable bowel syndrome.

The only consistent finding on examination is tenderness at discrete anatomic locations (Fig. 15-1). Such locations are

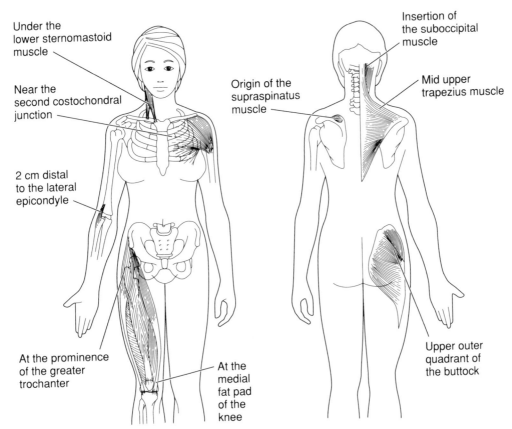

Under the
lower sternomastoid
muscle

Near the
second costochondral
junction

2 cm distal
to the lateral
epicondyle

At the prominence
of the greater
trochanter

At the
medial
fat pad
of the
knee

Origin of the
supraspinatus
muscle

Insertion of
the suboccipital
muscle

Mid upper
trapezius muscle

Upper outer
quadrant of
the buttock

Fig. 15-1. Tenderness at characteristic musculoskeletal locations establishes fibromyalgia as a consistent entity. The nine tender points depicted are important in diagnosis. Each is bilateral, for a total of 18 test sites widely distributed on the body surface. Tenderness on digital palpation of at least 11 sites in a patient with at least a 3-month history of diffuse musculoskeletal pain is recommended as the diagnostic standard for fibromyalgia. (From Hosp Pract, Sept 30, 1989, with permission.)

termed tender points, and their presence in multiple locations and the generalized pain pattern are sensitive and specific diagnostic criteria (Table 15-2).[3] Nevertheless, some training in the locations and techniques of a tender point examination is necessary for the diagnosis to be verified. The etiology and pathophysiology of fibromyalgia are poorly understood, and therefore treatment is empiric. Low doses of tricyclic medications, such as amitriptyline (Elavil) or cyclobenzaprine (Flexeril), have been moderately helpful in improving the sleep disturbances and the

myalgias. Simple analgesics or low doses of NSAIDs are often used for further pain relief. A team approach to management with physical therapy, rehabilitation specialists, and mental health professionals is often the most effective way to treat patients. Hands-on physical therapy, a structured low-impact cardiovascular fitness program, and a mind-body relaxation program can then be tailored to each patient.

Some authors have included myofascial pain syndrome as a more localized form of fibromyalgia, and there are many over-

Table 15-2. American College of Rheumatology 1990 Criteria for the Classification of Fibromyalgia*

1. History of widespread pain

    Definition. Pain is considered widespread when all of the following are present: pain in the left side of the body, pain in the right side of the body, pain above the waist, and pain below the waist. In addition, axial skeletal pain (cervical spine or anterior chest or thoracic spine or low back) must be present. In this definition, shoulder and buttock pain is considered as pain for each involved side. "Low back" pain is considered lower segment pain.

2. Pain in 11 of 18 tender point sites on digital palpation

    Definition. Pain, on digital palpation, must be present in at least 11 of the following 18 tender point sites:

    Occiput: bilateral, at the suboccipital muscle insertions

    Low cervical: bilateral, at the anterior aspects of the intertransverse spaces at C5–C7

    Trapezius: bilateral, at the midpoint of the upper border

    Supraspinatus: bilateral, at origins, above the scapula spine near the medial border

    Second rib: bilateral, at the second costochondral junctions, just lateral to the juntions on upper surfaces

    Lateral epicondyle: bilateral, 2 cm distal to the epicondyles

    Gluteal: bilateral, in upper outer quadrants of buttocks in anterior fold of muscle

    Greater trochanter: bilateral, posterior to the trochanteric prominence

    Knee: bilateral, at the medial fat pad proximal to the joint line.

Digital palpation should be performed with an approximate force of 4 kg. For a tender point to be considered "positive" the subject must state that the palpation was painful. "Tender" is not considered "painful."

* For classification purposes, patients are said to have fibromyalgia if both criteria are satisfied. Widespread pain must have been present for at least 3 months. The presence of a second clinical disorder does not exclude the diagnosis of fibromyalgia.[2]

lapping features in these two chronic forms of soft tissue rheumatism. However, myofascial pain syndrome has been traditionally defined as a regional pain disorder with identifiable "trigger points" limited to one anatomic area, such as the right neck and shoulder. Generally it is responsive to local therapeutic measures, such as "spray and stretch."

DISABILITY EVALUATION IN RHEUMATIC DISEASES

It is especially difficult to measure work capacity accurately in the context of rheumatic diseases. Work is most often limited by the patient's self-assessment of pain, which is a subjective phenomenon. In structural disorders such as RA, there is at least some anatomic basis for a patient's dysfunction. The extent of arthritis and tenosynovitis of the fingers, wrists, elbows, and shoulders can be visualized on physical examination and radiologically. Functional classification schemes for RA (class I–IV), although crude, provide some guidelines for disability determination. Nevertheless, pain, not structural anatomic abnormalities, is the most common cause of work loss in RA. Furthermore, in chronic musculoskeletal pain disorders, such as fibromyalgia, myofascial pain, or idiopathic low back pain, no "objective" disease severity measures or scales exist. Determination of disability in such conditions is especially difficult to standardize. For example, Carey et al.[4] presented a series of sample back pain patients applying for disability benefits to physicians, some of whom worked for the Social Security Administration. Physicians' ratings, which determined whether an individual patient met the criteria for compensation, varied tremendously. Those physicians who worked for the Social Security Administration were less likely to certify an individual as being eligible for compensation. Thus, the examiner's role in such situations may bias the determination of disability. On the other hand, there has been concern that patients with musculoskeletal pain apply and receive disability more often than their illness requires. However, most reports have not found that patients with chronic musculoskeletal pain are malingerers.[5]

The Social Security Administration defines an impairment as one that "results from anatomical, physiological, or psychological abnormalities which are demonstrable by medically acceptable clinical and laboratory diagnostic techniques. Statements of the applicant, including his own description of his impairment (symptoms) are, alone, insufficient to establish the presence of a physical or mental impairment" (Code of Federal Regulations 404.1501). Furthermore, the personal physician's assessment of the patient's functional capacity is not a primary consideration of disability. Thus, in conditions, such as fibromyalgia, myofascial pain, or idiopathic low back pain, in which "objective" clinical and laboratory abnormalities are not present and the patient's and personal physician's assessment are the basis of disability determinations, Social Security-assigned independent examiners are more likely to disallow disability than in such a condition as RA. It is unlikely that these physicians perform a tender point evaluation and apply current diagnostic criteria when evaluating disability claims for fibromyalgia, myofascial pain, and related soft tissue rheumatism.

DISABILITY IN RA

The indirect costs of arthritis due to work loss exceed the direct costs of medical care for arthritis. In one study, over 50 percent of patients who were working before the onset of RA stopped working within 10 years of the diagnosis.[6] Severity of illness correlated weakly with work disability, the strongest correlation was with the nature of the job held when RA developed. Yelin et al.[6] noted that characteristics of work and the work environment "profoundly alter the probability of work loss among persons with RA." Mitchell and co-workers[7] evaluated work disability and factors contributing to earnings loss in men and women with a symmetric polyarthritis (probable RA). Overall, 51 percent of women and 47 percent of men with polyarthritis were severely disabled, compared with 4.5 percent of women and 3.7 percent of men with no arthritis. The earnings of women were 27 percent and those of men were 48 percent of the earnings of individuals without arthritis. Only one-third of this earnings gap was explained by the arthritis itself, whereas two-thirds were explained by social factors and co-morbidity, such as hypertension, obesity, and gastrointestinal illness. Reisine et al.[8] also evaluated factors contributing to disability in employed women and homemakers with RA. The single most important causative factor of work disability was the characteristics of the job, such as autonomy in the pace and scheduling of work and the nature of the work. However, unlike Yelin's findings, disease factors did correlate strongly with functional disability. Homemaker role responsibilities had an effect on work status. Women with greater home responsibilities were more likely to be employed, suggesting that higher levels of family responsibility may enhance self-worth and provide a sense of greater control over the illness.

Hagglund et al.[9] evaluated factors that best predicted pain and functional impairment in RA patients. Such disease measures as the erythrocyte sedimentation rate and radiologic severity did not correlate with pain and functional outcome, although joint swelling scores did. Psychological variables, particularly depression, explained a substantial proportion of the variance in outcome, even after disease activity was taken into account. Another study found that patients with greater feelings of helplessness reported greater pain and impairment in performing activities of daily living.[10] Thus, job, social, and psychological factors are as important or more important than disease factors in determining disability in RA. Such factors must be evaluated and considered when a patient requests an informal or formal determination of their functional disability related to a chronic rheumatic condition.

DISABILITY IN OTHER RHEUMATIC CONDITIONS OF THE UPPER EXTREMITY

Approximately one-third of adults aged 18 to 50 and most adults older than age 50 have evidence of osteoarthritis. However, only about 30 percent of patients with osteoarthritis of the hands ever complain of pain or other symptoms. The association of occupational trauma with osteoarthritis of the hands is controversial, although there are a number of occupationally related activities that predispose to soft tissue and joint trauma (Table 15-3) and may contribute to osteoarthritis.[11] The other most important conditions related to the work place, including tenosynovitis, carpal tunnel syndrome, and other entrapment neuropathies, are discussed in other sections of the book. However, two rheumatic disorders, olecranon bursitis and reflex sympathetic dystrophy, do sometimes occur in work settings and are reviewed here briefly.

Olecranon bursitis is generally related

Table 15-3. Some Occupationally Related Disorders of the Upper Extremity That Potentially Cause Chronic Rheumatic Problems

Occupation	Chronic Condition
Pneumatic drill operator	CTS, osteoarthritis
Pipetter's thumb	Osteoarthritis
Boxer	MP osteoarthritis
Butcher, cobbler	Ulnar neuropathy
Carpenter	Olecranon bursitis

to repeated trauma or skin abrasions near the elbow. It is especially common in carpenters, construction workers, miners, and students. Generally, a sterile, traumatic bursitis is present, and symptoms range from asymptomatic swelling to quite intense pain and inflammation. Usually avoidance of trauma and the use of NSAIDs treat the condition effectively. Protection of the elbow by wearing some form of padding chronically may prevent recurrence. Sometimes, septic olecranon bursitis develops in this setting. In a series of 20 patients presenting with septic olecranon bursitis, occupational-related trauma was identified in 14 patients, including plumbers, janitors, bartenders, glass cutters, and a gymnastics instructor.[12]

Any potentially infected bursa should be aspirated immediately for diagnostic and therapeutic purposes. Most cases of septic olecranon bursitis are caused by *Staphylococcus aureus* and should be treated with parenteral antibiotics and appropriate drainage. Although some patients respond well to oral antibiotics, recent reports suggest that all patients with septic bursitis should initially receive parenteral antibiotics until there is evidence of significant improvement.

Reflex sympathetic dystrophy (RSD) may also develop in work place settings, and is usually related to minor or major trauma to the shoulder and arm. The etiology and pathophysiology of RSD are unclear, and therefore many potential precipitating factors have been postulated. In occupational disorders, soft tissue injury followed by prolonged immobilization with a splint or a cast has been the most common triggering event.[13] The classic clinical features of RSD include burning pain and exquisite tenderness in one extremity, swelling with pitting or nonpitting edema, vasomotor changes, and dystrophic skin changes in chronic conditions. Scintigraphy is the most helpful laboratory test, with increased (or sometimes decreased) uptake in more than 75 percent of cases.[14] Later, a patchy osteoporosis of the involved limb is present on plain x-rays. Early mobilization with appropriate physical therapy is the key aspect of treatment. NSAIDs or sometimes short courses of corticosteroids have been found to be beneficial in controlled studies.[14] Interruption of regional sympathetic tone by medications, sympathetic ganglionic blockade, or surgical sympathectomy has been done in many recalcitrant cases, although its use and effectiveness remains controversial.

DISABILITY IN FIBROMYALGIA AND MYOFASCIAL PAIN

Fibromyalgia is by definition a chronic pain disorder. However, until recently there have been few studies of the natural history or functional disability in this condition. Most descriptive studies of fibromyalgia report that the average duration of pain before diagnosis is 5 years. There have been three recent longitudinal studies of at least one year's duration after the diagnosis of fibromyalgia was made. Felson and Goldenberg[15] interviewed 39 pa-

tients being treated for fibromyalgia yearly for 3 years. More than 60 percent of patients had moderate or severe pain and globally felt fair or poor during each of the 3 years. More than 75 percent of patients were taking medications regularly for fibromyalgia. Less severe symptoms initially and a younger age were associated with better outcome at year 3, whereas the duration of symptoms and the presence of a psychiatric condition had no effect on outcome. Hawley et al.[16] surveyed 75 fibromyalgia patients during a 1-year period. The symptoms in individual patients were very stable, but there was a wide range of symptoms among the patients. This data contrast with the view of a stereotyped fibromyalgia patient with very high levels of pain, irritability, and distress. Pain was the most important determinant of severity, followed by depression. However, functional disability contributed independently to illness severity.

The impact of fibromyalgia on the work place is substantial. Cathey et al.[17] examined the work status of 156 fibromyalgia patients with a work survey questionnaire (Table 15-4). Sixty-four percent of the 156 fibromyalgia patients were employed. Disability scores measured by means of the Stanford Health Assessment Questionnaire (HAQ) were almost twice as high in the nonworking as the working group ($P < .001$). Among the working patients, there was considerable time lost from work because of fibromyalgia (about 5 days per 6 months). Nonworking patients reported an average of 13 days per 6 months when they were completely unable to do their usual activities. Ten percent of working-aged fibromyalgia patients reported themselves disabled, but only 6 percent had received disability payments for a musculoskeletal illness and none specifically for a diagnosis of fibromyalgia. Twenty-nine percent of patients reported that they had changed jobs

Table 15-4.   Work and Disability in Fibromyalgia and Rheumatoid Arthritis

Author	Year	Number of Patients	Currently Employed	Home-maker	Dis-abled	Receiving Disability	Changed Jobs	Missed Work In Past Month (>50 %)
Cathey	1988	156 (<65 yr.)	64%	27%	10%	6%	29%	Yes
Mason	1989	116 (<65 yr.)	63%	11%	22%	12%	33%	Yes
Cathey	1990	544	47%	22%	15%	11%	—	—
RA: Mason	1989	186	41%	21%	32%	—	17%	Yes

because of fibromyalgia, and among those not working, 42 percent had stopped working because of fibromyalgia.

Cathey et al.[17] also assessed the functional ability of 28 patients with fibromyalgia during the performance of five standardized work tasks and compared their performance with that of 26 RA patients and 11 healthy controls. The work testing was performed on a work simulator made up of changeable tools and pulleys that simulate various work tasks and a microprocessor that controls force and measures force, distance, and time. Specific tasks that involved pronation and supination, pushing and pulling, vacuuming and mopping, and lifting were evaluated. Overall, there was no difference between fibromyalgia and RA patients in their ability to perform standardized work tasks, but both differed from normals ($P = .05$). There were differences in individual tasks, such as wrist twist motion, which was most impaired in the RA patients. The fibromyalgia and RA patients had lower task completion rates and took longer to complete the tasks than controls. Work ability correlated with functional disability as measured by the HAQ; with psychological status, as measured by the SCL-90-R and the Arthritis Impact Measurement Scale (AIMS); and with pain, measured using visual analogue scales (VAS), a 10-cm scale rating pain from 0 (none) to 10 (most severe).

Mason et al.[18] compared the rheumatologic condition's impact on work in 116 fibromyalgia patients and 186 RA patients given a work questionnaire. Of the 73 fibromyalgia patients currently employed, 33 percent had changed jobs because of fibromyalgia and 33 percent missed work during the past month. Twenty-two percent of the fibromyalgia patients considered themselves to be currently disabled from work or from their ability to take care of a household, and 81 percent of those considered the disability to be due primarily to fibromyalgia. Of the 76 currently employed RA patients, 26 percent had changed jobs at least once and 7 percent missed work during the past month. Thirty-two percent of the RA patients considered themselves to be currently disabled from work or from their ability to take care of a household adequately.

A multiclinic North American study evaluated the service utilization and work disability of 544 patients with fibromyalgia.[19] Ninety percent of patients were women, with a mean age of 50 years. Forty-seven percent of fibromyalgia patients were employed, 22 percent were homemakers, 9 percent were retired, and 15 percent considered themselves disabled. Twelve percent were currently receiving disability payments, the majority from the federal government under the Social Security Disability Program. Work disability was most strongly correlated with HAQ functional disability, global severity, and pain. Male sex and being unmarried were also associated with disability.

McCain et al.[20] reviewed the Canadian experience with long-term disability payments and litigation in fibromyalgia. Unique problems in fibromyalgia litigation include the perceived subjective nature of the condition, as well as its uncertain duration, natural history, and optimal treatment. Nine percent of the disability payments of a major Canadian life insurance company in one year were related to fibromyalgia. Extrapolating to all disability claims in Canada, it was estimated that private disability insurers in Canada pay out over $200 million per year in long-term disability claims for fibromyalgia. Over 50 percent of the fibromyalgia disability claimants were out of work for over 2 years. Fibromyalgia also has been the subject of intense litigation because it has been temporally related to trauma at work or because it began in the wake of a motor vehicle accident.

The most striking example of the medicolegal impact of fibromyalgia or the related myofascial pain syndrome was the Australian "epidemic" of what was referred to as repetitive strain injury in the early 1980s.[21] This condition was initially considered to be a form of tenosynovitis in industrial workers. However, as more publicity attracted attention to this disorder, large numbers of workers from a variety of occupations reported symptoms of upper extremity pain attributed to their work. Up to one-third of workers in some industries were out of work because of RSI at the peak of the epidemic. Unions encouraged early symptom reporting, and many individuals were advised to stop working and seek compensation. Ergonomic factors were blamed for the condition. Standard treatments for soft tissue injury, such as rest, physical therapy, and injections, were generally not very helpful.

In retrospect, the majority of Australian workers diagnosed to have RSI most likely had localized fibromyalgia. Most had a history of aching or pain in the wrist, elbow, or shoulder that spread to the whole arm and neck. A chronic regional pain syndrome involving the arm, shoulder, neck, and upper chest wall then developed with dysethesias and poor grip in the hand. Tender points were present in the involved region, and there was no evidence of neurologic abnormality, synovitis, or tenosynovitis. Some patients developed reflex sympathetic dystrophy and others the more generalized pain and tender points characteristic of fibromyalgia. Miller and Topliss evaluated 229 consecutive patients who were referred with a diagnosis of RSI.[22] All the patients were receiving workers' compensation. Twenty-nine of the 229 patients fulfilled criteria for a specific rheumatic condition, including 15 with fibromyalgia. The demographic, clinical, and psychological characteristics of the other 200 patients were similar to those in fibromyalgia, except the pain and tender points were usually confined to one anatomic region. Littlejohn[21] postulated that fibromyalgia that occurs in the context of the work place or is related to injury is amplified by compensation systems. Clinical features are exaggerated, and appropriate therapy is often negated by medicolegal issues. The epidemic spread of RSI in Australia has also been viewed as an example of mass hysteria fueled by widespread public acceptance that an "injury" was the cause of the symptoms. Social acceptability thus may play an important role in the clinical expression of musculoskeletal pain problems.

If the medicolegal system is unintentionally promoting incapacity in these situations, how can the system respond more appropriately? McCain, et al.[20] suggest that rehabilitation rather than litigation be the focus of disability claims. In the long run, insurers would gain greatly if patients could be placed back to work earlier with a sophisticated but compassionate rehabilitation program. The short-term costs of the rehabilitation program would be acceptable if insurance companies anticipated that patients would return to work sooner and would be less likely to have a recurrence of their functional disability. Nevertheless, time and fiscal restraints should be incorporated into such a rehabilitation program. Since experience with low back and other chronic pain syndromes indicates that the longer patients are out of work, the less likely it is that they will return to work, it is important that patients receive optimal treatment, including specific rehabilitation, as soon as possible.

SUGGESTIONS FOR EVALUATION AND TREATMENT OF RHEUMATIC CONDITIONS IN THE WORK PLACE

Any discussion of disability related to rheumatic disorders in the work place should begin with a discussion of prevention. Unfortunately, we do not know how to prevent RA or fibromyalgia, nor do we know how to prevent progression of the disease. However, we may be able to prevent disability from the condition if we can modify the work place (Table 15-5). Ergonomic issues that are easy to identify include instruction in lifting, avoidance of prolonged immobility, assessment of optimal chair and desktop height, and provision for some physical and psychological break during the work day. Physically demanding jobs may be more obviously injurious to the patient with chronic rheumatic pain conditions, but, psychologically stressful work, although more difficult to assess, may promote equal impairment. As suggested above, in studies of RA some control over the work

Table 15-5. Recommendations for the Evaluation and Treatment of Rheumatic Conditions in the Work Place

Evaluation of the job
  Physical demands
  Correlation with patient's dysfunction
  Correlation of ergonomic problems
Evaluation of the rheumatic disorder
  Use validated diagnostic criteria
  Measure disease severity, with appropriate instruments
Rehabilitation and treatment program tailored to the patient's condition and the job limitations

schedule appears to be especially important. Job satisfaction is more important than disease severity in determining the ability to work.

However, many of these items are difficult to control in the work place, and even in an optimal job environment, some workers will not be able to continue because of their chronic pain and dysfunction. At that point the patient should undergo a careful evaluation either by the patient's physician or another physician who has significant experience with diagnosis and treatment of the condition. The diagnosis should be validated according to published classification criteria (Table 15-1 and 15-2) and the activity of the condition assessed. This evaluation may include such "objective" measures as a tender joint count, review of x-rays, and blood tests in RA and a tender point count in fibromyalgia. However, just as importantly, instruments that measure the patient's pain experience and psychological state should be administered. They can be as simple as self-administered 10-cm visual analogue scales or as detailed as formal psychiatric and neuropsychological testing, depending on the situation. A team evaluation approach would not only be helpful in documenting the extent of disability but also in designing a specific treatment plan for each patient. For example, the focus of evaluation of a patient with RA who has a severe deformity and loss of power of the hand would be on the dynamics of hand function and its relation to the patient's occupation. Another RA patient with no deformities but severe pain and fatigue may be best evaluated by measures of depression, pain, and sleep.

The results of such evaluations would document the specific impairments that interfere with work, grade their severity, and compare the results to other patients. Most importantly, specific treatment recommendations would be based on the results of the evaluation. Patients would be told openly what their basic limitation is and how they could be treated. If after optimal treatment the patient still cannot return to work, a specific rehabilitation program would be established, taking into account the job and the relationship of the patient's condition to work dysfunction (Table 15-5). For example, the above-mentioned RA patient with limited mobility and decreased strength from arthritis and tenosynovitis of the hand and wrist would be provided with optimal local therapy, possibly including splinting, hand exercises, and corticosteroid injections. Job retraining to decrease the physical demands of the occupation that might be provoking further symptoms would be initiated. In contrast, an RA or fibromyalgia patient unable to work because of generalized pain, fatigue, and stress would be treated with a multidisciplinary approach, including physical therapy, cardiovascular fitness training, cognitive-behavior training, analgesics, and medications, to reduce sleep disturbances, depression, and anxiety.

I work directly with a psychiatric clinical nurse specialist and a psychiatrist and one or both of them see each of my patients with a chronic painful disorder. This is very helpful for diagnostic purposes to formally determine levels of anxiety, stress, and depression. These professionals form the nucleus of a mind-body treatment program that emphasizes relaxation techniques and coping skills. As mentioned, the rehabilitation program must be initiated as soon as possible, and the focus of the medicolegal issues should be on getting the patient back to work, not on proving that disability is persistent and that one is entitled to compensation.

SUMMARY

In conclusion, occupational aspects of chronic rheumatic disorders are difficult to evaluate and often defy traditional treatment approaches. Most of these disorders fall into the second category mentioned in the introductory chapter of this book: "Diagnosis is established, but treatment for the condition is not always successful and the prognosis for returning to the job is unclear." Two such chronic rheumatic conditions, RA and fibromyalgia, were selected as models for the development of recommendations for the evaluation and treatment of rheumatic disorders in the work place. Despite their clinical and pathophysiologic differences, both of these chronic painful disorders cause significant and similar loss of work productivity and time. Psychosocial, demographic, and specific job characteristics are as important or more important than disease severity in determining disability in chronic rheumatic conditions. Therefore, the evaluation process and rehabilitation recommendations must assess each of these factors carefully if we are to lessen the impact of such chronic illnesses on the worker.

REFERENCES

1. Harris ED Jr: The clinical features of rheumatoid arthritis, p. 643. In Kelley WN, Harris ED Jr, Ruddy S, Sledge CB (eds): Textbook of Rheumatology. 3rd Ed. WB Saunders Co, Philadelphia, 1989

2. Goldenberg DL: Fibromyalgia syndrome. JAMA 257:2782, 1987

3. Wolfe F, Smythe HA, Yunus MB et al: The American College of Rheumatology 1990 criteria for the classification of fibromyalgia. Arthritis Rheum 33:160, 1990

4. Carey T, Hadler N, Gillings D, Stinnett S, Wallston T: Medical disability assessment of the back pain patient for the Social Security Administration: the weighting of presenting clinical features. J Clin Epidemiol 41:691, 1988

5. Tait R, Margolis R, Krause S, Leibowitz E: Compensation status and symptoms reported by patients with chronic pain. Arch Phys Med Rehabil 69:1027, 1988

6. Yelin E, Meenan R, Nevitt M, Epstein W: Work disability in rheumatoid arthritis: effects of disease, social, and work factors. Ann Intern Med 93:551, 1980

7. Mitchell JM, Burkhauser RV, Pincus T: The importance of age, education, and comorbidity in the substantial earnings losses of individuals with symmetric polyarthritis. Arthritis Rheum 31:348, 1988

8. Reisine ST, Grady KE, Goodenow C, Fifield J: Work disability among women with rheumatoid arthritis. Arthritis Rheum 32:538, 1989

9. Hagglund KJ, Haley WE, Reveille JD, Alarcon GS: Predicting individual differences in pain and functional impairment among patients with rheumatoid arthritis. Arthritis Rheum 32:851, 1989

10. Nicassio PM, Wallston KA, Callahan LF, Herbert M, Pincus T: The measurement of helplessness in rheumatoid arthritis: the development of the Arthritis Helplessness Index. J Rheumatol 12:462, 1985

11. Radin EL: Mechanical aspects of osteoarthrosis. Bull Rheum Dis 26:862, 1975

12. Ho G Jr, Tice AD, Kaplan SR: Septic bursitis in the prepatellar and olecranon bursae. Ann Intern Med 89:21, 1978

13. Schwartzman RJ, McLellan TL: Reflex sympathetic dystrophy. Arch Neurol 44:555, 1987

14. Kozin F: Reflex sympathetic dystrophy syndrome. Bull Rheum Dis 36:1, 1986

15. Felson DT, Goldenberg DL: The natural history of fibromyalgia. Arthritis Rheum 29:1522, 1986

16. Hawley DJ, Wolfe F, Cathey MA: Pain, functional disability, and psychological status: a 12-month study of severity in fibromyalgia. J Rheumatol 15:1551, 1988

17. Cathey MA, Wolfe F, Kleinheksel SM: Functional ability and work status in patients with fibromyalgia. Arthritis Care Res 1:85, 1988

18. Mason JH, Simms RW, Goldenberg DL, Meenan RF: The impact of fibromyalgia on work: a comparison with RA. Arthritis Rheum (suppl), 32:S36, 1989

19. Cathey MA, Wolfe F, Roberts FK, et al: Demographic, work disability, service utilization and treatment characteristics of 544 fibromyalgia patients in rheumatologic practice. Arthritis Rheum, suppl. 33:S10, 1990

20. McCain GA, Cameron R, Kennedy JC: The problem of longterm disability payments and litigation in primary fibromyalgia: the Canadian perspective. J Rheumatol, suppl. 19. 16:174, 1989

21. Littlejohn G: Medicolegal aspects of fibrositis syndrome. J Rheumatol, suppl. 19. 16:169, 1989

22. Miller MH, Topliss DJ: Chronic upper limb pain syndrome (repetitive strain injury) in the Australian workforce: a systematic cross sectional rheumatological study of 220 patients. J Rheumatol 15:1705, 1988

16

Psychological Factors in Upper Extremity Disorders: Pain as a Paradigm

Theodore Nadelson, M.D.

All physicians are trained to deal primarily with infirmity bounded by the skin, within the *body*, as opposed to the *mind*. This mind versus body dualistic construct is the background against which even the most rigorous physicians ask their psychiatric consultant, "Is this condition organic or functional"? For the clinician a major question is,"Do the complaints derive from a *disease state* within the body, or to a greater degree are they a manifestation of *sickness* derived from the psychosocial factors and secondarily referred to the body?" This question is frequently asked about in occupational injury to the upper extremity because of the recognized complexity of the forces that add up to disability, and most experienced clinicians accept most complaints as potentially deriving from a mixture of organic and psychosocial factors.

All physicians, including psychiatrists, are committed to not missing physical disease when it is present. Bodily and emotionally derived complaints are also mixed in varying degrees. The patient may have symptoms and signs indicating real disease, but these seem out of proportion to the intensity of complaint. Some groups of patients create symptoms and also magnify them.[1] Many surgeons have greatest difficulty with this very common occurrence. They feel deceived, manipulated, and misused.[2] Frustration and anger toward the patient may interfere with treatment.

It has long been recognized that patients frequently seek physicians for psychological reasons while presenting with bodily complaints. Estimates vary, but internists report that, although patients may have disease within their body space, 40 percent come to an appointment because of emotional disequilibrium.[3–5]

THE PATIENT: THE SICK ROLE

A person grows up bounded by a culture that shapes family and individual behavior, perception, and expectations.

That which is acceptable as social behavior is one society is not in another. All societies clearly define, but in widely varying ways, that which is socially acceptable. In every cohesive human society without exception, there are people designated as healers/doctor for the sick. (Indeed that is one of the factors that defines a particular society as cohesive). Members of every society recognize the needs of members, who in falling ill and seeking help, become patients and then take on a different role.[6]

As a socially defined role, patienthood has implicit yet fairly clear expectations. If societal expectations are met, the person who has become ill is granted special consideration. Consider the man who is drunk, sitting unnoticed on the curbstone. He suddenly lurches forward and becomes a patient the instant that a car hits him. he is taken to the nearby hospital, where he is treated with the respect assigned to patients. A patient has a recognized disturbance of capacity that is the result of accident; that is, the patient cannot be held responsible for the incapacity. The sick person is further exempted from the usual obligations. Within this legitimate state, the sick person is expected

(only) to cooperate with caretakers to shed patienthood as quickly as possible. There is an implied obligation to prevent further illness as well.[7]

It is to be understood that this description does not hold for every patient; on the contrary, this definition describes only expected societal norms. Many patients deviate from such expectations.

A SPECTRUM OF DISEASE PRESENTATION

The Real Patient

From within the understanding of the social norm for patienthood, there can be arrayed a spectrum of disease presentation, starting with those patients who are conventionally seen as having "real" disease (Table 16-1). Those are the patients defined above under patienthood. Such patients are placed in a purely medical category and are the primary focus of medical training, yet this group of patients should best be viewed as *ideal*, rather than as usual and expectable. Many such patients, at another time, with or

Table 16-1.   The Spectrum of Disease Presentation

The Real or Ideal Patient	Psychological Factors Contributing to Disorder ("Psychosomatic" or "Psychophysiologic")	Abnormal Illness Behavior
Infection, trauma, metabolic disease, cancer	Obesity, gastric ulcer, dysmenorrhea, asthma, tension headache, etc.	False patients Munchausen (primary gain) Malingerers (secondary gain)
	Somataform: industrial syndromes (e.g. "RSI") and chronic pain disorders	
	Volitional production of symptoms and signs	
No psychic factors	Unaware of wish for sickness	Aware of production of symptoms? Signs of illness

without awareness, may take part in producing their illness.

The Abnormal Illness Spectrum of Behavior

A category designated "abnormal illness behavior"[8] does not occupy a formal position in the pantheon of diagnostic categories. It is helpful, however, for our present purpose, to use this broad and general category for the varied presentation of patients who somatize psychological issues.

Munchausen and Malingering

Many patients use physical symptoms to obtain emotional rewards for past emotional hurt or as a way of compensating for a chronic sense or conviction of past personal injustice. This is often termed "primary gain". At the far end of the spectrum are those we designate as disease simulators or as having the Munchausen syndrome, which is designated more officially as Factitious Disorder. For reasons about which they have only the barest recognition, these patients have as the center of their life a preoccupation, approaching on addictive drive, with confusing the physician by false complaints of bodily symptoms. Such patients also may secretly take medications, inject foreign substances, or use any other means (limited only by the imagination) to produce the signs that will validate the complaint. The Munchausen patient, although aware that a deception is practiced, is mostly unaware of the underlying motivation. That lack of awareness follows for only a quasi-legitimization by society of such behavior. Munchausen patients are barely within acceptable limits of psychiatric diagnosis.[9]

A further distinction is drawn regarding malingerers, who are placed in the category of "conditions not attributable to psychiatric disorder." Such people are motivated by secondary gain: monetary gain, "avoidance of duty, evading criminal prosecution, obtaining drugs, and securing better living conditions."[10] Such patients are really nonpatients and are neither in the medical category nor in a psychiatric one. Malingerers have been called "false patients" as well.[5]

Abnormal illness behavior lies between the "ideal patient" and the malingerer. It is found, in widely varying degrees, among all people. There is a common human tendency to claim sickness as a means of avoiding emotionally troubling situations or relationships or burdensome work, if not chronically then at times when one is feeling "down." (Perhaps some readers may have wished for a little sickness so as to be cared for, in bed, for a day. Parents may indulge such a wish as a means of comforting a child in the midst of transient despondency or disappointment). It is inaccurate to view the occasional use of the sick role as an example of psychopathology or moral turpitude. Psychological categorization is earned when there is a continuous reflexive presentation of bodily illness without a bodily source for the complaint or when such complaints are disproportionate to the objective findings.

> Mr S, a 45-year-old drill press operator, had seen the same internist for many years. His physician had long recognized that his patient sought medical help often for seemingly trivial reasons. His doctor identified the patient as a very dependent person, resenting social and work obligations. When the physician left on vacation, the patient usually responded with a downturn in health. The patient would call often, for very little "real" reason.
>
> He was similarly dependent on family members. When his wife was about to

leave on a trip to visit her ill mother in Canada, he presented with a very painful shoulder. He said that it had been "coming on for a while," that it was in some way related to work but that he had managed to bear it. While at work, performing the familiar task of lifting a box of metal parts up to his work station, he experienced a "sharp pain," which exacerbated the more chronic ache. He was unable now to function at work, and he was severely restricted with regard to his ability to perform household chores.

The internist referred the patient to an orthopaedist surgeon he knew, who specialized in occupational disorders, with the suggestion that perhaps the patient "really needed a psychiatrist." The orthopaedist, also feeling the problem was psychosomatic, suggested a psychiatric consultant as well. The patient did not see the psychiatrist, but later called his internist and asked resentfully if the orthopaedist "thought he was "crazy." The orthopaedist had asked some questions about the connection between the complaint and his wife's absence.

Somatoform Disorder

The term "somatization of psychological problems" is also used, and patients who habitually present with complaints about their body without objective findings are categorized as Somatoform Disorder. These patients feel that their symptoms are real and that such strongly felt symptoms must arise from some definite disturbance or injury to their body; they are not aware of any personal attempt at deception. They either seek or welcome illness, disability, or patienthood. Patients who present with somatic disorder, when there are underlying psychological or social issues motivating them, tend to be "attached" to the somatic presentation. *They are, again, often refractory to attempts directed toward erasing the physical manifestation.* Even when there are recognized psychiatric symptoms, such as

depression the effective treatment may alter mood positively without at all affecting somatization.[11]

The largest group of patients seen by orthopaedists, however, are those patients with some tissue damage, with a specific bodily reason for complaint, but who magnify symptoms out of all proportion to the more objective signs elicited and observed. These patients can be placed on the spectrum between psychosomatic patients and those who manifest abnormal illness behavior. They often have less than adequate coping skills, and in the case of industrially related complaints they are often angry (perhaps for valid enough reason), at those in authority toward whom they simultaneously feel dependent. In their hopelessness and frustration they regress to a presentation of sickness or disability to claim attention or money or as a way of manifesting resentment from within the relatively safe haven of victim. Such patients complain then of what psychiatrists call "equivalents"; that is, pain as an equivalent of hopelessness, frustration, or depression. Rather than complaining of psychological problems as such, these patients complain of bodily symptoms.

In occupational injuries the orthopaedist may be the first echelon of care receiving patients and may see a greater number of somatoform patients. The usual impetus for the sick role—dependent wishes found in greater or lesser degree in everyone—is often compounded by anger at the employer or the family for being tied to labor that is burdensome and unrewarding. There is another usual human motivation: the injured worker feels supported and justified in seeking money when injury is perceived as coming out of onerous work. That feeling reinforced by social forces that compensate psychologically driven behavior deriving from the past and a sense of injustice, rather than from anatomical injury.

For some personality types, all work leads to the perception of being used. Patients with life-long histories of dependence on others, a spotty work history, or prior claims for disability should alert the physician to the possibility (possibility only) that they have an "agenda" other than relief from pain or dysfunction in seeking medical help. Deep understanding of such personal motivation may not be available to the patients' consciousness; indeed a large portion of their psychological defenses is arrayed against such self-awareness. That state of affairs is both common and frustrating to physicians who early on recognize that they are not struggling with natural occurrence or accident but rather, with a facet of human nature.

PSYCHIATRIC ISSUES IN CLINICAL MANAGEMENT

An Empathic Approach to Surgical Care

When patients' complaints fail to yield an etiology within the body after the usual methods of clinical or laboratory assessment are completed, orthopaedists may correctly say, "We cannot yet find the physical cause for your (fatigue, pain, disability). Sometimes, such conditions are very much affected as well by psychological factors." In other words, physicians "hedge their bets"; to do otherwise can be damaging to their patients who may angrily respond to a perceived attack with the reply, "So you think that it is *all* in my head?"

W. B. was a 44-year-old lineman with 15 years of good work record at the telephone company. When he was initially seen, the orthopaedist noted classic signs and symptoms of lateral epicondylitis and treated the patient with a wrist splint and ibuprofen and then recommended light duty for 3 weeks. The patient returned improved in the doctor's judgment, but still complaining of pain. The orthopaedists further questioning revealed, in an emotional statement, that the "supervisor was hassling [him]." The patient started rehabilitative therapy, was taken off work, but symptoms persisted. A cortisone injection provided only temporary relief.

With time and subsequent visits, it became increasingly clear to the orthopaedist that the patient was magnifying the degree of pain; he was overly dramatic in his grimace as he grasped the lateral side of his arm. He claimed that he could not hold a glass of milk and indeed demonstrated that by dropping a glass in front of the surgeon. He repeatedly stated his wish to go back to work, but re-emphasized that his supervisor was "on him all the time" and would be quick to blame and fire him. He stressed that he wanted an operation for cure.

The orthopaedist sensed that the patient felt unvalued and vulnerable at work and that the patient's supervisor gave him little credit for his effort. While indicating that the patient would not gain from an operation, the surgeon underscored the positive potential of physical therapy. In addition, realizing that the patient felt troubled by a supervisor who did not value him, the doctor was direct in his support; he suggested that he might intervene on behalf of the patient with the supervisor. He further supported the value the patient placed in being hard working. The orthopaedist allowed the patient to borrow some of his own strength in identifying with him: "You are a hard-working man, like me, not laid back." He convinced the patient, along with support from the patient's wife, of the necessity of physical therapy as opposed to therapy. The patient made a recovery and went back to work.

In this case, the orthopaedist made use of his own feelings regarding the patient's needs. He sensed that there was an emotional component to the patient's persistent symptoms and dramatic presentation and saw the failure of the rehabilitation procedure as related in a major way to the patient's diminished self-esteem. His intervention lent to the patient that which the patient needed during a time of emotional vulnerability. The orthopaedist was *psychotherapeutic* in his attention after he had made a correct surgical anatomic diagnosis. Although not all orthopaedists may feel inclined toward such activity, it is demonstrably valuable for the patient. There are patients for whom the physician's psychological support is far more important than that which can be given by a psychiatrist. *For any patient and at any time, the sense of respect, value, and of being understood are valuable adjuncts to any surgical diagnosis or intervention.*

An *empathic* response by a physician does not contest the patient's subjective experience and initiate a struggle. Rather the physician sees the situation from within the patient's psychological framework and responds to the patient from that perspective. From that position, it is less awkward and more convincing to suggest a visit to a psychiatrist when such consultation is appropriate. For those occasions when referral to a mental health professional is appropriate, try the following statements when referring a patient whom you see as resistant to psychiatric intervention:

- "This pain is a burden to you; it would be to anyone. You might be helped by seeing someone who can help you bear the pain, and possibly help your functioning."
- "I frequently ask a psychiatric colleague of mine for consultation in cases like your own where the patient has an extra burden of pain. Sometimes their particular insight can be helpful;

sometimes they help by suggesting medication. You are having a really difficult, painful time."

Pain

Pain is endemic in the United States where $100 billion is spent on chronic pain syndromes annually. This represents 25 percent of the annual health care budget.[12]

A generally accepted definition of pain comes from the International Association for the Study of Pain (IASP): **An unpleasant sensory and emotional experience associated with actual or potential tissue damage or described in terms of such damage.**[13]

Pain is best viewed as an individual perception, a subjective experience that has origins in pathophysiology, development, and personality and the patient's social context as well. Conceptually separable but interacting forces designated as biologic, psychological, and social are incorporated into the biopsychosocial model. This interaction is viewed as the modern meaning of the "psychosomatic concept."[14] Afferents from the brain to an injured limb mediate the perception of pain at the spinal cord level and possibly at the periphery as well. The modulation of such pain and its perception stem from a multiconvergence of sources.

Six components of pain can be a useful guide for a clinical description.[13]

1. *Pain sensation*: The actual experience of the pain as reported by the patient.
2. *Pain behavior*: The mode or manner in which the experience is conveyed; restriction of movement, grimaces, groans, and use of and requests for medication are behaviors related to pain.
3. *Functional status at work*: How does the patient function at work? How is

that related to muscle strength and endurance as assessed by testing?

4. *Functional status at home*: How does the pain patient function at home in relation to physical tasks? To the prior role in the family? What is the role and relationship with the children? With the spouse socially and sexually?

5. *Emotional state*: Does the pain follow an extremely anxious state, or does the pain state precede affective change? Often, patients have an increased sensation of pain after specific stresses that result in emotional shifts. Such emotional change is often expressed somatically. Depressed people may express their affect as a somatic equivalent, i.e., as pain or fatigue. Anxiety may also alter pain perception and increase or decrease it. (At times of extreme stress one can see a diminution of pain perception. A woman carried an infant out of a wrecked automobile, carefully laid the child safely on the ground. She did not complain of pain until it was noticed that she was bleeding. A physician found comminuted fractures of both arms).

6. *Somatic preoccupation*: Somatic preoccupation is the degree of sensitivity or attention to the pain. The patient who is continually attentive to any bodily discomfort is often refractory to change, and complaints remain high whatever treatment is instituted. *Patients who have a high level of this part of the pain picture should be told that the pain can be reduced, not usually eliminated.* Pain is often just one component of hypochondriacal concerns, as in this case example.

A 51-year-old woman complained of multiple aches and pains with an almost "entirely positive review of systems." Her main complaint was "soreness in the shoulders," which she said made it impossible to work at her household jobs; mopping up floors had just "completely worn out her shoulders." Moving her upper arm caused great pain, and as she rotated her shoulder she grimaced. She had just finished a 3-day "bout of the flu" (with no temperature elevation). She had an entirely full range of motion and no tenderness in her upper extremity. During the examination she made frequent references, however, to "pain in the ribs," "ear pain," "headache," and "fatigue." The examining physician indicated that she might have "post-flu syndrome," and asked a psychiatrist to see her before she left the clinic.

The psychiatrist started by saying that the patient "seemed burdened." The patient immediately spoke about the recent death of her son-in-law (a "big strong man who was very care taking of her now-widowed daughter) and of the necessity of helping in the care of his children. She worked as a domestic because her husband "never made a large enough salary" and placed "all the responsibility on me." She then said loudly, emphasizing her words with a pounding fist on the table, "Do you know, I was wishing they would put me in the hospital today, so that I could just stay in bed and not have to get up!" She left the office feeling "a bit better." "You know it feels good to talk to someone, sometimes," was her final remark.

Although the patient may have had a viral illness with attendant muscular ache, her long-standing grievance with her husband was being presented somatically. The psychological functions of such presentation are multiple:

- The patient can get rest and care, somewhat free of the guilt attendant on not meeting her obligations.
- She can covertly register her objections against a husband who has not provided her with wished-for caretaking.
- She avoids direct confrontation and the stress of directly presenting her own anger, which she psychologically de-

fends against by denial and avoidance and, now, somatization.

- She attempts to legitimize her position by seeking patienthood. She is then in the more respectable position of victim of somatic injury, rather than an aggressive, demanding woman.

Types of Pain

Acute Pain.   Psychological or psychiatric understanding of pain is not usually applicable to acute pain, although psychiatrists are sometimes consulted with regard to failure in analgesic control of acute pain or about concerns regarding addiction to narcotic analgesics or adjunctive anxiolytics (see section on Acute Pain Management).

Chronic Pain.   Chronic or intractable pain differs from acute pain in that there is no value to the individual in the pain; it is "useless, malevolent and destructive."[12] Rather than having its origins solely in somatic injury, it is an imperfectly understood entity deriving from both somatic and psychosocial forces. Tissue damage that may have been present at the initiation of the syndrome ceases to be the continuing generator of behaviors that are personally and socially maladaptive.

The orthopaedist trying to arrest this ongoing pernicious situation must realize the following:

- Chronic pain behavior is complex and derives from multiconvergent causes that include probably, tissue injury as well as equally strong psychosocial factors.
- The orthopaedist did not create the situation; the exercise of skill, talent, tools, experience, and his or her own need to repair will be limited by the patient's capacity.
- The patient's anger is important in that it often makes the patient unavailable to further help.

- The orthopaedist should first discuss the somatic etiology of the pain. Patients always fear that the physician will tell them that it is "*all* in their head."

For example, do *not* say: "You really cannot have the pain (or amount of pain) of which you complain," or "This all seems more psychological than physical. I will refer you to a psychiatrist/shrink." Rather, it is better to say the following:

> We know that you have suffered from the burden of pain, and we are not able to pinpoint a cause. Given the results of the extensive examinations we may not be able to do so. There are ways to live with burdens, even if we cannot eliminate them. We should strive for bringing back some of your *function*, helping your family/social life by therapy of various forms.

This introduction can be followed by a general outline of forms of rehabilitation. Among those approaches the potential for help from psychiatry may be included.

"Six D's", have been defined by Engelberg,[12] any two of which should be considered to characterize chronic pain:

- *Duration*: A diagnosis of chronic pain can be made within 2 or 3 weeks (rather than at 6 weeks as more usually indicated)
- *Dramatization*: dramatic gestures and vocal mannerisms (moaning, posturing)
- *Drugs*: use of multiple drugs
- *Despair*: the patient is close to surrendering hope; the ability to cope has deteriorated; the patient becomes bitter and irritable
- *Disuse*: the patient protects the extremity by not using—by self-splinting which can result in secondary pain that is exacerbated rather than helped by physical therapy
- *Dysfunction*: with increasing disuse and secondary pain, the patient may withdraw from normal activities; "bereft of social contacts, shunned by loved

ones. . .isolated. . .and deprived of financial sustenance, the patient becomes an. . .invalid in the physical, emotional, social and economic sense"[12]

Somatoform Pain Disorder. Psychological factors are always present in any situation of chronic pain. Indeed, such features are to be viewed as a component in the multiconvergence of forces resulting in pain perception and chronic pain behavior. The somewhat rare somatoform pain disorder is discussed here because of the understandable clinical confusion regarding this category.

The essential features characterizing the somatoform disorders are physical symptoms for which there is no demonstrable organic finding and/or known physiologic mechanism, with positive evidence or a strong presumption that the complaint is linked to psychological factors. Such psychological factors include the predisposition to somatizing (i.e., presenting psychological needs in the form of a somatic complaint), obvious dependency needs, the primary and secondary gains attendant on physical symptoms, identification with important others who have pain, and chronic low levels of despondency (a characteristic that may "run in the family"), which blooms into major depression at times. Psychiatrists use the term "masked depression" to describe a patient's presentation to the physician with pain as an "equivalent" for the basic emotional distress. Such patients characteristically feel despondent because they are "getting less than they deserve." Unaware that they are in pursuit of their idiosyncratic view of what is equitable, they then may present to the orthopaedist with chronic pain from an industrial trauma. Because they have a need to demonstrate the extent of their victimization and distress, they present symptoms far in excess of what the orthopaedist would expect from such anatomic stress.

Repetitive Strain Injury (RSI). Some clinical investigators hold the view that repetitive activity (usually at an occupation) may cause strain and attendant physical injury resulting in pain and dysfunction; this disorder is termed repetitive strain injury (RSI) or overuse syndrome.[15] RSI is often presented as localized form of fibromyalgia (or fibrositis), but there has been continuing evidence of the effect of psychosocial forces enhancing an individual's adoption of abnormal illness behavior.

RSI symptoms may be shaped by the social acceptability of financial gain from employment in the form of workers' compensation benefits. Such symptoms have been characterized as the "golden wrist" or "kangaroo paw," both indicating the motivation and the epidemic extent of the complaint in Australia.[16] One view, presented after a systematic study in which specific rheumatologic diagnoses were ruled out, suggests the primary and overwhelming (almost 90 percent) etiologic influence of social factors in chronic rheumatic syndrome, such as RSI. The authors temper what could be explicit criticism of the patients: the "great majority", they conclude, "are not defrauding the workman's compensation system."[17] Rather they are to be seen as victims themselves because the compensation system, initially directed toward helping the injured in the work force, has become the largest factor in promoting incapacity. Eliminating the terms "RSI" and "overuse syndrome" is suggested to curb the tendency of more susceptible workers to convert "soft tissue discomfort into a chronic traumatic pain syndrome.[17] Other Australian investigators have commented earlier than the social system supports dysfunction and "compensation neurosis."[18,19] Suggestions have been made for rehabilitation programs to offset the enormous costs of such disabilities, instead of the delivery of rewards to patients (and lawyers) through litigation.[20]

Medication Use, Chronicity and Abuse

Although a usual response to pain is to seek pharmacologic relief, the relationship of the prescriber to the patient is extremely important. The manner in which medication is dispensed is a long recognized and powerful factor in its effectiveness. An understanding of the patient's psychological social context and relationship to family and occupation should be imbedded in a treatment plan that includes physical rehabilitation, education counseling, and *medication as an adjunct* to the goal of increased functioning.

When the pain is acute, or when adequate trials of NSAIDs been tried, the question is raised about the use of the opiates, centrally acting analgesics. There is often concern regarding addiction. It should be said that all patients who are appropriately prescribed controlled substances are not on a collision course toward addiction. The prescribing physician, aware of the pitfalls of overmedication, should also be aware of the dangers of its opposite.[21]

Management of Acute Pain

The management of acute pain is not usually within the psychiatrist's arena. However, consultation is sometimes requested regarding the use of centrally acting analgesics (i.e., opiates or tranquilizers because of potential addiction problems), when there is a lack of pain relief with what is judged to be adequate amounts of medication, or when a patient seems to be feigning acute pain and seeking such controlled substances. There is understandably a great deal of concern on the part of the physicians, patient, family, and insurance companies regarding the use of narcotic analgesics. The potential use of analgesic medications for pleasure—for a high or a "buzz"—is bound to make the prescriber concerned.

If strong medication is to be used it should be tried as an adequate dosage in which it is presumed to have an effect and the dosage should be increased, short of toxicity, until it is effective. (That does not imply "pain-free"; only that the pain is manageable). Medication should also be given at a regular dosage, with *only adjunctive use on an as-needed basis.* Prescribing on a PRN basis leads to "ping-ponging" the patient between pain and sedation.

Management of Chronic Pain

The pharmacologic management of chronic pain is best shifted toward the antidepressants. Morphine derivatives alone are not effective in chronic pain management. The older group of tricyclic antidepressants (TCAs)—imipramine and amitriptyline and its derivatives—in relatively smaller amounts than used for depression are often effective in restoring function. However, it should not be assumed by the patient or the physician that these medications will ease all painful sensation. The newer, nontricyclic antidepressants—trazodone (Desyrel), fluoxetine (Prozac), bupropion (Welbutrin)—are probably equally effective in reducing chronic pain and often, but not invariably, have fewer side effects.

TCA side effects can be severe for many patients and, even in relatively low doses for chronic pain (compared to their use in depression), can cause anticholinergic side effects—dry mouth, constipation, excessive sweating, decreased libido and impotence. The negative effect on sexual function is exerted by trazodone and fluoxetine. Dose can be regulated, up or down, and different medications tried in order to achieve an acceptable balance.

Chronic use of a medication does not imply addiction or habituation. Medications in the benzodiazepine category—alprazolam (Xanax), lorazepam (Ativan), and diazepam (Valium)—given to calm anxiety and as an adjunct to pain management are effective and safe within the boundaries of the usual prescribed dose. Although some patients with addictive tendencies overuse medications and attempts to get more, the typical patient tries to avoid overuse. The chronically anxious patient usually does not overuse medication, but often uses less than is needed.[22]

There are times when physicians out of concern for iatrogenic addiction will try a clinical trial of placebo dosing. The general experience of this author and others is that such an attempt is not worth the risk of the patient perceiving the medical deception. If the placebo does work, very little information is garnered because a placebo works ordinarily and routinely. Why else do drug manufacturers commit themselves to the great expense of double-blind studies? Important questions revolve around use, chronic use, abuse, and habituation/addiction. Orthopaedists, in an attempt to deliver their patients from pain, have no wish to become a part of an iatrogenic addiction. The ethical *and* legal responsibility looms large. Some surgeons do not prescribe needed strong analgesics because of concern about being identified as a doctor who "gives highs." Triplicate prescriptions and other means of tracking controlled substances similarly make the orthopaedist concerned with legal investigation. No one wants the reputation of being a major dispenser of addictive drugs.

Chronic pain should be managed according to these guidelines:

- Never tell the patient that the pain is all in his or her head.
- Never tell the patient that the medication will make pain disappear *or* even that the medication will lessen the pain. Rather tell the patient that the medication is an adjunct to a general plan of rehabilitation, the important goal of which is restoration of function. The patient may be able to live with some pain. Your purpose is not to eliminate pain totally, because even if you could, the patient would then not achieve the primary goal; restoration of as much function as is possible.

Be wary of the patient with a history of substance abuse when prescribing any analgesic that affects mood as well. This does not mean that you cannot use such drugs at all. Some patients have a minor addiction problem, or they have recovered from it. The most successful recovered substance abusers often avoid any controlled narcotic medications. All physicians do well to heed their patients in such cases. They may know the limits of their own ability to withstand temptation better than the prescriber.

REFERENCES

1. Barsky A, Klerman G: Hypochondriasis, bodily complaints and somatic styles. Am J Psychiatr 140:273, 1983
2. Lipsitt DR: Medical and psychological characteristics of "crocks." Psychiatr Med 1:15, 1970
3. Hoeper E, Nycz G, Regier D et al: A diagnosis of mental disorder in adults and increased use of health services in four outpatients' settings. Am J Psychiatr 137:207, 1980
4. Ford CV: The Somatizing Disorders. Elesevier, New York, 1983
5. Nadelson T: False patients/real patients: A spectrum of disease simulation. Psychother Psychosom 44:175, 1985
6. Henderson S: Care eliciting behavior in man. J Nerv Ment Dis 159:172, 1979
7. Parsons T: Social Structure and Personality. Free Press, New York, 1964

8. Pilowsky I: Abnormal illness behavior. Br J Med Psychol 42:347, 1969

9. Nadelson T: The Munchausen spectrum: borderline character features. Gen Hosp Psychiatr 1:11, 1979

10. American Psychiatric Association: The Diagnostic and Statistical Manual of Psychiatric Disorders. 3rd Ed. rev. American Psychiatric Press Inc, Washington, 1987

11. Katon W, Ries R, Kleinman A: A prospective DSM II study of 100 consecutive patients. Compr Psychiatr 25:305, 1984

12. Engelberg AL: Guides to Permanent Evaluation of Permanent Impairment. American Medical Association, Chicago, 1988

13. Feuerstein M: Definitions of pain, p. 2. In Tollison CD (ed): Handbook of Chronic Pain Management. Williams & Wilkins, Baltimore, 1989

14. Leigh H, Reiser M: Major trends in psychosomatic medicine: the psychiatrist's evolving role in medicine. Ann Intern Med 87:233, 1977

15. Browne CD, Nolan BM, Faithfull DK: Occupational repetition strain injuries: guidelines for diagnosis and management. Med J Aust 140:329, 1984

16. Auerbach M: RSI or kangaroo paw (letter). Med J Aust 142:237, 1984

17. Miller MH, Topliss DJ: Chronic upper limb pain syndrome repetitive strain injury in the Australian workforce: a systematic cross sectional rheumatological study of 229 patients. J Rheumatol 15:1705, 1988

18. Ellard J: Psychological reactions to compensable injury. Med J Aust 2:349, 1974

19. Rickarby G: Compensation neurosis and the psycho-social requirements of the family. Br J Med Psychol 52:333, 1979

20. McCain GA, Cameron R, Kennedy JC: The problem of longterm disability payments and litigation in fibromyalgia: the Canadian perspective. J Rheumatol, suppl. 19. 16:174, 1989

21. Marks RM, Sachar EJ: Undertreatment of medical patients with analgesics. Ann Intern Med 78:174, 1973

22. DuPont RL: Thinking about stopping treatment for panic disorder. J Clin Psychiatr, suppl A. 51:38, 1990

17

Unique Upper Extremity Disorders of Musicians

Michael E. Charness, M.D.

INSTRUMENTAL MUSICIANS AS A UNIQUE OCCUPATIONAL GROUP

Musicians constitute a unique occupational group. Training often begins in early childhood, and professional activity may be sustained throughout life. Arthur Rubinstein, the legendary pianist, began playing at the age of 3 and continued to delight audiences until the age of 90, when macular degeneration forced his retirement. For hours daily, musicians maintain bizarre postures and bear the weight of instruments on their hands while their fingers strike keys repetitively or depress strings with remarkable accuracy and rapidity. Not surprisingly, musicians are subject to a variety of upper extremity disorders that arise from playing.[1-8] Although in some respects, musicians resemble workers in other occupations that require sustained, repetitive use of the hands, they stand alone in the demands, longevity, and competitiveness of their careers.

The financial loss from even mild disability can be enormous for musicians. Salaries in the music profession are high for a very small group; the starting pay for major American symphony orchestras was just under $60,000 in the 1990-1991 season[9] and up to 200 musicians may compete for a single orchestral position. There are few comparable jobs in music for orchestral players whose talents are eroded by injury. Moreover, many musicians, who have devoted their lives to their art, bring few skills to a new occupation.

To lose the ability to play is to lose more than one's livelihood. For professionals or amateurs, making music is a lifelong joy (there are few amateur meatpackers or check-out clerks), and its potential loss is a source of profound anxiety and depression. Moreover, playing provides an important release from stress, which is lost when most needed. Thus, occupational injury in musicians affords little secondary gain and engenders a fierce drive to return to health and work. Issues of litigation or malingering are rarely prominent, distinguishing musicians from office or assembly line workers, whose occupational injury might be associated with considerable secondary gain.

Musicians are also unique in the degree to which mild dysfunction can produce disability.[3,10] There are pieces in the repertoire of virtually every instrument that are unplayable by all but a few virtuosi. Even within the mainstream of the repertoire, musicians, from celebrities to amateurs, are required to execute feats of neuromuscular learning and performance that would be unimaginable for a professional athlete or high-speed typist. Consequently, extremely mild degrees of hand dysfunction quickly expand the repertoire of unplayable pieces and rapidly invade the performance of easier literature. Some disorders, such as cubital tunnel syndrome or occupational cramp, can disable musicians before they would be recognized by nonmusicians.[3,8,11] This fact poses unique problems in both diagnosis and management.

When symptoms occur only with playing, the history will be presented in the language of music: difficulty with octaves, rapid passage work, intonation, trills, and double stops. More familiar complaints related to gripping pots, opening jars, or manipulating coins appear later—sometimes too late to prevent disability. Familiarity with musical jargon can be invaluable, but any physician can gain considerable insight by taking a detailed performance history.

Physical findings may be unimpressive compared to subjective complaints because playing is often a more sensitive bioassay than the physical examination or electrodiagnostic studies.[3,11] It is therefore particularly helpful to watch an injured musician play. Very slight neuropathic weakness may produce instability at certain joints, rendering clumsy the normally rapid, efficient, and effortless finger movements of a skilled performer. Minor interosseous weakness may cause a violinist to play out of tune. The occupational cramps may be evident only during particular passages; for example, ascending but not descending scales. A musician's performance may also reveal technical idiosyncrasies that contribute to the disorder, such as excessive wrist flexion in carpal tunnel syndrome. In many instances, the appropriate treatment may be a prosthesis for the instrument, rather than for the patient, or a referral to a good teacher, rather than to a good surgeon.

Musicians interpret and recreate the great range of human moods and emotions. As artists, they are sometimes regarded by their audiences and physicians as mercurial, volatile, and sensitive. Although it might be tempting to invoke psychosomatic explanations for symptoms that dwarf findings, emotional problems appear to play a small role in the genesis of playing-related upper extremity disorders.[5,6]

Thus, music is set apart from all other occupations by the early training, career longevity, unique demands on the upper extremity, requirement for neuromuscular perfection, and susceptibility to mild dysfunction. Recognition of this uniqueness has spawned a new field of arts medicine, and a dedicated journal, *Medical Problems of Performing Artists*, has appeared to address the occupational disorders of musicians. This chapter focuses on the occupational upper extremity disorders of instrumental musicians, which are divided into three broad categories: the overuse syndromes, peripheral nerve disorders, and occupational cramps or focal dystonias.

EPIDEMIOLOGY

Published Studies

Information about the prevalence, distribution, and type of upper extremity disorders in musicians derives from two sources: population-based question- naires and clinical reports from various performing arts clinics. Data from clinical series are subject to the bias of ascertain- ment, since there may be peculiarities in the referral pattern to individual clinics or physicians. Hence, although clinical series vividly portray the spectrum of per- formance-related upper extremity disor- ders, they tell little about their incidence. A small number of population-based studies have attempted to estimate the in- cidence or prevalence of hand problems in secondary school music students,[12,13] piano students,[14] university-level music students,[15,16] amateur participants at a music conference,[17] and professional or- chestral musicians.[4,18]

Music Students and Amateur Musicians

Fry et al.[13] used a questionnaire to esti- mate the prevalence of playing-related hand pain in orchestral musicians at a boys' and girls' secondary school in Aus- tralia. Pain with playing had occurred in 63 percent of the girls and 49 percent of the boys, and persistent pain was present in 53 percent of the girls and only 14 per- cent of the boys. By contrast, less than 14 percent of nonmusicians from the same schools noted pain from hand use. They concluded that adolescent girls are par- ticularly vulnerable to playing-related in- jury. Similar findings were obtained in a questionnaire study of British secondary schools.[19]

Lockwood[12] surveyed 113 American secondary school musicians aged 14 to 18 years. These students were serious mu- sicians who played an average of 19 hours per week. About half had experienced playing related pain, although in many (32 percent), symptoms were mild and did not interfere significantly with play- ing. In 10 percent of the musicians, pain, mild weakness, or loss of control signifi- cantly impaired playing and other daily

activities. Female students reported a sig- nificantly higher problem rate than male students, as did players of large instru- ments, such as cello or double bass, com- pared to players of small instruments, such as violin or viola. Hand size, as de- termined from tracings, did not correlate significantly with the prevalence of play- ing-related problems.

Manchester and Flieder[15,16] treated 305 episodes of performance-related upper extremity injury in 246 students at an American university-level music school. Because all enrolled students par- ticipated in the same prepaid health plan, it was possible to estimate the incidence of performance-related injuries in the en- tire student population. Two studies of consecutive 3-year periods showed an in- cidence of 8.5 episodes per 100 perform- ance majors per year. The incidence of problems in women was twice that in men, and the incidence in keyboard and string players was three times that in woodwind and brass players. Only among string players was one side (the left) in- volved disproportionately. Most students presented with pain involving the hand, wrist, or forearm, resulting most fre- quently in the diagnosis of muscle over- use syndrome (50 percent) or tendonitis (16 percent).[16] A variety of precipitating factors were identified in 71 of 100 epi- sodes, including an increase in playing time; a change in technique, teacher, or repertoire; and, in a small number, stress. The incidence of injuries was greatest in the fall, after a return to school, and in the spring, before performance examinations.

The relation of increased playing to the development of overuse injuries was studied using a questionnaire that was circulated at a music conference attended by serious amateur musicians.[17] The con- ference participants played an average of 7 to 8 hours daily, in contrast to 1 hour daily throughout the year and somewhat more during the preceding month. New performance problems, most commonly focal pain or muscle spasm, developed in 57 of 79 (72 percent) respondents, including all 11 musicians who increased their practice time by more than three-fold.

Symphony Orchestras

Major American orchestras require eight services (2- to 3-hour rehearsals or performances) per week through most of the year.[9] Orchestral musicians maintain rigorous schedules of practice, rehearsal, performance, and recording, and many play additionally as soloists, chamber players, or teachers. Musicians often win their first orchestral job in their early twenties, and many remain in orchestras into their sixties. It is therefore not surprising that many orchestral musicians succumb to playing-related upper extremity disorders.

Fry[4] interviewed members of eight orchestras in Australia (4), the United States (3), and England (1) and examined those musicians reporting symptoms of upper extremity pain. Musicians suspected of having nerve entrapment, tenosynovitis, or osteoarthritis were excluded. Symptoms were graded as follows[4]:

- Grade 1: Pain in one site is induced consistently by playing and ceases after stopping.
- Grade 2: Pain in multiple sites is induced by playing and is sometimes associated with weakness or loss of control.
- Grade 3: As in Grade 2, pain persists after playing and is induced by other hand activities.
- Grade 4: As in Grade 3, pain is induced by use of the hand in all activities of daily life.
- Grade 5: As in Grade 4, severe pain prevents use of the hand.

The overall prevalence of painful overuse was 64 percent with 42 percent having grade 2 symptoms or higher. Symptoms were most commonly mild (grades 1-2) and had been present in a majority of affected players for more than 2 years. The prevalence of painful overuse was highest in the 25 to 35 year age group, possibly because these younger musicians are most involved in auditions and extracurricular musical activities.[4] The most common affected sites were the hand and wrist (41 percent), neck (38 percent), shoulder (35 percent), forearm (11 percent), and elbow (10 percent). Some players had weakness or performance impairment with minimal pain, and it is possible that some of these had unrecognized nerve entrapment syndromes.[3,11]

In 1986, the International Conference of Symphony and Opera Musicians (ICSOM), an affiliate of the American Federation of Musicians, conducted a detailed survey of its 48 member orchestras on the prevalence of various medical problems.[18,20] Questionnaires were returned by 2,212 of 4,025 (55 percent) ICSOM members, constituting the largest inventory of medical problems of performing artists. Fifty-eight percent of the respondents reported musculoskeletal problems that severely affected performance. These were more common among women (70 percent) than men (52 percent) and among string players (66 percent) than woodwind (48 percent) or brass (32 percent) players. By contrast, the prevalence of nonmusculoskeletal problems was not strongly related to gender or instrument.[20] Severe musculoskeletal disorders occurred most frequently in the neck, shoulders, and back; however, a surprising 10 percent of ICSOM musicians reported sever problems in the left hand, again with a higher prevalence among women (13 percent) than men (8 percent) and among string players (12 percent) than woodwind (7 percent) or brass players (2 percent).

A detailed analysis of 1,378 string players suggested that the occurrence of some musculoskeletal problems was governed by a complex interaction among gender, type of string instrument, and side and location of involvement.[20] For example, the prevalence of severe musculoskeletal problems in the fingers and hand was two to three times greater on the left than on the right. This may reflect the fact that the left hand of a string player is constantly engaged in rapid, repetitive movements upon the fingerboard, whereas the right hand merely holds and guides the bow. By contrast, the demands placed on the wrist, forearm, and elbow are less severe and more symmetric than those placed on the hand, and not surprisingly, problems in these locations were less prevalent than hand problems and occurred equally on the two sides. Severe neck and shoulder problems were more prevalent among violinists and violists than among cellists and bass players, perhaps because the violin and viola are held between the chin and left shoulder, whereas the cello and bass rest on the ground. There were gender differences (women greater than men) in the prevalence of left neck problems among violinists but not among violists or cellists. By contrast, there were no gender differences in the prevalence of left hand problems among violinists, but significant differences among cellists (again women greater than men). Thus, playing certain string instruments appears to result in particular musculoskeletal problems, only some of which occur more commonly in women. These selective gender effects are better explained by gender-determined differences in hand size or neck proportions than by differences in pain threshold, readiness to report, or other psychosocial factors.[20] Caldron and colleagues[21] reported that women were more likely than men to report or seek treatment for playing-related injuries, but their questionnaire had only a 30 percent response rate.

Epidemiologic and Demographic Data from a Personal Series

Demographic data were retrieved on the first 200 musicians with upper extremity disorders examined by the author. The name, telephone number, age, sex, instrument, side of involvement, and primary, secondary and tertiary diagnosis of all musicians had been entered prospectively into a computerized data base beginning with the second patient. Patients were seen from 1984 to 1989 at the Health Program for Performing Artists at the University of California, San Francisco and from 1989 to 1991 at the Performing Arts Clinic at Brigham and Women's Hospital in Boston.

The data base was first analyzed by telephone area code. Patients came predominantly from the San Francisco Bay and Boston areas (75 percent), with the remainder from elsewhere in California, the Western and Northeast United States, Canada, and Europe. This was largely a local group of musicians referred by word of mouth or by physicians for primary care of an upper extremity disorder. All were examined personally, and most were seen repeatedly for follow-up care.

Figure 17-1 shows the breakdown for patient subgroups. The series is dominated by professional, classical musicians. Freelance professionals (46 percent) made their living by teaching and playing irregularly in solo recitals, chamber groups, shows, studio recordings, restaurants, and social events. Some supplemented their incomes with part-time jobs, such as word processing. Orchestral musicians (23 percent) were members of symphony, ballet, and opera orchestras, with most playing in full-time symphony orchestras. Twenty-one percent of the patients were conservatory students, mostly at the college and graduate levels, and 10 percent were serious amateur musicians.

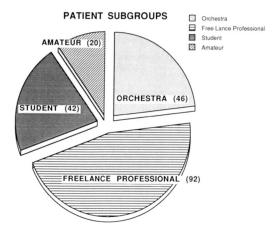

Fig. 17-1. Distribution of cases according to professional activity of 200 musicians with upper extremity disorders.

The average age was 33 years, and many were approaching the prime of their careers. This young age has been a feature of other series.[21-23]

Virtually all instruments were represented (Table 17-1). These instruments were grouped in categories based on similarities in hand use (Table 17-2): keyboard (organ and piano), strings (violin, viola, cello, and bass), flute, plucked instruments (guitar, banjo, mandolin, lute),

woodwinds (oboe, clarinet, English horn, bassoon), and others (brass, harp, drums, bagpipes, and one 21-dealer from Reno). A consideration of the side of involvement suggested some specific occupational hazards of certain instrument groups (Fig. 17-2).[5,22,23] For example, 75 percent of the problems in keyboard players were right sided, and 34 percent were bilateral. This predominance of right-sided involvement may reflect the fact that, although the upper extremities of a pianist are positioned symmetrically, the piano literature places far greater technical demands on the right hand. Upper extremity problems for string players were overwhelmingly left sided (75 percent), and only 13 percent showed bilateral involvement. This incidence mirrors the asymmetry of the burden borne by the left hand of string players. Flutist and pluckers were affected about equally on the two sides, and woodwind players showed mainly (79 percent) right-sided problems. The woodwinds are held vertically and balanced on the right thumb, whereas the flute is held transversely and supported by both hands. Although the left hand of the guitar and that of string instruments do similar work, the pluck-

Table 17-1.   Distribution of Instruments in 200 Musicians with Upper Extremity Disorders

Instrument	Number of Musicians	Instrument	Number of Musicians
Piano	69	Organ	2
Violin	28	Conductor	2
Flute	25	Harp	2
Guitar	17	Fife	1
Cello	13	English horn	2
Clarinet	6	French horn	1
Viola	6	Trumpet	1
Bass	6	Trombone	1
Saxophone	4	Banjo	1
Drums	4	Mandolin	1
Oboe	3	Bagpipes	1
Bassoon	3	"21" card dealer	1

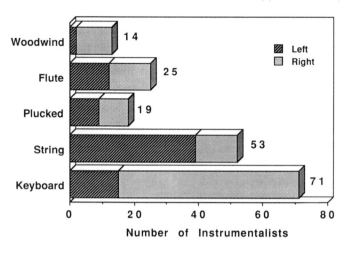

Fig. 17-2. Distribution of cases according to instrument and side of involvement.

ing, right hand of guitarists is challenged far more than the relatively passive bowing, right hand of string players.

The prevalence of upper extremity disorders in musicians is higher among women than men,[4,18,20–22] particularly among string players.[18,20] In my series the female to male ratio was 1.3:1; however, women were significantly overrepresented in certain instrument groups (Table 17-3). For example, women accounted for 75 percent of all string players, 76 percent of all flutists, but only 51 percent of all pianists. By contrast, in the ICSOM population there were fewer women than men string players and only slightly more women then men flutists.[18] These data support the contention that

string instruments are particularly hazardous for women.[20]

Many musicians had more than one upper extremity disorder, but each was assigned a primary diagnosis that accounted for their worst symptoms. Entrapment neuropathy was the primary diagnosis in 96 (48 percent) musicians, overuse injury in 57 (29 percent) and occupational cramp or movement disorder in 31 (16 percent). Taking secondary and tertiary diagnoses into account, 192 cases of nerve entrapment were diagnosed in 117 musicians, 89 cases of overuse injury in 68 musicians, and 41 cases of occupational cramp or movement disorder in 37 musicians. Women predominated among patients with overuse injury or nerve entrapment, whereas men predominated among patients with occupational cramp.

Table 17-2. Instrument Category as a Percentage of the Total Number of Patients

Instrument Category	Percentage of Total Patients
Keyboard	36
Strings	27
Flute	13
Plucked instruments	10
Woodwinds	7
Other	7

OVERUSE INJURIES IN MUSICIANS

Clinical Features and Pathophysiology

Lederman and Calabrese[24] define overuse as "the damage that occurs when a tissue is stressed beyond its anatomic or

Table 17-3. Distribution of Patients by Gender and Instrument

	Personal Series			ICSOM Membership[a]		
Instrument[b]	Female	Male	Female:Male	Female	Male	Female:Male
Keyboard	35	36	0.97			
Strings	40	13	3.07	1027	1489	0.69
Flute	19	6	3.17	85	75	1.13
Woodwinds	10	5	2.00	102	469	0.22
Plucked	6	13	0.46			
All instruments	113	87	1.30			

[a] ICSOM data are from Fishbein et al.[17]
[b] Some miscellaneous instruments are not listed separately.

physiologic limits, either acutely or chronically." The most common manifestation of upper extremity overuse is pain, with patterns of involvement depending on the instrument and the inciting activity. In some patients there may also be weakness, loss of dexterity, muscle fatigue, and numbness, although how often these symptoms represent mild, undiagnosed nerve entrapments is not clear. Fry believes that damage occurs predominantly in muscle, ligaments, and the joint capsule, with true inflammation of tendons or tendon sheaths being uncommon. He frequently found tenderness of the intrinsic muscles and articular regions of the hand among musicians with overuse injuries.[25,26] Lederman and colleagues[24] emphasize a "musculo-tendinous overuse syndrome" characterized by pain over the muscle belly and tendon attachment that is often increased during stretching or contraction against resistance. By contrast, Hochberg and colleagues[5,23] have described signs of tendinitis and tenosynovitis in a large number of injured musicians.

There are no pathologic studies of overuse injuries in musicians; hence, the pathophysiology of these disorders remains obscure. Pathologic findings in nonmusicians with overuse injuries are relatively nonspecific and include glycogen depletion, degeneration and edema of muscle fibers, and vascular changes.[1] To learn more about the overuse injury of small hand muscles, Dennett and Fry[27] performed a biopsy of the first dorsal interosseous muscle of 29 patients (mostly keyboard operators) with painful overuse syndromes and 8 normal volunteers. Changes observed, including an increase in type I fibers, hypertrophy and a decrease in type II fibers, mitochondrial abnormalities, and central nuclei, were proportional to the severity of clinical symptoms.[27]

The pathophysiology of muscle fatigue, a common complaint of musicians with overuse injury, is an area of active investigation. Maximal voluntary contraction (MVC) in the adductor pollicis declines rapidly after sustained contraction.[28] The decline in MVC and its rapid recovery are not associated with a drop in muscle ATP, as measured by NMR spectroscopy, but does correlate well with levels of $H_2PO_4^-$.[28] A more enduring phase of fatigue is associated with a slowly recovering defect in excitation-contraction coupling.[29] Application of these quantitative techniques to the study of overuse injury in musicians could be particularly fruitful.

Predisposing Factors

The majority of upper extremity disorders in musicians are precipitated by playing.[5,22] In a minority of patients, upper limb injury is induced or exacerbated by carrying heavy instruments, participating in sports or hobbies, and doing a variety of second jobs that sustain many students and freelance professionals. Traumatic injuries are more frequent than overuse syndromes in individual physician practices.[30] Why one musician and not another develops playing-related problems is determined by the interplay of extrinsic and intrinsic factors.[2,5,6,22,24] Extrinsic factors include the time and intensity of playing and the work performed by individual muscle-tendon units. The instrument itself determines the distribution of work among many muscle-tendon units.[2,26] Intrinsic factors include the strength, flexibility, size, and anatomic variations of the back, neck, or upper limbs.

The most common antecedent of a playing-related injury is an increase in the time and intensity of playing.[12,13,15–17,21,22,31] It may be an increase from no playing to the usual amount of playing time after a layoff or vacation or a rapid, several-fold increase over the usual playing time in preparation for a recital or audition. The stress associated with preparing for important public performances may contribute further to overuse by diffusely increasing muscle tone in the limbs ("playing tightly"). Unaccustomed burdens may be placed on individual muscle-tendon units when musicians change technique, begin studying with a new teacher, or change instruments. I have seen several pianists injured when trying to learn to play with flat fingers, as Horowitz did, or with their wrist below the instrument, as advocated by some French teachers. Excessive muscular tension, suboptimal hand position, poor posture, or unnecessary elevation of the shoulders are all technical risk factors that are remediable by good teachers. A change in repertoire or excessive repetition of a difficult passage may produce injury. A pianist accustomed to the close finger positions of Mozart may experience difficulty when switching to the wide stretches of Brahms or Liszt. I treated several members of one opera orchestra who were felled by the repetitious finger work of a new minimalist opera.

Intrinsic factors are also important in determining injury. Long necks may be problematic for violinists and violists, who must support their instruments between the neck and the shoulder. Clearly, small hands are a burden for players of large instruments, such as the viola, cello, and double bass. Small hands have also been injured playing the works of Rachmaninoff, Paganini, Brahms, and Liszt—composers who wrote for their own extremely large hands and hyperextensible joints. Hyperextensible joints, although arguably an advantage to Paganini's violin playing, may also be a risk factor for overuse injury,[2,26,32] perhaps because increased muscular effort is required to stabilize the small joints of the fingers and hands.[33] The presence of one overuse injury may predispose to another as uninjured muscles overwork to compensate for the pain or dysfunction of injured muscle-tendon units.[2,23] Anatomic variants, such as small passageways,[34] constricting fascial bands,[35] or anomalous muscles,[36] may predispose to various nerve entrapments. Poor general conditioning or more focal weakness of the shoulder girdle muscles may increase the risk of distal upper limb injury, as described below.

Treatment of Overuse

For more than 100 years, rest has been the cornerstone of therapy for the overuse syndromes of musicians.[37] Mild syndromes of upper limb pain can be treated by reducing playing schedules or modifying harmful performance practices (see below).[2,26,38] There is some disagreement over the management of patients with the more serious overuse injuries that render playing difficult and limit daily activities. Fry[26,38] advocates complete abstention from all activities that initiate or worsen upper limb pain. Rest is continued, often for as long as 12 months, until the injured limb is pain free and nontender for several weeks, at which time a graded return to playing is attempted.[26] This radical rest approach is reported to be effective in a majority of musicians with severe overuse injuries[38]; others report similar success with less prolonged rest.[23] The amount of rest required to produce improvement may be related to both the severity and duration of the symptoms.[22,23]

Management of the return to playing after prolonged rest is particularly important; some musicians resume playing with the passion of a lost lover and suffer early setbacks. During the period of rest, the upper limbs may become poorly conditioned, increasing the risk of new or recurrent injuries if playing time is accelerated too quickly.[15,17] It may therefore be helpful to initiate a program of progressive strengthening, stretching, and conditioning of the upper limb coincident with a return to playing. There follows a period of vulnerability during which a small amount of playing (5 to 10 minutes) is well tolerated, whereas longer or more intense playing is harmful. A slow, incremental return to playing allows these limits to be explored cautiously without incurring serious reinjury. Playing schedules must be tailored to the severity of the injury and the duration of rest. For absences longer than 12 weeks, I have recommended resuming playing of easy literature for 1 minute the first day, increasing by 1 to 2 minutes per day in three divided sessions. The pace can be accelerated quickly (increasing by 2 to 3 minutes per day) if the patient can play 15 to 30 minutes without symptoms

and needs to be reduced if symptoms recur. I share the belief that previously injured and healthy musicians should try to avoid playing more than 25 minutes at a time without a 5-minute break.[25,26]

A radical rest program is feasible for symphony musicians and other professionals whose contracts include workers' compensation and disability benefits. However, many other musicians, whether for psychological, professional, or financial reasons, will not stop playing completely. Freelance professionals may depend entirely on playing for their livelihood and usually do not pay into the workers' compensation system. Some musicians present with overuse injuries in the weeks leading up to a major recital, audition, or recording engagement and are reluctant to forego an important career opportunity that has been years in the making. In this instance I suggest a short period (1 or 2 weeks) of complete rest, often with splinting, followed by a graded return to reduced activity. Anti-inflammatory medications are employed during the rest and intermittently during periods of heightened activity. Patients are advised to stretch and warm up before performances and to apply ice to painful areas for at least 10 minutes after playing. Instrument modifications,[25,26,39] elimination of maladaptive playing styles, and physical therapy may all hasten recovery while important playing obligations are met.

Empiric data support the adjunctive use of anti-inflammatory medications in the treatment of some playing-induced overuse injuries. Nonsteroidal anti-inflammatory drugs (NSAIDs) are particularly helpful for acute injuries associated with marked focal tenderness and some signs of inflammation, such as lateral epicondylitis or tendinitis. There is, however, considerable discrepancy in the observation of physical signs of inflammation among physicians who care for musicians with overuse injuries. Those who tend to find signs of inflammation[5,23,40] are more enthusiastic about the use of anti-inflammatory medications than those who believe that the primary lesion is noninflammatory.[38] A small double-blind study found topical salicylates (Aspercreme) to be beneficial in decreasing the severity and duration of symptoms in musicians with painful upper limbs.[40] Local injection of corticosteroids may be helpful for certain focal inflammatory disorders, such as lateral epicondylitis, de Quervain's disease, intersection syndrome, and flexor carpi ulnaris tendinitis.[41] Rarely, I have used a 1-week course of prednisone to treat diffuse and severe overuse symptoms refractory to other measures.

A number of musicians with overuse injuries of the hand, wrist, or forearm have ipsilateral weakness of muscles of the shoulder and scapula. These large, tonically active muscles normally help support the weight of the arm and instrument. Small, rapidly contracting distal muscles may be injured when they take on large static loads from weakened proximal muscles. Electromyographic studies of the shoulder girdle in several of these patients have been normal, and presumably, these muscles have become weak through disuse. Exercises to strengthen the trapezius, rhomboids, supraspinatus, and serratus anterior have helped resolve distal injuries.[6]

Nontraditional therapies, such as the Alexander technique[42] and the Fleldenkrais method,[43] are frequently employed by musicians before or while they are cared for by physicians. The language and theory of these approaches are foreign to most physicians, but are reassuring to many musicians. These modalities attempt to improve posture and economize muscle action in movement and may help reduce or eliminate unnecessary muscle contraction during performance.

Both approaches have appeared to benefit patients with chronic spasm and tenderness of neck and shoulder muscles.

Surgery is rarely indicated for painful overuse syndromes. By contrast, conditions of true inflammation, such as De Quervain's tenosynovitis or tendon triggering, should be treated surgically if conservative measures are not effective quickly.[44] Overall, between 70 and 90 percent of musicians with overuse injuries are able to return to full performance schedules,[22,23,38] leaving a small minority who must seek other careers.

Prevention of Overuse Injuries

The identification of common circumstances that precede overuse injury in musicians suggests certain commonsense approaches for their prevention.[25,45,46] None of these measures has been tested scientifically, but they are appealingly simple and rational. Table 17-4 lists suggestions for preventing injury that I provide to both injured and noninjured musicians.

NERVE ENTRAPMENT SYNDROMES OF THE UPPER EXTREMITY

Epidemiology

Until recently, there were only rare reports of upper extremity nerve entrapment in musicians, including posterior interosseous nerve palsy,[47–49] pronator teres syndrome,[50,51] digital neuropathy,[52] thoracic outlet syndrome,[53] cervical radiculopathy,[10] and compression of the posterior cutaneous nerve of the arm.[54] With the advent of clinics for performing artists, peripheral nerve disorders have

Table 17-4.   Suggestions for the Prevention of Playing-Related Injuries

1. Begin to increase practice time weeks to months in advance of recitals or auditions. Start with small increments (e.g., add 5 minutes per day to the usual schedule), and leave the largest increments for the few weeks before the performance.
2. Compensate for increased playing intensity (for a recording session, more difficult program, stress, new instrument, or new technique) by reducing the total playing time.
3. Return to work gradually after a layoff. If you have not played for a few weeks, begin with only 10 to 20 minutes the first day and build up gradually. Longer layoffs require an even slower build-up to normal playing times.
4. Increase gradually the extracurricular use of your hands. Some musicians have been injured in the first 2 hours of gardening, bicycling, weight training, or raquetball.
5. Intersperse the repetitive practice of isolated passages throughout a practice session to avoid overworking one particular muscle group.
6. Stretch, warm up, and work gradually into a practice sessions.
7. Avoid playing more than 25 minutes without a 5-minute break.
8. Avoid unnecessary muscle contraction. Excessive shoulder elevation or neck twisting may result in muscle spasm and reduce the fluidity of movement in adjacent muscles. The burden of supporting the weight of instruments can be reduced by straps, posts, pegs, shoulder pads, and chin rests.
9. Be attentive to posture. Slouching in a chair for hours daily over a lifetime will eventually take its toll in back and neck problems. Good posture will reduce the work of small forearm and hand muscles by enabling large shoulder and back muscles to support the combined weight of the arms and the instrument.
10. Do not neglect your general physical and mental health. A happy, well-tuned, and fit individual will survive the rigors of a musical career better than an anxious, flabby, "couch potato."

been shown to be common among musicians with upper extremity complaints. Lederman[55] encountered peripheral nerve disorders in 29 percent of 226 musicians and Hochberg[6] in 18 percent of 1,000 musicians. The prognosis for recovery in this patient populations is quite favorable, with 74 percent of Lederman's patients describing a satisfactory outcome 1 to 8 years after presentation.[55]

In my practice, which is biased toward peripheral nerve disorders, entrapment neuropathy was the primary problem of 48 percent of 200 consecutively examined musicians with upper extremity disorders. Several musicians had more than one nerve entrapment syndrome. Figure 17-3 shows the distribution of 192 cases of nerve entrapment in 117 musicians. The ulnar nerve was affected most commonly, usually at the elbow. Thoracic outlet syndrome (TOS) was diagnosed in 59 limbs of 40 patients, including 21 who

were felt to have concomitant entrapment of the ulnar nerve at the elbow. There were 24 musicians with carpal tunnel syndrome, 12 bilateral, and a smaller number with entrapment of the posterior interosseous nerve, digital nerves, cervical roots, or miscellaneous other nerves. This series differs from others in which carpal tunnel syndrome[5] or TOS[7] was diagnosed more frequently than ulnar neuropathy.

Unique Aspects of Nerve Entrapment in Musicians

The maintenance of certain postures while executing rapid finger movements may predispose musicians to entrapment of various nerves. The elbow flexion test,[56] which is used in the diagnosis of cubital tunnel syndrome, is reproduced

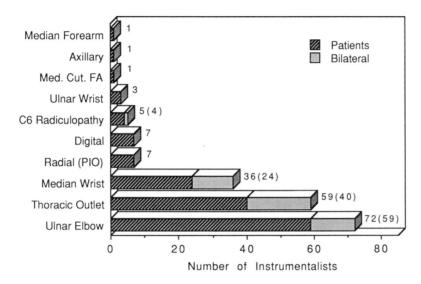

Fig. 17-3. Anatomic distribution of 192 nerve entrapment syndromes in 117 musicians.

daily for hours at a time by string players, flutists, woodwind players, guitarists, and keyboard players. Flexion-induced entrapment of the ulnar nerve under the aponeurosis of flexor carpi ulnaris[35] may be potentiated by static loading of the flexed arm by musical instruments and by forceful abduction of the little finger, which requires synergistic contraction of flexor carpi ulnaris (Fig. 17-4). Although the degree of elbow flexion required to play many instruments cannot be decreased readily, one can sometimes reduce static loading and minimize the contraction of forearm muscles. Two English horn players with cubital tunnel syndrome were treated successfully using a simple instrument prosthesis that unweights the partially flexed right arm (Fig. 17-5).

Sustained wrist flexion with rapid flexion-extension movements of the fingers is the daily lot of many string players, guitarists, and some pianists. Management of carpal tunnel syndrome in these musicians should include efforts to modify playing technique or the position of the instrument. Much of the weight of the flute is borne by the radial side of the left

index finger; compression of the underlying digital nerve[52,55] can be treated with small instrument prostheses that redistribute the weight of the instrument. Thoracic outlet syndrome in flutists may occasionally be managed by reducing hyperabduction of the right shoulder or internal rotation of the left shoulder during performance. Newmark[57] treated thoracic outlet syndrome successfully by lowering the high-hat cymbal of a drummer and shortening the end-pin of a cellist. A composer who spent long hours leaning his forearms against the edge of a table while copying scores developed numbness in the distribution of his medial cutaneous nerve of the forearm. This numbness resolved with forearm padding and a change in writing position.

Cervical Radiculopathy

Lederman[55] described eight cases of cervical radiculopathy in six musicians, with most showing involvement of the seventh and eighth cervical roots. Blau and Henson's[10] three musicians had sus-

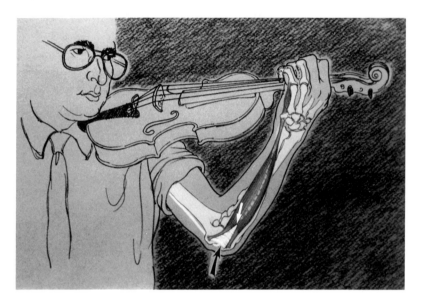

Fig. 17-4. Anatomy of ulnar nerve entrapment during violin playing. The ulnar nerve may be entrapped by the aponeurosis of flexor carpi ulnaris (*black arrow*) or fascia underlying flexor carpi ulnaris (*white arrow*), which is caused by elbow flexion and little finger abduction. Abductor digiti quinti arises from the tendon of flexor carpi ulnaris and must recruit this muscle to contract forcefully. (Drawing by Wayne Emery, reproduced with permission from the Network for Continuing Medical Education. Occupational Disorders in Performing Artists, Secaucus, NJ)

pected involvement of the fifth or multiple cervical roots. Four musicians in my series, three string players and one pianist, had radiculopathy of the sixth cervical root. Although the numbers are small, it is noteworthy that all three string players had left-sided symptoms whereas the pianist had symptoms on the right.

A 35-year-old female symphony violinist presented with a 1-year history of left neck pain and numbness of the left thumb for 1 month. For about 1 month she also noted difficulty lifting pots and playing the piano. Rest and physical therapy had improved her symptoms incompletely. She had a long neck and an inadequate shoulder pad, resulting in a 10° to 20° forceful tilt of her head toward the left shoulder when she held her violin. There was mild weakness of the

left supinator and pronator and decreased sensation to pin and light touch over the distal aspect of the left thumb. The left biceps tendon jerk was diminished. Cervical spine x-rays showed focal narrowing of the left C5-6 neural foramen. A teacher corrected her head tilt with a wider shoulder pad, and her numbness and weakness resolved over the next 4 weeks. She returned to a full performance schedule.

This violinist maintained a forceful neck tilt for 4 to 6 hours daily over many years. It is interesting to speculate whether her abnormal posture played a role in the development of focal cervical osteoarthritis and cervical radiculopathy. In support of this concept, Bard and colleagues[58] described radiologic evidence of realignment, degenerative

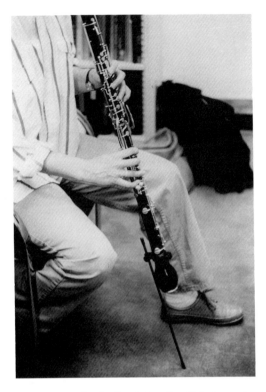

Fig. 17-5. The bell of the English horn has been fitted with a peg that transfers the weight of the instrument from the right thumb to the floor.

changes, and mechanical remodeling in the hands of 20 pianists whose mean age was 34 years. They attributed this osteoarthropathy to the stresses and strains of playing the piano over many years.

Ulnar Neuropathy

We have encountered a large number of musicians with ulnar nerve entrapment at the elbow.[3,11] Most patients were in their twenties and thirties and were, on average, about 20 years younger than nonmusicians with ulnar neuropathy.[59] The ratio of women to men was about 2:1. Elbow trauma was rare and contributed directly to the neuropathy in only two

musicians. The left side was preferentially involved in string players and the right or both sides in pianists. The selective involvement of the left hand in the string players with ulnar neuropathy suggests that sustained elbow flexion with finger movement (fingerboard, left side) is more important than flexion-extension (bow, right side) in the pathophysiology of this disorder.[11,55]

Most musicians experienced pain in the medial elbow radiating along the medial forearm into the hand and occasionally into the axilla. Some first noted pain in the ulnar aspect of the hand, but the medial elbow eventually became painful in most of these patients. Ulnar paresthesias were common, and burning along the course of the ulnar nerve occurred less frequently. Transient or enduring mild ulnar distribution numbness tended to occur later. Pain, paresthesias, and numbness were initially provoked by prolonged playing and resolved with rest. In time, symptoms occurred after less playing and, in some instances, merely with holding the instrument or at rest.

Few musicians complained of weakness in daily activities, whereas performance impairments were common and sometimes severe. Playing was initially effortful and then audibly impaired, first to the musician, next to colleagues, and finally to audiences. Complaints were focused on the control, strength, and endurance of the little and ring fingers, but to some degree all of the fingers were affected, perhaps because of mild interosseous weakness. Performance impairments occurred in the absence of sensory deficits and were probably related to mild degrees of weakness appreciated on examination. Pain, numbness, and ulnar paresthesias were absent in several musicians who presented the diagnostic challenge of performance impairment with subtle ulnar weakness and no localizing findings.

The site of entrapment in most patients could be localized to the elbow region based on elbow pain, an asymmetrically positive Tinel's sign, local tenderness over the nerve, usually at the cubital tunnel, a positive elbow flexion test, and the pattern of weakness or sensory loss. Routine EMG and nerve conduction studies were abnormal in less than half of the patients,[11] attesting to the potential for mild ulnar neuropathy to produce disabling symptoms in musicians.[3] The near nerve technique[60,61] has produced a much higher rate of abnormal findings than surface studies in musicians with ulnar neuropathy and has provided the sole source of localizing information in some studies (unpublished observations).

Treatment has consisted of rest, nocturnal splinting of the elbow in extension, avoidance of elbow flexion or external compression, instrument modification, changes in technique, and physical therapy to correct a coexisting thoracic outlet syndrome. Attempts to strengthen hand muscles tended to worsen the disorder, perhaps by recruiting contraction in flexor carpi ulnaris. Surgery was recommended to patients who failed these measures or developed career-threatening performance impairments. In most instances, the ulnar nerve was compressed by the aponeurosis of flexor carpi ulnaris or by its underlying fascia.[11] Nerve compression was mild, consistent with the clinical and EMG findings; however, compression increased intraoperatively when musicians reproduced their position of performance.[11] A total of 30 operations, approximately half simple decompressions and half submuscular transpositions, have been performed. Both procedures have produced significant improvement in symptoms and signs, and the majority of operated patients have been able to return to full performance schedules.[11] Lederman has reported similar favorable results in a smaller number of patients[55]

The occupational nature of ulnar neuropathy in musicians is suggested by the young age of the patients, the preferential involvement of a particular side among players of different instruments, the onset of symptoms with increased playing, and the improvement of symptoms with rest. Our experience with this neuropathy highlights the challenge of treating mild nerve entrapment syndromes in musicians. Disability can result from nerve lesions that would be asymptomatic in nonmusicians, and diagnosis must depend on careful examination, sensitive electrodiagnostic studies, and the observation of performance. Decisions regarding surgery rest more on the occupational demands and performance deficit than on the absolute severity of the lesion.

Ulnar entrapment at the wrist has been reported in two flutists.[62] Our experience and that of others[55] suggest that musicians develop entrapment of the ulnar nerve at the wrist much less commonly than at the elbow.

Thoracic Outlet Syndrome

Thoracic outlet syndrome (TOS) in musicians is a common, controversial disorder.[5,6,55,63] Lederman[55,63] has summarized his experience in 27 instrumental musicians. All were diagnosed with the "symptomatic" form of TOS, characterized by positional pain and paresthesias, primarily in the medial forearm and ulnar hand, and none of the features of the rare "true neurogenic TOS," which includes objective weakness, sensory loss, electrodiagnostic abnormalities, and cervical rib or elongated transverse process of the seventh cervical vertebra.[63,64] Symptoms occurred commonly while playing the instrument and could be reproduced or intensified most effectively by downward traction of the arm with internal rotation of the shoulder.[55] Half of the patients had the droopy shoulder configuration associated with TOS.[65]

The diagnosis of symptomatic TOS cannot be confirmed reliably by any electrophysiologic test, including conduction velocity across Erb's point or somatosensory evoked responses.[35,55,63,66-68] Electrodiagnostic tests in symptomatic TOS have been used primarily to exclude other conditions.[63] Physical therapy was successful in most of Lederman's patients, and two underwent first rib resection with postoperative improvement.[63] Overall, 81 percent of the patients have done well[55] Hochberg[6] recommended surgery in 10 percent of 70 musicians with TOS,[6] and Roos[69] operated with good results on 11 string players with severe TOS.

My experience with 40 musicians with TOS (19 bilateral) resembles that of Lederman[55,63] and Hochberg.[6] Included among my patients were 21 who had strong clinical or electrodiagnostic evidence of cubital tunnel syndrome, 4 with carpal tunnel syndrome, and 1 with pronator syndrome. The separate existence of TOS in these patients was based on the elicitation with different maneuvers.[6,63] of numbness or paresthesias in the forearm and hand, tenderness or a positive Tinel's sign over the symptomatic brachial plexus, or marked blanching of the symptomatic hand. Surgery of the concomitant distal neuropathy improved distal symptoms, such as elbow pain or ulnar hand numbness, without modifying symptoms attributable to TOS, such as positional numbness of the medial forearm and entire hand. In several patients the major site of brachial plexus compression appeared to be under the tendon of pectoralis minor. One patient, an amateur guitarist and word processor, had true neurogenic TOS from anterior subluxation of the humeral head. Her electrodiagnostic studies demonstrated focal slowing of ulnar motor conduction across the

elbow, no median nerve delay across the carpal tunnel, and denervation of both median and ulnar hand muscles. The occurrence of ulnar or median neuropathy in half of the patients with thoracic outlet syndrome supports the hypothesis that proximal nerve compression may predispose to distal entrapment.[70,71]

Conservative therapy improved TOS in most of the patients, but has ameliorated the distal neuropathies infrequently. In some patients with concomitant ulnar neuropathy, TOS exercises, especially those that require elbow flexion, exacerbated elbow pain and ulnar sensory symptoms. Surgical correction of the distal neuropathy facilitated more aggressive rehabilitation of the TOS, with subsequent resolution of both the distal neuropathy and TOS.

Median Nerve Disorders

Carpal Tunnel Syndrome

Carpal tunnel syndrome in musicians presents less of a diagnostic problem than cubital tunnel syndrome. Most of our patients presented with typical complaints of wrist, hand, or forearm pain along with median-distribution numbness and paresthesias. Playing was limited primarily by pain or unpleasant paresthesias, and few of the patients had demonstrable weakness. Routine electrodiagnostic studies were abnormal more often than in patients with cubital tunnel syndrome and occasionally revealed problems in asymptomatic limbs. Symptoms often began in association with increases in playing time or changes in instrument or technique. However, not all cases were occupational. A bass player developed carpal tunnel syndrome from carrying heavy pieces of concrete in his back yard, and a keyboard player experienced her first symptoms while pregnant. Once present, though, symptoms were made worse by playing and improved with rest.

The incidence of carpal tunnel syndrome in other professions may be a function of the size of the carpal tunnel.[34] Carpal tunnel dimensions have not been measured in musicians, but natural variations in carpal tunnel size may help determine which musicians develop carpal tunnel syndrome. One cellist with right carpal tunnel syndrome had an anomalous muscle, a proximal origin of a lumbrical, within the carpal canal. This anatomic variant may have rendered dangerous the normal use of her lumbricals in gripping the bow.

The challenge of carpal tunnel syndrome in musicians has been to identify reversible, occupational origins of the disorder. Correction of excessive flexion in the left hand of violinists and guitarists and excessive gripping of bows or strings, and obtaining more ergonomic cases for carrying heavy instruments have all been important adjuncts in the nonsurgical management of these patients. Rest, splinting, nonsteroidal anti-inflammatory medications, injection of the carpal tunnel with corticosteroids, and surgery have been employed in the same manner as in nonmusicians.[35] Postoperative recovery has been handled carefully, including a graded return to full playing, to avoid the overuse injuries caused by sudden increases in playing after a layoff. The outcome of surgery has been good in most patients, in agreement with Lederman.[55]

Pronator Syndrome

A 21-year-old cellist presented after an initially successful surgical procedure for pronator syndrome with recurrent mid-forearm pain, numbness of the thumb, and a positive Tinel's sign over the pronator muscle. There was no muscular hypertrophy of the forearm. She also had TOS and had previously undergone anterior transposition of her right ulnar nerve. This combination of thoracic outlet syndrome, ulnar neuropathy, and pronator syndrome may be another example of a double crush syndrome.[72] Lederman[55] described a harpist who developed pronator syndrome after tuning several harps, and examples of pronator syndrome in a fiddler[50] and a pianist[51] have also been described. The combination of finger flexion and forceful pronation may be important in the pathophysiology of this condition.[35]

Posterior Interosseous Nerve Syndrome

Entrapment of the posterior interosseous nerve is of historic importance to both musicians and physicians. The great composer and pianist, Robert Schumann, developed partial paralysis of his right hand, particularly the long and index fingers, which he attributed to "overdone technical studies."[48] Henson and Urich,[48] after sorting through contradictory historical documents, speculated that the composer suffered from entrapment of his posterior interosseous nerve. Deprived early in life of a career as a piano virtuoso, Schumann turned his energies to composition. The only secondary gain he derived from his affliction was an excuse from military service.[48]

The first documented case of posterior interosseous nerve compression involved a conductor.[47] Subsequent cases have been described in a flutist,[55] violinist,[49] and two pianists.[48] Forceful supination-pronation movements of the forearm are thought to provoke the disorder in anatomically susceptible individuals.

We encountered seven musicians whose symptoms were consistent with entrapment of the posterior interosseous nerve. One, a disabled pianist, had clear EMG abnormalities and underwent surgery with a return to active performance. A flutist with progressive, painless loss of performance dexterity had mild weakness of finger extensors and denervation of radial forearm muscles. Surgical exploration revealed compression of the posterior interosseous nerve by a thickened arcade of Frohse with conduction block at this site.[3] Surgery arrested his deterioration, but significant performance impairment persisted because of a concomitant occupational cramp. Heroic efforts by the patient at instrument redesign have diminished the focal dystonia, and he continues to play professionally. The remaining patients included a pianist, flutist, oboist, bassoonist, and drummer. Their diagnoses were established by combinations of forearm pain, marked asymmetric tenderness over the radial tunnel, mild weakness of finger extensors, and abnormal EMGs in two patients.

Digital Neuropathy

I diagnosed digital mononeuropathy in seven patients. Six conditions resulted from pressure of the flute, violin, viola, cello, oboe, or trombone against a digital nerve, and all recovered after rest, changing instrument position, or padding the instrument or finger. Several patients had a positive Tinel's sign at the point of instrument contact. A pianist developed a digital mononeuropathy after striking a key while attempting to pull back her arm forcefully; EMG did not reveal carpal tunnel syndrome, and the mechanism underlying her neuropathy remains unclear. Lederman[55] described compressive digital mononeuropathies resulting from pressure of a cello bow on the right thumb, a flute on the left index finger, and a marimba mallet on the left middle finger. A violinist with benign hypermobility of the fifth metacarpophalangeal (MCP) joint developed compression of the radial digital nerve of the little finger from contact of her hyperextended fifth MCP joint against the body of the violin. Splinting of the fifth MCP joint prevented joint subluxation and allowed fully recovery.[73]

OCCUPATIONAL CRAMPS AND MOVEMENT DISORDERS

Occupational Cramps as a Form of Focal Dystonia

Dystonias are movement disorders characterized by "involuntary sustained muscle contractions, causing twisting, repetitive movements, or abnormal postures."[74] They are classified as generalized, affecting all limbs and axial structures; segmental, affecting contiguous body parts, such as the arm and trunk; and focal, affecting one body part. Focal dystonias commonly affect the neck (torticollis), the facial muscles (blepharospasm, Meige's syndrome), and the limbs. Some focal dystonias are task specific, the most common of these being writer's cramp.[75] Writer's cramp, which is uncommonly painful, refers to stereotyped, involuntary spasms of the fingers, wrist, and forearm elicited by attempts to write.[74] Focal dystonias, including writer's cramp, occur with increased frequency among family members of affected individuals, and some individuals with inherited generalized dystonias or other degenerative neurologic diseases may present with writer's cramp.[74,76] The majority of patients with writer's cramp or musician's cramp have no demonstrable brain lesions,[74] and psychiatric disorders are uncommon.[8,74,75]

Tasks-specific dystonias are elicited by the skilled, stereotyped, repetitive movements of numerous different occupations, giving rise to the term "occupational cramp."[77] Occupational cramps can be subdivided into simple cramps, initiated by a single task; dystonic cramps, initiated by several skills tasks, such as writing and playing an instrument; or progressive cramps, denoting a transition from single cramp to dystonic cramp.[75] The first accounts of musician's cramp date back 150 years.[7]

Symptoms and Findings in Musician's Cramp

The disorder often develops insidiously, first manifesting as a loss of speed, dexterity, or accuracy in performance. A common early complaint is the uncharacteristic effort required to perform previously automatic technical feats. In the absence of overt spasms, these symptoms may be difficult to distinguish from ulnar or posterior interosseous neuropathy (above). Involuntary movements are, at first, often task specific; for example, a pianist may have difficulty playing ascending scales, but be unimpaired in playing descending scales, typing, or writing. In about half of our cases, involuntary movements generalized to other tasks, most commonly writing and typing. Similar generalization has been reported by others.[8,78] A variety of stereotyped patterns of involuntary movements are seen, with some representing compensation for the primary movement. Curling of the ring and little fingers into the palm and extension of the index finger are two frequent patterns of involuntary movement, and tremor may accompany some of these patterns.[79] The movements are not painful, although many patients develop uncomfortable tightness in their hand, forearm, and arm in attempting to overcome the dystonic movements. Newmark and Hochberg[8] identified stereotyped patterns of movement for particular instruments; for example, flexion of the ring and little finger in pianists, extension of the middle finger in clarinetists, and flexion of the middle finger in guitarists. By contrast, Lederman[78] found a variety of patterns of abnormal movement within instrumental groups. In my patients, the pattern of dystonic movements appeared to correlate best with the site of concomitant nerve entrapment or previous soft tissue injury.

The examination is usually normal, except in cases associated with nerve entrapment or antecedent injury. Subtle neurologic abnormalities, including tremor, are sometimes seen.[74,75,79–82] The movement disorder may be entirely task specific, and it is therefore imperative to watch the musician play. A pattern of abnormal hand movements may be difficult to discern in mild musician's cramp[7]; in these cases, it may only be apparent that the hand is stiff and somewhat awkward or that the performance is much less than expected for a given level of accomplishment. However, in most patients, careful observation reveals obvious dystonic movements during playing.

ELECTROPHYSIOLOGIC STUDIES

Polygraphic EMG recording during simple cramps reveals multiple abnormalities: long-duration bursts of co-contraction in agonist and antagonist muscles, tremor, failure of expected activation, and lack of selectivity in moving individual fingers.[81,83] Dystonic cramps are characterized by sustained co-contraction of agonists and antagonists, similar to the pattern of generalized dystonia.[81,84] Strong evidence for a central abnormality of the motor system in hand cramps comes from studies of the limbs at rest. The affected side shows decreased reciprocal inhibition of the H reflex, suggesting a failure of spinally mediated inhibition of antagonist motor neurons by agonist contraction.[85]

Relationship of Peripheral Injury to Focal Dystonia

More than 100 years ago, Gowers[80] described a seaman who developed writer's cramp while recovering from an injury to his thumb. Since that time, there have been many reports of focal dystonias following local trauma or peripheral neuropathy.[6,8,78,81,82,86–91] Newmark and Hochberg[8] elicited a history of antecedent trauma, inflammation, or overuse in 37 of 59 musicians with occupational cramp, and Lederman[78] identified 14 antecedent conditions in 21 musicians with occupational cramp.

How a peripheral injury activates a centrally mediated movement disorder is the subject of great speculation and uncertainty.[7,17,78,92–96] Perhaps the most perplexing aspect of this relationship is the persistence of the occupational cramp for years after the upper extremity injury resolves. To learn more about this phenomenon, I determined prospectively the prevalence of overuse injury, trauma, and nerve entrapment in 41 cases of occupational cramp in 39 musicians.[82] Men outnumbered women by a ratio of 2:1, as reported by others.[8,78,94]

Trauma to the affected limb preceded the development of musician's cramp by less than 1 year in seven patients. In most instances, the cramp first became apparent while playing during the resolution of an injury. The injuries were not trivial. A violinist developed involuntary extension of the left index finger while recovering from a puncture wound of the left wrist and an associated carpal tunnel syndrome. A saxophonist developed playing-induced dystonic extension of the index finger while recovering from an infected dog bite of the first web space. Cramps usually involved the region of the prior soft tissue injury and, in all seven patients, endured, long after the resolution of the injury. None of the patients had reflex sympathetic dystrophy, which sometimes antedates focal dystonias.[86,91–93]

Overuse preceded the development of occupational cramp in eight patients. This was, again, often quite dramatic. A pianist transposed to the left hand a difficult passage from the Chopin etude opus 10, #2 (which isolates and exercises the right long, ring, and little fingers) and practiced this single figure repetitively for several hours daily until he developed involuntary curling of the little and ring fingers. The dystonia later generalized to typing and writing.

Three musicians with occupational cramp had pre-existing neurologic abnormalities,[93] including childhood blepharospasm, resolving posttraumatic hemiparesis, and ipsilateral essential tremor. A total of 21 musicians had a coincident nerve entrapment syndrome, including 13 with ulnar neuropathy. The neuropathy was sometimes subtle, making it difficult to determine whether the onset of the occupational cramp preceded, accompanied, or followed the neuropathy. The affected peripheral nerve often predicted the pattern of the dystonic movement; for example, most patients with ulnar neuropathy had playing-induced curling of the little and ring fingers. In several patients, occupational cramp and peripheral neuropathy waxed and waned together. Five patients have shown substantial improvement of long-standing occupational cramps from a combination of successful therapy of a coincident neuropathy and slow relearning of nondystonic motor programs. Lederman[78] also described improvement of a musician's cramp following carpal tunnel surgery.

Occupational cramp developed in the absence of trauma, overuse, nerve entrapment, or preexisting neurologic disorders in only 3 of the 41 cases (7 percent). The strikingly high incidence of peripheral abnormalities may reflect the prospective ascertainment of cases and our recent use of near nerve recording[60,61] and quantitative EMG to identify subtle peripheral neuropathies. The possibility of treating a centrally mediated movement disorder by peripheral nerve surgery[78,82] is intriguing and merits further study.

Treatment

Occupational cramp has devastated the careers of many performing artists, including the great pianists, Gary Graffman and Leon Fleisher.[97] Spontaneous remissions of musician's cramps are rare[74] and restoration of a great career would require a virtual cure. Rest and long periods away from playing, the mainstay of treatment in overuse injury, are uniformly unhelpful in musician's cramp[8,24]; indeed, Lederman[7] described a French horn player whose oral dystonia recurred immediately when he resumed playing after a hiatus of 12 years. Anticholinergic and dopaminergic medications, which can improve segmental and generalized dystonias, are relatively ineffective in the occupational cramps and are poorly treated.[8,78,98]

Isolated instances of improvement in musician's cramp have been attributed to hypnotherapy, biofeedback,[99] and motor retraining,[96,100] but many patients have tried these and other treatment modalities without success.[8,24,95] Attempts at strengthening antagonist muscles may be helpful in a small minority of patients.[8,95]

Despite the few successes described above, we still undertake peripheral nerve surgery only when peripheral nerve symptoms merit treatment independently.

The most recent therapeutic approach to occupational cramp has been the use of botulinum toxin to weaken cramping muscles selectively and reversibly.[101,102] The toxin is injected through hollow EMG needles that are first used to identify target muscles. Significant improvement in the occupational cramp can be achieved for 1 to 6 months at a time, although usually at the expense of mild, functionally significant weakness.[101] Botulinum toxin does not alter the abnormal pattern of co-contraction, correct the failure of other muscles to contract, or restore selectivity of individual finger movements, suggesting that there is no change in the physiologic mechanism underlying the focal dystonia.[81,101] The functional improvement resulting from the reduction in dystonia usually exceeds the deterioration due to botulinum toxin-induced weakness, and improvements may sometimes be dramatic.[101] One patient of mine, a guitarist with a severe occupational cramp of the left hand, has been able to resume some public performance while receiving botulinum toxin.

REFERENCES

1. Lockwood AH: Medical problems of musicians. N Engl J Med 320:221, 1989
2. Brandfonbrener AG: Epidemiology of the medical problems of performing artists, p. 25. In Sataloff RT, Brandfonbrener AG, Lederman RJ (eds): Textbook of Performing Arts Medicine. Raven Press, New York, 1991
3. Charness ME, Parry GL, Markison RE et al: Entrapment neuropathies in musicians. Neurology, suppl. 35:74, 1985

4. Fry HJH: Incidence of overuse syndrome in the symphony orchestra. Med Probl Perform Art 1:51, 1986

5. Hochberg FH, Leffert RD, Heller MD, Merriman L: Hand difficulties among musicians. JAMA 249:1869, 1983

6. Hochberg FH: The upper extremity difficulties of musicians, p. 1197. In Hunter JM, Schneider LH, Mackin EJ, Callahan AD (eds): Rehabilitation of the Hand. Surgery and Therapy. CV Mosby Co, St. Louis, 1990

7. Lederman RJ: Neurological problems of performing artists, p. 171. In Sataloff RT, Brandfonbrener AG, Lederman RJ (eds): Textbook of Performing Arts Medicine. Raven Press, New York, 1991

8. Newmark J, Hochberg FH: Isolated painless manual incoordination in 57 musicians. J Neurol Neurosurg Psychiatr 50:291, 1987

9. Torch D: 1991–91 wage chart of ICSOM orchestras. Senza Sordino February:2, 1991

10. Blau JN, Henson RA: Neurological disorders in performing musicians, p. 300. In Critchley M, Henson RA, Charles CT (eds): Music and the Brain. William Heinemann, London, 1977

11. Charness ME, Barbaro NM, Olney RK, Parry GJ: Occupational cubital tunnel syndrome in instrumental musicians. Neurology, suppl. 37:115, 1987

12. Lockwood AH: Medical problems in secondary school-aged musicians. Med Probl Perform Art 4:129, 1988

13. Fry HJH, Ross P, Rutherford M: Music-related overuse in secondary schools. Med Probl Perform Art 1988

14. Revak JM: Incidence of upper extremity discomfort among piano students. Am J Occup Ther 43:149, 1989

15. Manchester RA: The incidence of hand problems in music students. Med Probl Perform Art 3:15, 1988

16. Manchester RA, Flieder D: Further observations on the epidemiology of hand injuries in music students. Med Probl Perform Art 6:11, 1991

17. Newmark J, Lederman RJ: Practice doesn't necessarily make perfect: incidence of overuse syndromes in amateur instrumentalists. Med Probl Perform Art 2:142, 1987

18. Fishbein M, Middlestadt SE, Ottati V et al: Medical problems among ICSOM musicians: overview of a national survey. Med Probl Perform Art 3:1, 1988

19. Fry HJH, Rowley GL: Music related upper limb pain in schoolchildren. Ann Rheum Dis 48:998, 1989

20. Middlestadt SE, Fishbein M: The prevalence of severe musculoskeletal problems among male and female symphony orchestra string players. Med Probl Perform Art 4:41, 1989

21. Caldron PH, Calabrese LH, Clough JD: A survey of musculoskeletal problems encountered in high-level musicians. Med Probl Perform Art 1:136, 1986

22. Knishkowy B, Lederman RJ: Instrumental musicians with upper extremity disorders: a follow-up study. Med Probl Perform Art 1:85, 1986

23. Newmark J, Hochberg FH: "Doctor, it hurts when I play": painful disorders among instrumental musicians. Med Probl Perform Art 2:93, 1987

24. Lederman RJ, Calabrese LH: Overuse syndromes in instrumentalists. Med Probl Perform Art 1:7, 1986

25. Fry HJH: Overuse syndrome in musicians. Prevention and management. Lancet 2:728, 1986

26. Fry HJH: Overuse syndromes in instrumental musicians. Semin Neurol 9:136, 1989

27. Dennett X, Fry HJH: Overuse syndrome: a muscle biopsy study. Lancet 1:905, 1988

28. Miller RG, Boska MD, Moussavi RS et al: 31P nuclear magnetic resonance studies of high energy phosphates and pH in human muscle fatigue. Comparison of aerobic and anaerobic exercise. J Clin Invest 81:1190, 1988

29. Moussavi RS, Carson PJ, Boska MD et al: Nonmetabolic fatigue in exercising human muscle. Neurology 39:1222, 1989

30. Dawson WJ: Hand and upper extremity problems in musicians: epidemiology and diagnosis. Med Probl Perform Art 3:19, 1988

31. Fry HJH: Prevalence of overuse (injury)

syndrome in Australian music schools. Br J Indust Med 44:35, 1987

32. Hoppman RA, Patrone NA: Musculoskeletal problems in instrumental musicians, p. 71. In Sataloff RT, Brandfonbrener AG, Lederman RJ (eds): Textbook of Performing Arts Medicine. Raven Press, New York, 1991

33. Bird HA, Wright V: Traumatic synovitis in a classical guitarist: a study of joint laxity. Ann Rheum Dis 40:161, 1981

34. Bleeker ML, Bohlman M, Moreland R, Tipton A: Carpal tunnel syndrome. Role of carpal canal size. Neurology 35:1599, 1985

35. Dawson DM, Hallet M, Millender LH: Entrapment Neuropathies. Little, Brown and Co, Boston, 1990

36. Lahey MD, Aulicino PL: Anomalous muscles associated with compression neuropathies. Orthop Rev 15:199, 1986

37. Poore GV: Clinical lecture on certain conditions of the hand and arm which interfere with the performance of professional acts, especially piano-playing. Br Med J 1:441, 1887

38. Fry HJH: The treatment of overuse syndrome in musicians. Results in 175 patients. J Roy Soc Med 81:572, 1988

39. Markison RE: Treatment of musical hands: redesign of the interface. Hand Clin 6:525, 1990

40. Hochberg FH, Lavin P, Portney R et al: Topical therapy of localized inflammation in musicians: a clinical evaluation of Aspercreme versus placebo. Med Probl Perform Art 3:9, 1988

41. Stern PJ: Tendinitis, overuse syndrome, and tendon injuries. Hand Clin 6:467, 1990

42. Rosenthal E: The Alexander technique—what it is and how it works. Med Problem Perform Art 2:53, 1987

43. Nelson SH: Playing with the entire self. The Feldenkrais method and musicians. Semin Neurol 9:97, 1989

44. Eaton RG, Nolan WB: Diagnosis and surgical treatment of the hand, p. 205. In Sataloff RT, Brandfonbrener AG, Lederman RJ (eds): Textbook of Performing Arts Medicine. Raven Press, New York, 1991

45. Hoppmann RA, Patrone NA: A review of musculoskeletal problems in instrumental musicians. Semin Arthritis Rheum 19:117, 1989

46. Brandfonbrener AG: The epidemiology and prevention of hand and wrist injuries in performing artists. Hand Clin 6:365, 1990

47. Guillain G, Courtellemont M: L'action du muscle court supinateur dans la paralysie du nerf radial. Presse Medicale 13:50, 1905

48. Henson RA, Urich H; Schumann's hand injury. Br Med J 1:900, 1982

49. Silverstein A: Progressive paralysis of the dorsal interosseous nerve. Arch Neurol Psychiatr 38:885, 1937

50. Morris HH, Peters BH: Pronator syndrome: clinical and electrophysiological features in seven cases. J Neurol 39:461, 1976

51. Kopell HP, Thompson WAL: Pronator syndrome: a confirmed case and its diagnosis. N Engl J Med 259:713, 1958

52. Cynamon KB: Flutist's neuropathy. N Engl J Med 305:961, 1981

53. Lascelles RG, Mohr PD, Heary D, Bloor K: The thoracic outlet syndrome. Brain 100:601, 1977

54. Makin GJ, Brown WF: Entrapment of the posterior cutaneous nerve of the arm. Neurology 35:1677, 1985

55. Lederman RJ; Peripheral nerve disorders in instrumentalists. Ann Neurol 26:640, 1989

56. Buehler MJ, Thayer DT: The elbow flexion test. A clinical test for the cubital tunnel syndrome. Clin Orthop 1988

57. Newmark J: Thoracic outlet syndrome. Can symptoms a diagnosis make? Classical Overtones 2:11, 1989

58. Bard CC, Sylvester JJ, Dussault RG: Hand osteoarthropathy in pianists. J Can Assoc Radiol 35:154, 1984

59. Odusote K, Eisen A: An electrophysiological quantitation of the cubital tunnel syndrome. Can J Neurol Sci 6:403, 1979

60. Shefner JM, Dawson DM: The use of sensory action potentials in the diagnosis of peripheral nerve disease. Arch Neurol 47:341, 1990

61. Shefner JM, Buchthal F, Krarup C:

Slowly conducting myelinated fibers in peripheral neuropathy. Muscle Nerve 14:534–542, 1990

62. Wainapel SF, Cole JL: The not-so-magic flute: two cases of distal ulnar nerve entrapment. Med Probl Perform Art 3:63, 1988

63. Lederman RJ: Thoracic outlet syndrome. Review of the controversies and a report of 17 instrumental musicians. Med Probl Perform Art 2:87, 1987

64. Gilliat RW, LeQuesne PM, Logue V, Sumner AJ: Wasting of the hand associated with a cervical rib or hand. J Neurol Neurosurg Psychiatr 33:615, 1970

65. Swift TR, Nichols FT: The droopy shoulder syndrome. Neurology 34:212, 1984

66. Lederman RJ: Nerve entrapment syndromes in instrumental musicians. Med Probl Perform Art 1:45, 1986

67. Veilleux M, Stevens JC, Campbell JK: Somatosensory evoked potentials: lack of value for diagnosis of thoracic outlet syndrome. Muscle Nerve 11:571, 1988

68. Wilbourn AJ: The thoracic outlet syndrome is overdiagnosed. Arch Neurol 47:328, 1990

69. Roos RB: Thoracic outlet syndromes. Symptoms, diagnosis, anatomy and surgical treatment. Med Probl Perform Art 1:90, 1986

70. Narakas AO: The role of thoracic outlet syndrome in the double crush syndrome. Ann Chir Main Memb Super 9:331, 1990

71. Upton ARM, McComas AJ: The double crush in nerve-entrapment syndromes. Lancet 2:359, 1973

72. Narakas A, Bonnard C, Egloff DV: The cervico-thoracic outlet compression syndrome. Analysis of surgical treatment. Ann Chir Main 5:195, 1986

73. Patrone NA, Hoppman RA, Whaley J, Schmidt R: Digital nerve compression in a violinist with benign hypermobility: a case study. Med Probl Perform Art 4:91, 1989

74. Marsden CD, Sheehy MP: Writer's cramp. TINS 13:148, 1990

75. Sheehy MP, Marsden CD: Writer's cramp—a focal dystonia. Brain 105:461, 1982

76. Waddy HM, Fletcher NA, Harding AE,

Marsden CD: A genetic study of idiopathic focal dystonia. Ann Neurol 29:320, 1991

77. Hunter D: The Diseases of Occupations. Vol. 6, Hodder and Stoughton, London, 1978

78. Lederman RJ: Occupational cramp in instrumental musicians. Med Probl Perform Art 3:45, 1988

79. Rosenbaum F, Jankovic J: Focal task-specific tremor and dystonia: categorization of occupational movement disorders. Neurology 38:522, 1988

80. Gowers WR: A Manual of Diseases of the Nervous System. Vol. 2. Churchill, London, 1888

81. Cohen LG, Hallet M: Hand cramps: Clinical features and electronmyographic patterns in a focal dystonia. Neurology 38:1005, 1988

82. Charness ME: The relationship between local injury and focal dystonia in performing artists. Neurology, suppl. 39:246, 1989

83. Hughes M, McLellan DL: Increased co-activation of the upper limb muscles in writer's cramp. J Neurol Neurosurg Psychiatr 48:782, 1985

84. Rothwell JC, Oeso JA, Day BL et al: Pathophysiology of dystonias, p. 851. In Desmedt JE (ed): Motor Control Mechanisms in Health and Disease. Raven Press, New York, 1983

85. Panizza ME, Hallet M, Nilsson J: Reciprocal inhibition in patients with hand cramps. Neurology 39:85, 1989

86. Marsden CD, Obeso JA, Traub MM et al: Muscle spasms associated with Sudeck's atrophy after injury. Br Med J 288:173, 1984

87. Scherokman B, Husain F, Cuetter A et al: Peripheral dystonia. Arch Neurol 43:830, 1986

88. Schott GD: The idiopathic dystonias. A note on their orthopaedic presentation. J Bone Joint Surg 65:51, 1983

89. Schott GD: The relationship of peripheral trauma and pain to dystonia. J Neurol 48:698, 1985

90. Schott GD: Induction of involuntary movements by peripheral trauma: an analogy with causalgia. Lancet 27:712, 1986

91. Schwartzman RJ, Kerrigan J: The movement disorder of reflex sympathetic dystrophy. Neurology 40:57, 1990

92. Lockwood AH, Lindsay ML: Reflex sympathetic dystrophy after overuse. The possible relationship to focal dystonia. Med Probl Perform Art 4:114, 1989

93. Jankovic J, Van Der Linden C: Dystonia and tremor induced by peripheral trauma: predisposing factors. J Neurol Neurosurg Psychiatr 51:1512, 1988

94. Jankovic J, Shale H: Dystonia in musicians. Semin Neurol 9:131, 1989

95. Hochberg FH, Harris SU, Blattert TR: Occupational hand cramps: professional disorders of motor control. Hand Clin 6:417, 1990

96. Wilson FR: The acquisition and loss of skilled movement in musicians. Semin Neurol 9:146, 1989

97. Graffman G: Doctor, can you lend an ear? Med Probl Perform Art 1:3, 1986

98. Lang AE, Sheehy MP, Marsden CD: Anticholinergics in adult-onset focal dystonia. Can J Neurol Sci 9:313, 1982

99. LeVine WR: Behavioral and biofeedback therapy for a functionally impaired musician. A case report. Biofeedback Self Regul 8:101, 1983

100. Hays B: "Painless" hand problems of string pluckers. Med Probl Perform Art 2:39, 1987

101. Cohen LG, Hallett M, Geller BD, Hochberg F: Treatment of focal dystonias of the hand with botulinum toxin injections. J Neurol Neurosurg Psychiatr 52:355, 1989

102. Jankovic J, Brin M: Therapeutic uses of botulinum toxin. New Engl J Med 324:1187, 1991

18

Therapy and Work Hardening for Upper Extremity Disorders

Elaine LaCroix, MHSM, OTR/L, CHT
Susan A. Emerson, M.Ed., OTR/L, CHT

Occupational and physical therapists have been a vital part of the hand management team since Paul Brand, M.D., in India in the early 1950s, and Earl Peacock, M.D., John Madden, M.D., and H. Irene Hollis, OTR, in South Carolina in the late 1950s founded the first clinics specializing in surgery and rehabilitation of the hand and upper extremity.[1] Orthopaedic surgeons realized that the outcome of their efforts in the operating room was influenced by these paraprofessionals. Hand therapists skilled in evaluation, splinting, and the therapeutic use of exercise and activity and who have an understanding of work skills and activities of daily living have become essential to achieving maximal recovery after an injury or disease process.

The professions of occupational and physical therapy were first organized in the wake of World War I. Their involvement in the epidemic of infantile paralysis provided alternate means of dealing with the devastating effects of this dread disease. Federal funds began to supplement private financing of programs and services to rehabilitate the disabled when federal mandates, such as the Vocational Rehabilitation Act of 1920, were enacted.[2] Disabled veterans of World War II, motivated to live productive lives, demanded programs to assist their return to economic independence. Occupational and physical therapists were greatly involved in the rehabilitation of these veterans and other such disabled individuals.

The 1943 and 1954 amendments to the Vocational Rehabilitation Act facilitated program development for rehabilitation centers.[3] In the 1950s and 1960s, occupational and physical therapists began to work more aggressively in rehabilitation hospitals with a wide variety of physically and emotionally handicapped individuals.

Over the past two decades there has been a dramatic increase in the incidence first of hand injuries and now of cumulative trauma disorders in the work place. As these problems have escalated, the need for highly trained therapists who are specialized in the evaluation and treatment of occupational disorders has increased. In addition to traditional evaluation methods and treatment modalities, therapists have begun to understand and use approaches that have been developed specifically to deal with the problems of the injured worker. These approaches include patient and employer education, work hardening programs, and physical capacity evaluations (PCE).

One of the first reports to quantify upper extremity difficulties related to the work place was a 1974 study entitled *Upper Extremity Disorders—A Survey of Their Frequency and Cost in the United States* by Jennifer Kelsey.[4] She stated that at least one-third of work-related injuries involve the upper extremity. Since then, other authors have verified her contention. Some authors have found that in certain segments of the labor market an even higher percentage of work-related injury involves the upper extremity.[5-7]

The management of upper extremity conditions has become a subspecialty of both occupational and physical therapy. The American Society for Hand Therapists was founded in 1974. Its members have begun to promote more timely intervention and to verify or disprove the value of a number of commonly practiced therapeutic approaches. In May 1990, occupational therapists and physical therapists experienced in the treatment of upper extremity conditions were able to take the first nationwide examination to become Certified Hand Therapists.[8]

The purpose of this chapter is to provide the reader with an overview of the broad spectrum of therapy methods used by hand therapists to treat the injured worker population. Traditionally, therapy has followed a course beginning with an initial evaluation and treatment with periodic re-evaluations. These aspects of care are part of the medical management phase of care given to an injured worker following the injury and surgical procedure.

It is now recognized that successful return to work frequently requires the attainment of maximal strength and functioning.[1,3,9] Thus, a course of work hardening may be appropriate. As the work place changes and cumulative trauma disorders become more recognized, a large percentage of patients, regardless of their problem, will require therapy that is based on their specific job duties and uses treatment methods to reach their goal of returning to gainful employment.[10] The sections of this chapter—evaluation, treatment, work hardening, work site evaluation, physical capacity evaluation, and consultation—address both acute injuries (e.g., a flexor tendon laceration) and cumulative trauma disorders (e.g., flexor tendon synovitis) (Figs. 18-1 and 18-2).

EVALUATION

Examination of the upper extremity must be comprehensive. Only after baseline information has been recorded and a re-evaluation of the patient has been performed is it possible for the therapist to assess the effectiveness of the treatment program. Evaluation methods and instruments used should be standardized and results recorded accurately.[11-14] Observations, as well as objective information, need to be recorded throughout the course of the treatment program. A patient's inability to perform the recommended technique should be documented. Those with acute disorders may be unable to withstand a full evaluation. Patients who are symptomatic from a nerve compression in the arm may only be able to give one or two responses on the dynamometer or pinch gauge before noting an increase in dysesthesias. Modifications to the evaluation must be documented. As improvement occurs, the

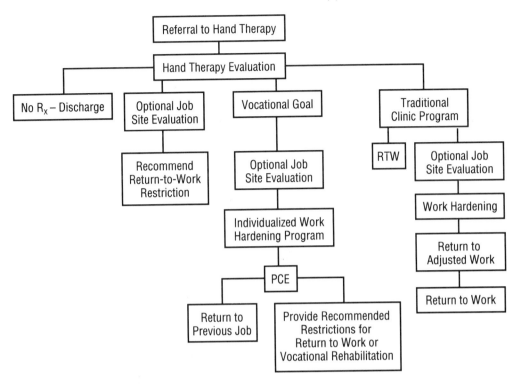

Fig. 18-1.

more standardized assessment approach can be pursued.

With any condition, improvements should be detectable within the first few days of care, and reproducible increases should occur within the first 2 to 3 weeks. Progress should continue throughout the treatment course. When no change is seen in objective measurements from one week to the next, the question must be asked: Is the patient's condition or compliance a factor in the lack of progress, or is it the therapy program?

Whether referred for traditional therapy or initiation of a work hardening program, the patient's status must be assessed before treatment begins. All too often, individuals arrive for their initial treatment with a physician's referral that indicates only the primary diagnosis and the preferred treatment modalities. The details of the incident or onset of symp-

toms can generally be gained through discussion with the patient. However, the specifics of the medical intervention and any precautions related to surgical procedures must be obtained through communication with the referring physician's office. Plans for further reconstruction or repair should be clarified. Pertinent medical information, such as high blood pressure, previous back injury, arthritis, or balance disorders, must be identified. Any gaps in the medical history could present a hazard in the planning and implementation of the initial treatment, subsequent therapy, and the work hardening program. In addition, the mechanism of injury should be fully understood so that secondary conditions, such as imbalance of the shoulder musculature following the amputation of a fingertip in a conveyor belt, can be assessed and treated from the onset.

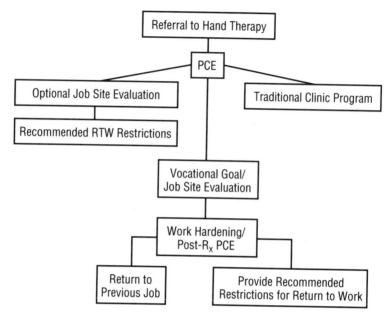

Fig. 18-2.

Trophic Assessment

First, hand posturing should be observed.[11] Vascular changes, bony or soft tissue abnormalities, and scar or wound conditions should be assessed. Muscle wasting, skin tone, or evidence of use (e.g., calluses or embedded dirt) confirm or contradict patients' description of their dysfunction or use.

Initially, the wound site may present with marked swelling. A volumeter,[15] tape measure, or circumferential gauge can document the degree of swelling, and its resolution or continuation can be charted. Even after the objective measurements indicate stabilization of the swelling, the individual may still perceive swelling in the involved site. This is a common complaint from a patient with an acute trauma or a cumulative trauma disorder and may persist for months.

Any inflammatory response to activity should be assessed since an evaluation should not cause an exacerbation of the symptoms. When assessing strength, ask the patient to go to the point of pain and not beyond. If this guideline is used during reassessments, then progress can be assessed without causing a recurrence of inflammation.

Sensibility Assessment

Documentation of pain and dysesthesias can serve to track recovery or assist in identifying the source of pathology. The peripheral nerves may be compressed at the neck, shoulder, or more distally. Localization of the compression is crucial for correct treatment. Carpal tunnel syndrome causes paresthesias in the middle finger, as does nerve compression at C7.[16] Therefore, additional information may be needed to establish the diagnosis. If more proximal structures are involved, a therapeutic program that includes the upper trunk may result in a decrease in the more distal complaints.[17,18]

Light touch testing using the eraser end of a pencil can be performed to assess grossly the areas supplied by the three peripheral nerves. The Semmes-Weinstein monofilaments[19,20] are used for a more detailed assessment. These nylon threads are graded in size and assess the thresholds of light touch and protective sensibility. The aesthesiometer[19] is used to assess the ability to discriminate between one and two points of pressure. A tuning fork is often used to assess tolerance of vibration (256 cps vibration), but the value of the information obtained is still under investigation (Fig. 18-3A & B).[19,21]

Soft Tissue Assessment

The musculotendinous system should be examined to determine the status of the muscles, tendons, and joints. Nodules, crepitus, or snapping should be localized and identified. Specific tests such as the Finkelstein or superficialis glide, help indicate compromised areas. Active and passive motion discrepancies must be identified and measured.[22] Tightness in the extrinsic and intrinsic muscles should be assessed.[11] Return to work can be delayed if tight intrinsic muscles cause pain during grasping, thus reducing grip strength.

Strength Assessment

Muscle strength can be measured using a dynamometer, pinch gauge,[23,24] and manual muscle testing. In addition, a vast array of computerized equipment is available to assist in measuring motion and isometric and dynamic strengths, endurances, and resistances against torque motions. Those tests most frequently used

for the upper extremity are the Baltimore Therapeutic Equipment (BTE) Work Simulator (Baltimore Therapeutic Equipment Co., Baltimore), Valpar Work Samples (Valpar Corporation, Tucson), Lido (Loredan Biomedical, Davis, California), and WEST (Work Evaluation Systems Technology, Huntington Beach, California) (Fig. 18-4).[25]

Generally, with a right-handed individual, the force exerted by the dominant hand is equal to or 10 percent greater than the strength found in the left. With left-handed people, both sides often have equal strength because of the number of everyday objects that require right-hand operation. Normal gross grasp strengths using the second notch on a Jamar dynamometer are 30.4 to 70.4 kg (65 to 155 pounds) for men and 14 to 38 kg (30 to 85 pounds) for women. Approximately 4 kg (9 pounds) of grip is needed to perform the majority of daily tasks. One kg (2.5 pounds) of pinch strength is necessary for simple activities.[26]

TREATMENT

Hand therapy is a progressive process that enables individuals to move from the acute phase of injury to a program designed to return them to their place of employment. As their condition improves, the treatment program should be upgraded and modified. While waiting for the acute injury or flare to resolve, all other body systems can be kept at peak performance. A home program that includes guidelines to maintain lower extremity strength, cardiovascular endurance, and overall general body conditioning must be provided. For example, after a flexor tendon repair, the muscle groups of the shoulder, elbow, and forearm can be strengthened and used functionally throughout the rehabilitation phase. The

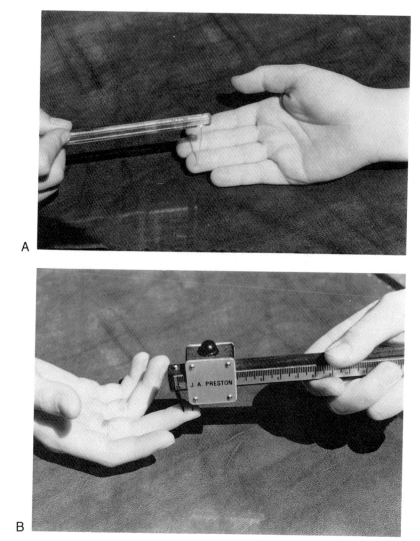

Fig. 18-3. (A) The Semmes-Weinstein pressure aesthesiometer is used to assess touch thresh-old through a system of nylon probes. **(B)** Similar aesthesiometers are used to assess discrim-inative (functional) sensibility.

tone of the intrinsic muscles can be main-tained by practicing finger abduction and adduction against resistance.

Although helpful, computerized and expensive equipment is not required for treatment. The resourceful therapist and patient can develop a program to fit any situation. Lower body conditioning can

be accomplished through stair-walking or walking up inclines in a local park. Sit-ups can be done anywhere. The hand specialist needs to be aware of the impact of these various systems on the injured worker. When unfamiliar with instructing patients in exercises for other areas of the body the therapist should consult with a

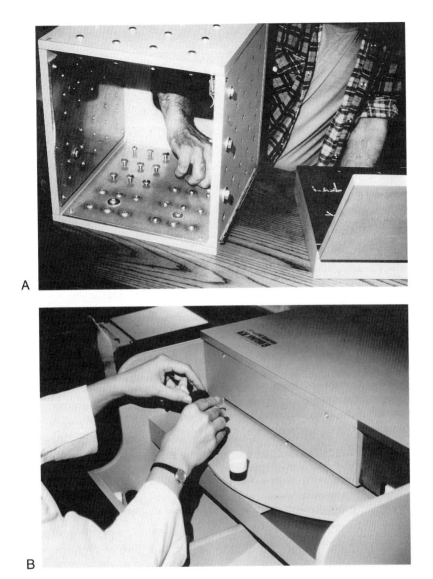

Fig. 18-4. (**A**) Valpar Component Work Sample No. 1 (small tools mechanical). (**B**) Valpar Component Work Sample No. 8 (simulated assembly). Both of the above are used in the assessment and in work hardening to simulate various skills needed at the work place.

colleague who has more expertise in this area.

The therapist should make every effort to use treatment modalities based on the physical findings; for example, a whirlpool may be appropriate to debride a healing wound,[27] but is often thought to be contraindicated for someone with carpal tunnel syndrome or tenosynovitis. Ultrasound may be indicated for breaking down scar tissue after a metacarpal fracture is felt to be healed, but should be used for only 12 to 20 applications. Subtle changes should begin to be seen within the first 7 to 10 treatments. The application of cold may cause negative responses in the local tissues and be tolerated for a very short period of time. Quite often, when something cool is applied after an activity, it is tolerated and does decrease the perception of internal pressure. The use of extremes of temperature should be avoided.

Carpal Tunnel Syndrome

Carpal tunnel syndrome (CTS) is used in this chapter as a typical cumulative trauma disorder since it is a common work-related condition. The authors have found that, through the use of immobilization, reduction in swelling, and then gradual range of motion and strengthening, patients are often able to return to work without requiring a surgical procedure. For some patients, education about the biomechanics involved is sufficient. For others, job modification may be required. However, if the condition persists after these approaches, a surgical release is often sought.

A conservative management program should begin with an evaluation of the frequency and extent of symptoms, thenar atrophy, grip and pinch strengths, and sensation.[28] Attention should be given to the elements of the patient's job and recreational activities that may be aggravating the symptoms. A well-fitted wrist-support splint should be provided with instructions to be worn for all hand use activities and at night.[29] The splint should be removed three or four times daily for hygiene, range of motion to the wrist to prevent stiffness, and gentle finger exercises. Differential tendon gliding exercises improve tendon excursion through a synovitic carpal tunnel canal.

Strengthening and repetitive or resistive hand and wrist exercises should be avoided during the acute phase of conservative management. At least three times a day something cool should be placed against the volar wrist[30] to assist in reduction of tendon sheath edema. Two ways to provide cooling are to place a can of cold soda against the wrist or to place the wrist splint in a freezer for ten minutes and then reapply the chilled splint. As the symptoms resolve, the patient may begin more rigorous exercises, such as strengthening and work simulation. When this conservative treatment is initiated early, the authors have seen as many as 50 percent of the patients with CTS succeed in returning to employment without surgical intervention.

With many cumulative trauma disorders, if resolution is attained early enough, the need for prolonged disability and surgery may be avoided. However, as Calisto cited at the 30th annual meeting of the Human Factors Society in 1986, job modification is often necessary to prevent recurrence. Work site modifications may include decreased repetition of tasks, institution of on-site stretch exercise programs, intermittent splinting, or work station or tool redesign. For example, if an electronics assembler uses a short-handled pair of pliers in which the base of the handle rests against the distal end of the carpal tunnel, the constant compression from the handle can cause discomfort and lessen productivity. By changing to a plier design that has longer, padded handle ends, this problem could be avoided (Fig. 18-5).

If surgery is necessary for CTS, the patient should be referred for postoperative therapy when the sutures are removed. Early referral prevents the unnecessary development of the most frequent complications of carpal tunnel surgery: hypersensitive scars, wrist stiffness, and tendon adherence.

Goals of postoperative management of CTS include the following:

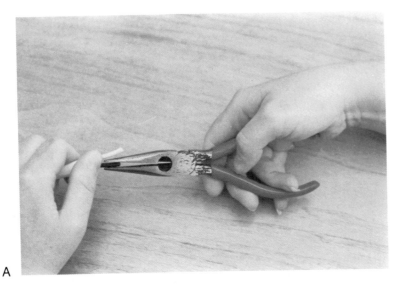

A

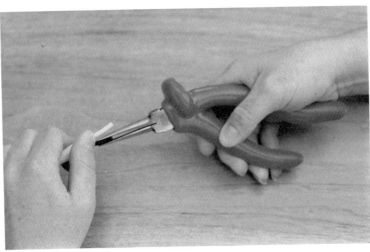

B

Fig. 18-5. (**A**) Needle-nose pliers used in wire assembly usually have short handles that compress the structures at the distal end of the carpal tunnel. To comfortably operate, the wrist is palmar flexed and ulnarly deviated. To enhance speed and efficiency, workers use the pressure of a digit to open them. Tendinitis in that digit often develops. (**B**) Ergonomically designed needle-nose pliers have longer padded handles and are self-opening.

- soften scar and prevent scar hypersensitivity
- regain full range of motion
- restore strength and endurance
- return to work

These goals must be discussed with the patient at the initial visit to ensure maximal cooperation and participation. A home program is designed and should be performed at least four times daily. Except for jobs that are highly repetitive or involve maximum strength for an entire shift, these goals can be achieved within 4 to 6 weeks.

Scar management includes light friction massage as soon as the wound is closed. Massage becomes progressively more rigorous and deep until full pressure is tolerated by the fourth postoperative week. If the scar remains hard and tender, ultrasound may be initiated at this time. The scar may be softened further by the pressure provided by one of the many catalyst-activated molding materials. The custom-fit mold may be worn intermittently over the scar under Coban wrap (Coban Self-Adherent Wrap, Medical-Surgical Division, 3M Health Care Group, St. Paul, Minnesota) or splints. Desensitization is a program of scar stimulation that decreases the patient's sensitivity and fear of tactile stimulation to the area. Desensitization should commence on the first day of therapy and be completed by the third to fourth postoperative week. Only mild sensitivity to deep pressure should remain by the fourth week.

If range of motion limitations do not resolve with simple traditional exercises, fluido therapy—a unit providing a dry whirlpool—can be used to heat deep tissues and relax muscles. Gentle joint mobilization may be beneficial. Full wrist range of motion and tendon excursion should be seen by the third week.

Strength and endurance are developed through the use of progressive resistive exercises beginning with coordination tasks, e.g., crumpling paper or turning over playing cards. By the second week, therapy putty is introduced for grip and pinch. Formal exercises and functional tasks are increased both in the clinic and at home. The authors have noted that, often within 2 or 3 weeks after a carpal tunnel release, 25 percent of the preop-

erative strength and endurance has been regained. By 4 weeks after surgery or after 2 weeks of therapy, grip strength should be at least 50 percent of that seen preoperatively. Some variation is seen, particularly if scar sensitivity is not resolved. The authors have found that approximately 50 percent of the patients who have undergone a release have regained their preoperative grip strength by the end of a 4-week therapy program or the sixth postoperative week.

Return to work should be considered in the sixth postoperative week, particularly if reduced or light work is available. Often, starting a patient back on regular duty but on a part-time basis facilitates successful re-employment by this date.[31] For someone who performs sedentary light work (e.g., a secretary or store clerk), a gradual return to full duty over a 1-month period of time is expected. A union carpenter may require several more weeks to increase strength and endurance enough to be able to return successfully to full duty.

Tenosynovitis

Management of tenosynovitis is much the same as conservative management of carpal tunnel syndrome. Careful assessment should be pursued, with attention to the exact tendon that is inflamed. Splinting must immobilize the involved structure. For example, a patient with de Quervain's tenosynovitis must be placed in a thumb spica splint involving wrist and thumb metacarpophalangeal joints and slightly limiting interphalangeal joint motion with the majority of the thumb pad free. A wrist support that leaves the entire interphalangeal joint free allows slight gliding of the involved tendons and may prevent resolution of pain. Ultrasound, phonophoresis (use of 10 percent hydrocortisone gel with ultrasound), or iontophoresis (use of pads impregnated with a variety of medications with or without electricity) to volar or dorsal wrist tendons may assist with edema reduction.[30] Oral anti-inflammatories or steroid injections may also be used in conjunction with the therapy program. Tendon excursion exercises prevent stiffness and facilitate restoration of normal tendon biomechanics. Assessment of home and work activities may identify tasks that can be modified to reduce stress to inflamed structures.

As symptoms diminish, weaning from the splint and increasing activities and resistive exercises should be introduced. Endurance is often an issue, particularly for patients performing highly repetitive assembly tasks. Attention should be directed to gradually increasing time spent on tasks or exercises to improve endurance in preparation for return to work.[29] To prevent recurrence, patients should be educated in the anatomic structures involved, postures to be avoided, and exercises to be performed. When strength and endurance have improved sufficiently, patients may be moved into work hardening or returned to work with job task modifications on a part-time basis, gradually increasing to full activity.

Epicondylitis

Lateral epicondylitis, or tennis elbow, and medial epicondylitis, or golfer's elbow, may be treated successfully with conservative therapy, eliminating the need for the less than optimal surgical procedure. Bands worn on the proximal forearm 24 hours a day, except for bathing, are designed to redirect the forces of muscle contraction from the muscle origins on the epicondyle. Thus, the inflammation and irritation of that area are reduced. If symptoms continue, stress on the muscle origins can be eliminated by the addition of a wrist splint. As inflammation and irritation resolve, gentle stretching of the involved muscles begins and continues until full, pain-free range is attained.

Recently, iontophoresis has been found to be a successful modality for reducing epicondylar inflammation, scar formation, and the resultant pain. This modality is less traumatic to tissues than traditional steroid injections. Iontophoresis involves the induction of topically applied ions into tissues by application of low-voltage direct galvanic stimulators.[27] Pads saturated with hydrocortisone, Lidocaine, and menthol are placed over the affected area, over which the low-voltage galvanic stimulator is applied. The patient may also wear the medication-impregnated pad for up to 8 hours at a time after the treatment. The ions of the medication are absorbed into the body by tissue penetration and osmosis. Thus, a rapid fluid built-up is avoided. The effects last longer than those obtained from an injection since a course of iontophoresis treatment lasts 2 to 3 weeks. Used in conjunction with splints and ice treatments, iontophoresis is another noninvasive treatment measure that helps reduce pain and localized edema.

As symptoms resolve, eccentric strengthening is introduced to increase muscle strength and tissue extensibility by controlled lengthening contractures,[32] rather than traditional shortening contractures. Generally, patients are started with only one-half pound of resistance. They build up to 30 repetitions. Then, the amount of weight is increased by another half-pound, and the number of repetitions is again gradually increased to 30. This system of strengthening has been shown to be particularly helpful in facilitating greater strength gain with less discomfort in the muscle group involved in epicondylitis.

Acute Injuries: Fractures

The management of fractures and acute trauma is initially quite different from that of cumulative trauma and soft tissue injuries. Early referral for a phalangeal fracture allows the therapist to use special skills to construct fracture braces or splints that leave all noninvolved joints free for range of motion while supporting and protecting the fractured bone and involved joints. If the fracture is pinned and stable, mobilization of adjacent joints may begin as early as 3 to 5 days postfracture. Rigorous handling should be avoided. Patients should be advised to keep the hand elevated and to apply something cool to the area every 2 to 3 hours to prevent excessive edema. If edema is a problem, Coban wrap should be used. Patients properly educated in the wrapping technique (e.g., wrapping distal to proximal using a single layer) can wear Coban wrap safely at all times except during skin care.

Gentle active range of motion helps reduce the swelling during the healing phase. Movement begins with the therapist supporting the fracture. If the fracture is stable and well aligned, the patient may be instructed in active unsupported range of motion at 3 weeks. By the fifth or sixth week, x-ray findings should indicate enough healing to permit a more rigorous joint mobilization and dynamic splinting program. When the motion is good to excellent, gentle strengthening begins. The most troublesome complication of the phalangeal fracture is development of a proximal interphalangeal (PIP) flexion contracture, caused by joint edema and soft tissue adhesions, or PIP extension lag, caused by injury to or attenuation of the extensor mechanism. If PIP flexion contracture occurs, PIP extension splints should be issued. Adjustments are then needed to stretch the shortened structures. If an extension lag is the problem, a night extension splint may be used for several months to allow for gradual retraction of the attenuated structures. Return to most job tasks should be expected after noncomplicated phalangeal fractures in 6 to 10 weeks with minimal restrictions or job modifications.

WORK HARDENING

Work-oriented treatment programs have been used as a part of rehabilitation for almost 200 years.[1] Initially used in psychiatric settings, disabled individuals were given work tasks as an alternative to custodial care.[2,3] Programs were titled "industrial therapy" and defined as "the prescribed use of activities inherent to the hospital operation, planned for the mutual benefit of patient and institution." These programs required the efforts of professional teams analyzing the skill level, physical and mental demands, and potential benefit of the job for the patient.[3]

With the increase in work-related injuries and workers' compensation claims in the 1970s and 1980s, work evaluation programs, vocational rehabilitation, prevocational programs, and work hardening programs emerged as major facets of the rehabilitation process.[3] Work hardening has been defined as an individualized work-oriented activity with simulated or actual work tasks.[10,33] This approach is not new to hand therapy programs as the majority of centers have always included this aspect of treatment.[29] As Lane[29] points out, it is, in reality, simply progressive resistive exercise. Sophisticated equipment and dedicated programs do not imply originality, although they offer significant benefits. Work hardening enables more consistent prediction of capacity and readiness for work after physical injury and better preparation of the injured worker for a successful return to gainful employment. Hand tools are often part of a traditional strengthening and coordination program. With a work hardening program, they are a small part of a more comprehensive reconditioning approach.

Definition

Several terms are used interchangeably with work hardening, including work conditioning, work tolerance, and work therapy.[9,34] All of these describe programs designed to provide a transition between acute care and return to the work force. These highly structured and individualized programs address issues of productivity, safety, physical tolerances, and work behaviors. Patients' performances are documented daily, and the rate of productivity should increase as endurance and tolerances improve. Safe methods of task performance are taught to the patient, such as correct postures for lifting and ergonomically correct positioning for work at a computer work station. Issues of pacing and alternating work with breaks and exercise, concepts particularly important to the population at risk for cumulative trauma, are stressed. By completion of the program specific tolerances for tasks, repetitions, and endurance are identified. Work behaviors and attitudes are observed and documented throughout the program. The emphasis is on adjusting to the injury and returning to the job market with increased strength and endurance and/or minimal physical limitations.[9]

Work hardening programs should include initial assessments, individual program development and implementation, and final evaluations, often in the form of a physical capacity evaluation (PCE). As is explained in more detail later, a PCE provides the physician and employer with specific recommendations for implementation of a safe return to work.[25] The therapists involved with the work hardening program must be knowledgeable in and consider the following elements when developing a specific program tailored to each individual[33]:

- the anatomy, diagnosis, and prior treatment of the patient's condition
- a comprehensive analysis of the job to which the employee will return
- the psychosocial aspects of the work place
- the patient's adjustment to residual disability
- family and work issues

Many work hardening programs are multidisciplinary and include occupational and physical therapists, rehabilitation specialists, psychologists, and other health care providers.[3,10] Alternatively, hand therapists in private practices may provide highly specialized work hardening programs for upper extremity injuries without the assistance of a large number of professional staff. These therapists coordinate care with the physician, insurance carrier, vocational specialist, and industry to form a team. In conjunction with the patient, they facilitate an efficient return to work.

CARF Standards

The Commission on Accreditation of Rehabilitation Facilities' (CARF) 1990 *Standards Manual for Organizations Serving People with Disabilities*[35] outlines the guidelines for establishing multidisciplinary work hardening programs. At the time of publication of this text, Florida, Ohio, Oregon, Iowa, and Washington had accepted these standards as necessary for reimbursement of services provided and titled as work hardening.[36] These standards are very specific about the space required, the numbers and range of professional staff, the comprehensive nature of work simulated, and the length of treatment allowed. The requirement of accreditation serves to regulate the services and attempts to ensure quality. The intent is admirable, but its effectiveness cannot be assessed at this time because of the limited number of facilities that have achieved the status of CARF accreditation. In addition, it is not clear if the CARF guidelines will truly become the standard as many facilities provide competent services with much less than is required by them. If the program is of high quality and the patient benefits by returning to work, the objective of any program is met, regardless of how large it is.

Referrals

Any worker is appropriate for referral to work hardening when there is concern about readiness for return to work particularly in terms of strength for heavy duty work and endurance for many assembly, clerical, and data entry positions. Referral may be made by a physician, rehabilitation nurse or counselor, occupational health nurse, or employer.[2,33,34] Occasionally, patients recognize the need for some type of work readiness program and request it themselves. A physician's prescription is usually required by the state's licensure law for therapists, and prior approval from the insurance carrier is required to ensure reimbursement. The patient's medical condition must be stable and must have reached a plateau with traditional modalities.

The patient must understand that the work hardening program should be treated as a job. The patient should arrive on time, focus on the program, and miss appointments only for valid reasons. Many programs allow a maximum number of excused absences after which the program is discontinued and the insurance carrier and physician notified of the patient's noncompliance.

In any program, the new patient must be evaluated for two reasons: to assess the appropriateness of the program and to establish baseline data for evaluating the patient's progress.[2,9,33]

All patients must have a vocational goal. Unless a specific job is available, they may lack the motivation necessary to succeed. If no job exists or alternative employment is not identified and the program is pursued, the patient, despite achieving maximal improvement at the completion of the program, may eventually regress.[37] In addition, if there is no job goal, readiness for return to work and specific job requirements cannot be assessed. In these cases, the therapist should make the recommendation to the insurance carrier that vocational services be considered first and work hardening pursued only when return to work goals have been established.

Elements of the Work Hardening Program

A work hardening program offers a way for the injured worker to regain confidence and improve areas that, during a PCE, tested below normal. A summary of the criteria for acceptance into the work hardening program is as follows.

- Patient is physically ready for work hardening.
- Therapist understands the work environment.

- A mutually agreed-upon work goal is established.
- A comprehensive evaluation has been completed.
- Critical physical factors have been identified.
- Work simulation tasks and activities have been implemented.

Work hardening programs usually run 4 or 5 days per week and initially may be as short as 2 hours per day depending on patient tolerance. Over the course of 6 to 8 weeks, the patient should increase time in the program to 4, 6, or 8 hours daily as the program, job requirements, and patient progress dictate. Work hardening programs should have specific time limitations. Premature discharge can lead to either of two scenarios. First, if the individual feels ready to return to work after two or three sessions but the job requirements have not been met and the job is not clearly appropriate for the worker's degree of readiness, the patient may fail the attempt to return to work. Second, if the patient feels unable to continue to participate because of pain or discomfort, early discharge may reinforce the perception of disability. Instead, the program demands should be lowered, and the patient encouraged to continue. On the other hand, a program with no end date fosters the patient dependence on the program or staff and the continued perception of the need for therapeutic management, rather than capacity for a work milieu. With any of the above situations, the cost to insurance carriers becomes exorbitant and the major objective of return to work is never met.

Most programs are limited to 8 to 10 weeks, with only extenuating circumstances allowing for extensions. An anticipated length of treatment in the program must be discussed, and upon completion, return to work must be the goal.

Evaluation for Work Hardening

The evaluation should include all issues of any initial upper extremity evaluation appropriate to the diagnosis.[9] In addition, work simulation should be attempted and endurance and postures observed. An example of a premature referral to work hardening might be the patient who is 3 weeks postcarpal tunnel release. This patient's strength and endurance are too poor to complete one half-hour of work. His problems—scar tenderness, dyscoordination, and decreased range of motion—should be addressed in traditional therapy. Therefore, the initial evaluation would indicate that this patient is a poor candidate for work hardening and the authors would recommend a course of appropriate traditional therapy before work hardening.

In contrast, the patient with epicondylitis who has been splinted, has completed iontophoresis, and has pursued eccentric strengthening may demonstrate grip strength at 50 percent of normal, poor endurance for work-related tasks, general body deconditioning, and some discomfort at the end of the evaluation. This patient is an excellent candidate for work hardening and should benefit maximally from its processes.

Each patient should be given an individualized program that uses the concepts of therapeutic exercises and progressive resistive exercising tailored to the specific job task demands. The patient's strength and endurance should increase gradually in preparation for return to the job. Several hand and arm strengthening tools may be used, including using pipe trees to simulate plumbing; carrying and emptying large boxes or trash cans for maintenance workers or warehousemen; typing, doing data entry and filing for secretaries; and sawing, hammering, and carrying lumber for carpenters.

When space is limited, either the BTE Work Simulator or the Work Cube (Advanced Therapy Products, Richmond) is of great assistance. The BTE Work Simulator is a computerized machine with an electronic breakhead and various exercise handles that may be used to simulate a wide variety of hand tasks, motions, or postures (Fig. 18-6). Resistance and speed of task performance are increased gradually. The data output from the computer gives information on force, distance, and work produced. The motivated patient can be challenged safely by this unit, and the symptom magnifier or malinger can be identified more objectively.

The Work Cube is a noncomputerized metal frame with attachments that enable the patient to perform fine coordination tasks by assembling nuts and bolts. Small hand tools can be used if desired. Patients can progress in lifting tolerance from 4 to 100 lb using weighted bars (Fig. 18-7).

Lifting should be assessed carefully, particularly if any wrist disorder is present. Schultz[38] has outlined the stresses on the wrist based on the different postures of the task, e.g., straight lift to knuckle keeps the wrist in neutral with minimal strain. She points out that lifting to the waist, chest, or overhead forces the wrist through a variety of postures. If the patient with wrist pain or who is recovering from a wrist injury is not evaluated correctly and strengthened in the required postures and sequences of motions, return to work may be jeopardized.

It is critically important that the tasks used in work hardening be sufficient to challenge the patient's interest, yet not be so difficult that reinjury or a flare-up occurs. Many patients in these programs

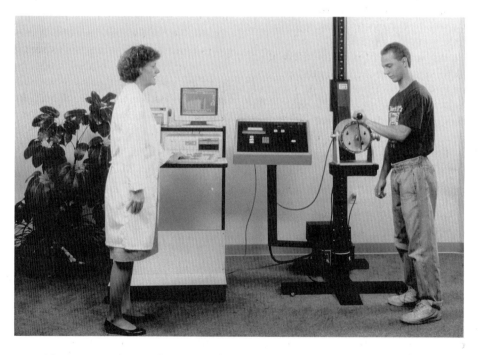

Fig. 18-6. The BTE Work Simulator with the Quest Computer System is used for assessment and work simulation.

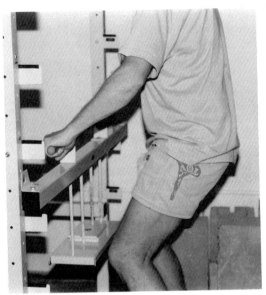

Fig. 18-7. Proper body mechanics can be taught and lifting strengths increased using the Work Cube.

tend to focus on their limitations, rather than on their capabilities. Until referral to work hardening, the aim of traditional therapy tends to be the management of the injury and reduction of the pain. In work hardening, when pain and limited use persist, the staff tries to assist the patient to focus on improving functional capacity, rather than on the pain. In all work hardening programs, a critical balance is needed to ensure that highly motivated patients learn to respect and respond to their limits, and patients who have been immobilized by fear and perceived disability receive encouragement to move beyond self-imposed boundaries.[39,40] Identifying valid limitations for either of these types of patients, helping them recognize those limits, and providing the opportunity to expand their capacity and manage their physical response to work are all key elements to work hardening. The patient who is motivated strongly by secondary gains to maintain a prework

hardening condition may not be able to benefit from this approach. The lack of progress or cooperation should be documented and addressed by other professionals.

WORK SITE EVALUATION

Work site evaluations, in combination with discussions with the patient, may range from informal and brief assessments to formal, comprehensive observation of the individual's job or of an entire assembly line.[25] In an informal evaluation, which is used primarily to develop a work simulated therapy program or a work hardening program, the therapist may ask the patient to describe a typical day on the job, identifying the tools used, motions performed, and postures assumed. Sometimes the employer is able to provide the therapist or physician with a job description. However, these descriptions are usually vague and do not identify specific hazards for the hand and arm.

If the informal "walk through" or employer-provided job description is deemed insufficient, the therapist, physician, employer, insurance carrier, or occupational health nurse may request a more formal on-site evaluation. The therapist performing this evaluation may make careful observation of some or all of the following:

- general environment: lighting, ventilation, temperature
- hours: work per day, number and frequency of breaks, quotas, rates of performance, bonuses
- general postures: sitting, standing, stooping, crawling, awkward or extreme positions
- specific arm/hand postures or motions: reaching, grasping, twisting

- tools: size, shape, texture, force required during use
- weights: held, lifted, carried

Of particular importance with regard to upper extremity cumulative trauma disorders are hand and wrist postures, static hold times, extremes of a range of motion, postures, grasp forces, and repetitions.[41,42] Repetitive jobs have been defined as those with tasks which have a cycle time of less than 30 seconds or where more than 50 percent of the time is spent performing the same motions.[7] Several authors[7] describe the wrist as a pulley on which greater forces increase exponentially as wrist arc increased beyond 30° in either flexion or extension. With these increased angles, the space available for the median nerve and the volar wrist tendons in the carpal canal is decreased. Repetitive tasks further aggravate the involved structures if volar wrist tenosynovitis exists.

The ergonomic literature repeatedly emphasizes that the static hold of tools, parts, or postures has been associated with decreased blood flow to musculoskeletal structures.[7,41,43] In a 1987 study, Rogers[41] developed charts indicating the amount of recovery time needed to prevent muscle fatigue for employees doing repetitive or heavy tasks. These charts are very helpful in identifying the need to slow rates of performance on industrial lines or redesigning assembly lines to reduce unnecessary stress.

The therapist must be aware of the patient's perception of the disability when developing the work hardening program. Visiting the work site and performing a job site evaluation enable the therapist to develop a "feel" for the job and work environment. Such visits help build additional confidence and trust between the worker and the therapist, especially for those workers who are fearful and apprehensive about returning to work.

After a work site evaluation, the therapist's recommendations should achieve the following aims:

- assist the physician in determining whether a patient should return to regular or altered work on a full- or part-time basis
- assist the company in adjusting or adapting the work place or a particular job
- assist the patient in acquiring a better understanding of safety techniques and preventive measures to avoid reinjury

Exercise programs are frequently instituted in industries both for individuals returning to work after injury and for workers at risk for injury because of the nature of their job.[44-46] Prework stretch programs are designed to improve flexibility and decrease the incidence of sprains and strains that occur when muscles are cold and tight. Through prestretch programs, J.M. Smuckers Co. of Woodburn, Oregon reduced its injury rate by 56 percent, saving 95 percent in workers' compensation costs for its employees in 1 year.[44] Hansford et al.[43] found that exercises done periodically during the work day produce an increase in blood flow. In their study, they demonstrated a significant improvement in blood flow during a break incorporating light stretch exercises.

PHYSICAL CAPACITY EVALUATION

Functional capacity evaluation, work capacity evaluation, work tolerance evaluation, and physical capacity evaluation are terms that are often used interchangeably. Assessment using simulated tasks was first introduced in 1972 at the Vocational Rehabilitation Service at Rancho

Los Amigos Hospital in Downing, California in its evaluation of workers with cardiovascular conditions. This program involved exercise physiologists, cardiologists, and vocational evaluators and resulted in a higher rate of return to work and increased safety and confidence. Over time, it was determined that a physical capacity evaluation (PCE) could reduce the permanent disability costs of workers by identifying viable skills in those who were once deemed totally disabled[34,47] and by providing safe return to work recommendations. In many incidences, the PCE is now considered a link between the clinic and the work place.[25,49] The injured worker is no longer viewed as a patient, but as a viable member of society.

Matheson,[48] who did much of the preliminary work in this area, in 1986 defined a work capacity evaluation as "a systematic process of measuring and developing an individual's capacity to dependably sustain performance in response to broadly defined work demands."

A PCE is most frequently given for one of the following reasons:

- resolution of a case
- identification of ongoing problems
- clarification of the worker's remaining abilities
- preparation for a work hardening program by establishing baseline information on work capabilities
- augmentation of information to be included in a physician's independent medical evaluation (IME)[50]

The format used for a PCE varies. Regardless of the length of the evaluation, the approach used by each center should be standardized and should include both objective and subjective data. The person administering the assessment has to be familiar with the data to be gained from the tests and also the patient's job re-

quirements. If not, very subtle yet crucial pieces of data may be overlooked.

Workers who are interested in returning to work will show maximum effort and a positive attitude throughout the entire PCE session. Concluding comments can state their levels of functioning and the probability of a safe and successful return to work. Evaluators must be alert to identify individuals in this category who might deny or minimize residual problems of pain and lack of endurance. A graduated return to their job may be the only modification required. Patients who are uncertain of their capabilities initially may be hesitant in performing tasks but by the conclusion of the session they usually attempt the various tasks and show improvement in strength. When pain is the overriding problem for the individual, the PCE has limited value. The performance seen on a "good day" may vary greatly from that seen on a "bad day." The PCE documents the patient's level of functioning at one particular point in time and is greatly influenced by a perceived level of discomfort.

Individuals who do not want to return to work for any variety of reasons will demonstrate limited effort and express pain, resulting in poor scores on the PCE. In these cases, objective data are recorded, but the evaluator's impressions based on nonverbal clues and inconsistencies in performance will be of greatest value to the other team members.[25]

PCEs are almost always scheduled by vocational specialists with the sanction of the insurance carrier. They may follow a physician's IME. The therapist's PCE is used to identify the person's level of functioning, whereas the physician's IME determines whether a medical end has been attained. Ideally, both the therapist and physician receive all previous medical and therapeutic information before making their assessments. A job description is particularly helpful. If specific work demands, such as lifting a certain amount of weight or maneuvering a specific sized object, are known, the therapist can duplicate those tasks and assess the person's capabilities. The performance on each test should be compared not only to what is known to be normal for the population in general but also to the individual's uninvolved side. Any trends in performance should be looked for throughout the assessment section.

Regardless of the intent of the assessment, all individuals should be asked to identify clearly their problems, disabilities, and levels of discomfort. It is helpful to have them document their usual patterns of pain by marking them on an illustration of the body. This information can be useful in clarifying any other physical conditions that may influence their functioning. At times, the authors have noted that those who are being evaluated for their function after a carpal tunnel release have indicated pain patterns that correlate with nerve compression in a more proximal area.

The evaluation begins with the traditional hand assessment. In addition, a pyramid grip check may be done. Pressure is applied to the dynamometer in three successive attempts on each of five handle settings; maximal effort is considered to be applied if the forces attained form a bell-shaped curve, e.g., 30, 36, 32, 30, 28 kg. When the same force is applied for all handle settings, the evaluator must question whether submaximal effort is being presented.[11] Alternatively, vast variations in the force exerted may occur. These variations may also indicate submaximal effort or the effect of pain. Only by noting verbal and nonverbal cues can the therapist make an educated, professional judgment. In addition, computerized equipment is beginning to be used for PCE assessment (EVAL Computer, Greenleaf Medical, Palo Alto and LIFE CORP, Lifestyle Enhancement Systems,

Inc., Tucson). However, only if the data collected are combined with the observations of the therapist overseeing the assessment can the recommendations be considered comprehensive. In addition to the usual areas of assessment—range of motion, strength, and sensibility—a PCE almost always includes comments on the patient's attitude; visual acuity; ability to read, write, and speak English; and general physical functioning, such as ability to walk, stoop, crawl, and reach. These observations, in combination with the amount of weight that can be lifted and carried, assist the vocational specialist in recommending the appropriate category of work for the person to consider.

The U.S. Department of Labor's published guidelines for work placement based on physical abilities are summarized as follows:

- *Sedentary Work:* Seated with occasional walking and standing; lifting a maximum of 10 lb with occasional lifting and/or carrying of job-related items
- *Light Work:* Seated tasks may include pushing and pulling with the arms and/or use of leg controls; a greater amount of walking and standing is anticipated; lifting up to 20 lb with more frequent handling of 10 lb items
- *Medium Work:* Lifting maximum of 50 lb with more frequent lifting and carrying of 25 lb
- *Heavy Work:* Lifting maximum of 100 lb with more frequent lifting and carrying of 50 lb
- *Very Heavy Work:* Lifting items of 100 or more pounds and lifting and/or carrying items of 50 or more pounds.[6]

CONSULTATION

The final area of practice to be addressed is that of a consultant. Hand therapists who specialize in work-related conditions are finding that the breadth and depth of knowledge required is seemingly endless. Requests for consultation may come from medical suppliers who wish to fabricate a newer and better "widget"; from insurance carriers, employers, and special interest groups who are seeking to better understand upper extremity conditions[51]; and from industries who wish to decrease the incidence of upper extremity injuries.[46,52,53] Hand therapists across the country are reporting increasing numbers of requests from physicians and therapists to assist them by evaluating a patient they have been treating but who has not responded as anticipated to the care given. Such intervention is often called "Second Opinion for Therapy."

More and more therapists who have knowledge of hand conditions and the industrial setting are asked to consult on the appropriate treatment modalities and to give recommendations on safe return to work conditions. For example, if a person is involved in a therapy program several times a week for a number of weeks without showing any true progress, hand therapists are frequently requested to give a second opinion for the insurance carrier. The treating therapist may be following the usual and customary treatment approach for that person's particular condition, but the injury may warrant a variation from the usual approach or the patient's attitude may be sabotaging the program. Preparing such second opinions usually entails reviewing the previous therapeutic approach, assessing the patient's current status, and determining which therapy interventions will be most effective at this point in the recovery phase. Generally, the treating therapist resumes the care based on these recommendations and the treating physician's sanction.

Businesses, whether the small local florist, the secretarial staff at a university, or

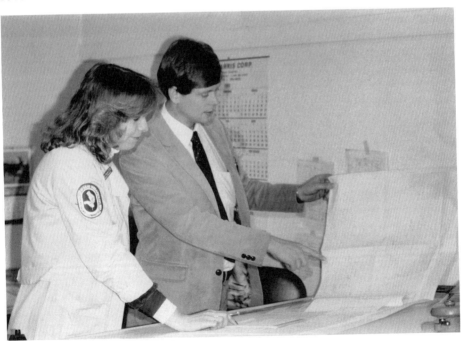

Fig. 18-8. The hand therapist consults with the industrial engineer during work place assessment and consultation for the ergonomic design of work tasks.

a large electronics firm, have become interested in reducing the incidence of cumulative trauma disorders. Therapists, especially occupational therapists, are trained in task analysis and adaptive approaches to tasks. Their expertise has been sought in lecturing on the biomechanics of cumulative trauma disorders, redesigning work stations to decrease the repetitiveness or force required to perform certain job functions, adapting existing equipment and tools, or finding alternatives to enable injured workers to reduce the likelihood of reinjury[54-58] (Fig. 18-8).

Some states have a more litigious climate than others. Therapists who work in states where lawyers are very active and influential in workers' compensation cases are frequently called upon to be expert witnesses[59,60] or have their comments included in PCEs challenged in court. Very often, therapists' medical records are subpoenaed to be used by the lawyers on either side of the case when attempting to settle a workers' compensation dispute. Participating in the legal arena requires significant experience and expertise in hand management, as well as a willingness to stand firm on what has been observed, measured, and documented.

Acknowledgement

The authors wish to thank Francesca Sullivan for maintaining a sense of humor during her numerous hours at the keyboard and proofreading.

REFERENCES

1. Ballard M, Baxter P, Bruening L, Fried S: Work therapy and return to work: Hand Clin 2:247, 1986
2. Commission on Practice: Work hardening. Am J Occup Ther 40:841, 1986
3. Matheson L, Ogden L, Violette K et al: Work hardening: occupational therapy in industrial rehabilitation. Am J Occup Ther 39:314, 1985
4. Kelsey JL, Pastides H, Kreiger N et al: Upper Extremity Disorders: A Survey of Their Frequency and Cost in the United States. CV Mosby, St. Louis, 1980
5. Seaton M, Feely C: OT team studies repetitive motion disorders in industrial settings. Occup Ther Week 4:4, 1990
6. US Department of Labor: Selected Characteristics of Occupations Defined in the Dictionary of Occupational Titles. US Government Printing Office, Washington DC, 1981
7. Armstrong T, Fine L, Goldstein S: Ergonomics considerations in hand and wrist tendinitis. J Hand Surg 12A:830, 1987
8. Hand Therapy Certification Commission, Inc., 1002 Vandora Springs Road, Suite 101, Garner, NC 27529 (919) 779-7342
9. Baxter-Petralia PL, Bruening LA, Blackmore SM: Work therapy program of the hand rehabilitation center in Philadelphia, p. 1155. In Hunter JM, Schneider LH, Mackin EJ, Callahan AD (eds): Rehabilitation of the Hand: Surgery and Therapy. 3rd Ed. CV Mosby, St. Louis, 1990
10. Wyrich J, Niemeyer L, Ellexson M et al: Occupational therapy work hardening programs: a demographic study. Am J Occup Ther 45:109, 1991
11. Aulicino PL, DuPuy TE: Clinical examination of the hand, p. 31. In Hunter JM, Schneider LH, Mackin EJ, Callahan AD (eds): Rehabilitation of the Hand: Surgery and Therapy. 3rd Ed. CV Mosby, St. Louis, 1990
12. Wolfe T, Diplacido M, Lubahn J: Unable to return to work—now what? p. 483. In Kasdan ML (ed): Occupational Hand and Upper Extremity Injuries and Diseases. Hanley & Belfus, Philadelphia, 1991
13. American Society for Surgery on the Hand: The Hand—Examination and Diagnosis. ASSH, Aurora. Churchill Livingstone, New York, 1987
14. Smith S, Cunningham S, Weinberg R:

The predictive validity of functional capacities evaluation. Am J Occup Ther 40:564, 1986

15. DeVore G, Hamilton G: Volume measuring of the severely injured hand. Am J Occup Ther 22:16, 1968

16. Hoppenfeld S: Orthopaedic Neurology—A Diagnostic Guide to Neurologic Levels. JB Lippincott, Philadelphia, 1977

17. Caillet R: Shoulder Pain. FA Davis, Philadelphia, 1966

18. Smith K: The thoracic outlet syndrome: a protocol of treatment. J Occup Speech Phys Ther 1(2):89, 1979

19. Fess EE: Documentation: essential elements of an upper extremity assessment battery, p. 53. In Hunter JM, Schneider LH, Mackin EJ, Callahan AD (eds): Rehabilitation of the Hand: Surgery and Therapy. 3rd Ed. CV Mosby, Philadelphia, 1990

20. Tomancik L: Directions for Using Semmes-Weinstein Monofilaments. North Coast Medical, Campbell, CA, 1987

21. Dellon A: Evaluation of Sensibility and Re-Education of Sensation in the Hand. Williams & Wilkins, Baltimore, 1981

22. American Academy of Orthopaedic Surgeons: Joint Motion, Method of Measuring and Recording. AAOS, Chicago, 1965

23. Mathiowetz V, Weber K, Volland G, Kashman N: Rehability and validity of grip and pinch strength evaluations. J Hand Surg 9A:222, 1984

24. Mathiowetz V, Kashman K, Volland G et al: Grip and pinch strength: normative data for adults. Arch Phys Med Rehabil 66:69, 1985

25. Schultz-Johnson K: Assessment of upper extremity injured person's return to work potential. J Hand Surg 12A:950, 1987

26. Swanson AB, Swanson G, Goran-Hagert C: Evaluation of impairment of hand function, p. 109. In Hunter JM, Schneider LH, Mackin EJ, Callahan AD (eds): Rehabilitation of the Hand: Surgery and Therapy. 3rd Ed. CV Mosby, Philadelphia, 1990

27. Mullins PA: Use of therapeutic modalities in upper extremity rehabilitation, p. 195. In Hunter JM, Schneider LH, Mackin EJ, Callahan AD (eds): Rehabilitation of the Hand: Surgery and Therapy. 3rd Ed. CV Mosby, St. Louis, 1990

28. Baxter-Petralia PL: Therapist's management of carpal tunnel syndrome, p. 640. In Hunter JM, Schneider LH, Mackin EJ, Callahan AD (eds): Rehabilitation of the Hand: Surgery and Therapy. 3rd Ed. CV Mosby, St. Louis, 1990

29. Lane C: Hand therapy for occupational upper extremity disorders, p. 469. In Kasdan ML (ed): Occupational Hand and Upper Extremity Injuries and Disease. Hanley & Belfus, Philadelphia, 1991

30. Poole B: Cumulative trauma disorder of the upper extremity from occupational stress. J Hand Ther 1:172, 1988

31. Randolf S, Dalton P: Limited duty work: an innovative approach to early return to work. AAOHN 37:446, 1989

32. Trombly CA: Occupational Therapy for Physical Dysfunction. 3rd Ed. Williams & Wilkins, Baltimore, 1988

33. Bear-Lehman J: Factors affecting return to work after hand injury. Am J Occup Ther 37:189, 1983

34. Ogden-Neimeyer L, Jacobs K: Work Hardening—State of the Art. Slack, Thorofare, NJ, 1989

35. Commission on Accreditation of Rehabilitation Facilities: Standards Manual for Organizations Serving People with Disabilities. CARF, Tucson, 1990

36. Work hardening accreditation. In Matheson LN (ed): Industrial Rehabilitation Quarterly. Vol. 2. Roy Matheson and Associates, Irvine, CA, 1989

37. Dortch H, Trombly C: The effects of education on hand use with industrial workers in repetitive jobs. Am J Occup Ther 44:777, 1990

38. Schultz K: Upper extremity factors in evaluation of lifting. J Hand Ther 3:72, 1990

39. Herbert LA: Living With C.T.D.—There is Life After Cumulative Trauma Disorder. IMPACC, Bangor, 1990

40. Raithel K: Chronic pain and exercise therapy. Physician Sports Med 17:203, 1989

41. Rogers S: Recovery time needs for repetitive work. Semin Occup Med 2:19, 1987

42. Rogers S: Job evaluation in worker fitness determination. Occup Med State of Art Rev 3:9219, 1988

43. Hansford T, Blood H, Kent B: Blood flow

changes at the wrist in manual workers after preventive interventions. J Hand Surg 11A:503, 1988

44. Allers V: Work place preventive programs cut costs of illness and injuries. OHS 58:26, 1989
45. Rystrom C, Eversmann W: Cumulative trauma intervention in industry: a model program for the upper extremity, p. 489. In Occupational Hand and Upper Extremity Injuries and Disease. Hanley & Belfus, Philadelphia, 1991
46. Lutz G, Hansford T: Cumulative trauma disorder controls: the ergonomics program at Ethicon inc. J Hand Surg 12A:863, 1987
47. Smith S, Cunningham S, Weinberg R: The predictive validity of functional capacities evaluation. Am J Occup Ther 40:564, 1986
48. Matheson LN: Work Capacity Evaluation—Systematic Approach to Industrial Rehabilitation. ERIC, Anaheim, 1986
49. Herbin M: Work capacity evaluation for occupational hand injuries. J Hand Surg 12A:958, 1987
50. Engleberg AL: Guides to the Evaluation of Permanent Impairment. 3rd Ed. American Medical Association, Chicago, 1988
51. Putz-Anderson V: Cumulative Trauma Disorders—A Manual for Musculoskeletal Diseases of the Upper Limbs. Taylor & Francis, Philadelphia, 1988
52. Collings G: The broader issue—health care management at the individual and systems level, p. 315. In Gentry WD et al (eds): Behavioral Medicine: Work, Stress and Health. Martinas Nijhoff Publishers with NATO Scientific Affairs Division, Boston, 1985
53. Melnek M: Comprehensive injury prevention programs in business and industry. Work Prog Special Interest Section Newsl, 4:3, 1990
54. Bartel J: View from the top. Visions. Nat Assoc Occup Health Prof 1:7, 1990
55. Randolph S, Dalton P: Limited duty work: an innovative approach to early return to work. AAOHN 37:446, 1989
56. Davis LM: Use whole-brain learning methods to control repetitive motion injuries. OHS 59:26, 1990
57. Johnson SL: Ergonomic design of hand-held tools to prevent trauma to the hand and upper extremity. J Hand Ther 3:86, 1990
58. Armstrong T, Foulke J, Joseph B, Goldstein S: Investigation of cumulative trauma disorders in a poultry processing plant. Indust Hyg Assoc J 43:103, 1982
59. Smith S: The Forensic Model of Occupational Therapy: The Changing Roles of Occupational Therapists. Haworth Press, Binghamton, NY, 1984
60. DeMaio-Feldman D: The occupational therapist as an expert witness. Am J Occup Ther 41:590, 1987

19

Rehabilitation Services

Evelyn R. Davis, M.S., CRC, CIRS

Rehabilitation is the restoration of good health and the ability to work.[1] When hard-working people are injured on their jobs, their lives change immediately. Suddenly they must deal with insurance benefits, legal advice, physician recommendations, physical therapy exercises, frustrated employers, and anxious family members. Concurrently they are coping with pain, confusion, fears, and anger. Left alone with a myriad of input *and* overwhelmed with feelings, they often become immobilized, depressed, or enraged. However, there is an anchor that can provide the stability to prevent unnecessary anguish and facilitate the successful use of professional input. The rehabilitation specialist is that anchor, the professional trained to coordinate services, simplify the complex maze of advice being given, and provide injured workers with viable future options so that they can resume a productive lifestyle.

The clients who have the opportunity to work with a rehabilitation specialist soon after their accident are more likely to have a successful outcome. They have had less time to focus on their disability, and the rehabilitation professional assists in capitalizing on their strengths, thereby creating an atmosphere for positive move-ment and future productivity. The ultimate goal is to enable the injured individuals to retain dignity and to make informed decisions that will result in productive lifestyles.

Consider this typical case example of an injured worker.

Mr. J. runs a printing press. His dominant hand was degloved when it was caught in the printing machine. He was rushed to the hospital where his wound was cleaned, and a hand surgeon treated him. After several surgical procedures the injured hand began to heal. At the appropriate time he began occupational therapy with a qualified hand therapist. He was cooperative and slowly regained motion and use of his hand. In fact, he regained sufficient function to be able to perform light duty responsibilities with his former employer. He was told by his physician and therapist that he had reached a medical end point and that he could return to work. His employer, who found an alternate and appropriate job for him, was willing, even eager, to rehire him. However, as Mr. J neared his maximum medical improvement, he began to complain of new pains, focusing on his more limited range of motion and an overriding feeling that he was not yet ready to return to work. All further medical tests were negative, and there were no objective findings to support his new complaints.

In this case example, the health care community has provided the best available services, and by all measurable standards it is their opinion that this individual should be able to resume a productive lifestyle. Why, then, does he not return to work and resume his preinjury activities? What are the factors that allow for a successful surgical outcome, but not a successful human outcome? This question has been of concern to the medical community for years. Only recently have physicians begun to work closely with rehabilitation specialists so that the overall outcome of a person's trauma is that the individual is able to maintain dignity and continue as a productive member of society. It is the interaction of various experts who contribute to this ultimate outcome that enables individuals to successfully go on with their lives after coping with an unexpected injury.

Rehabilitation services are an integral part of the overall care provided to an injured worker. *The goal of a rehabilitation specialist is to coordinate services so that an injured individual can gain maximum improvement within the limits of the physical impairment.* Rehabilitation specialists are case coordinators, highly trained professionals who can facilitate action among various experts. They are specially trained nurses and Masters-level counselors who establish ongoing, trusting relationships with clients. They are in the unique position to act as a liaison between the injured party, the employer, the attending physician, the insurance company, the attorney, and other involved parties. In fact, from a rehabilitation perspective, all the people who provide services to the injured worker create a team that can, by working together, provide the client with the greatest chances for future success. Additionally, rehabilitation specialists can offer a positive focus for a client who may feel fragmented by the many different people involved and services being offered for his care.

This chapter focuses on the role of the rehabilitation specialist, how it is integrated with the roles of the various other professionals who work with the injured worker, and how the specific expertise provided by the rehabilitation specialist enables the client to progress and eventually resume productivity.

RAPPORT WITH CLIENT

The key to successful rehabilitation is the development of a positive, working relationship with the client. Therefore, the rehabilitation specialist must be a highly skilled professional who has developed interviewing techniques that promote a climate of trust. Only the establishment of this positive rapport makes possible any hope of successful rehabilitation. The dialogue between the client and the rehabilitation specialist and their joint efforts to develop realistic goals are critical to the ultimate outcome.

REFERRAL FOR REHABILITATION SERVICES

Generally the rehabilitation specialist becomes involved with an industrially injured individual when the insurance company from whom the injured worker receives compensation benefits requests rehabilitation services. In some cases the insurance company makes the referral because state laws mandate rehabilitation services. Even without state mandates, many insurance carriers are aware that the involvement of rehabilitation services decreases the overall exposure of the case, resulting in lower overall costs. Therefore, they refer cases for rehabilitation services.

Physicians request rehabilitation services so that the rehabilitation specialist can free them from the pressures of dealing with the psychological and vocational aspects of the case, thereby enabling them to concentrate on medical issues.

UNDERSTANDING THE IMPACT OF DISABILITY

Sometimes a referral for rehabilitation is made within days of the accident. Other times, it can be months or even years after the injury before a rehabilitation specialist becomes involved. At the initial client visit, the rehabilitation specialist is unaware of exactly how the client is coping with the situation. The client must cope not only with physical pain and/or limitations but also with a new self-image based on the disability and its influence on overall functioning. A client progresses through five stages of acceptance similar to those described by Kubler-Ross in her book, *On Death and Dying.*[2]

1. Initially injured individuals focus primarily on coping with a myriad of medical problems. It is unlikely that they think beyond the acute phase of their recovery. Most often they follow carefully and closely their doctor's instructions, paying little attention to the long-range impact of their situation. They dwell heavily on specific symptoms.
2. As they begin to heal, clients have more time to reflect, making them increasingly aware of the long-term effects of their injury. Some grossly deny

their situation, unable to face future lifestyle changes. Others become enraged. (In both cases the rehabilitation specialist must be sensitive to the clients' feelings. Professional support and encouragement are crucial.)
3. Becoming discouraged, clients constantly stress what they *cannot* do. (The rehabilitation specialist identifies with them their remaining capabilities so that they can build on them.)
4. As clients come to grips with their new selves (accept their disability), they must "mourn" the loss of their former bodily function. During this time they readjust to a new body image, a different pace of life, and/or alternate activities.
5. Once clients have begun to accept their situation, rapid progress—physically, psychologically, and vocationally—can occur as they mobilize and develop a new lifestyle within the limitations imposed by their impairment.

At any point clients can become "stuck" by disappointment, anger, and fear that can prevent medical progress. The impact of the injury can be altered with the consistent professional counseling and coordination provided by a rehabilitation specialist.

ATTORNEY REPRESENTATION

Injured workers retain legal representation to understand better what their benefits are and to ensure that they receive all the services to which they are entitled. They often retain attorneys when they are angry and do not feel that they have an advocate to whom they can express their angry feelings. Early referral to rehabilitation professionals can often eliminate the need for lengthy and costly legal involvement. If an attorney has already been retained when a rehabilitation referral is made, the lawyer is contacted and informed of the request for services by the rehabilitation specialist.

A rehabilitation specialist focuses primarily on a client's capabilities. While developing a rehabilitation plan with injured individuals, the rehabilitation specialist encourages them to utilize their remaining abilities so that they can ultimately become productive in a timely manner. Identifying viable, realistic vocational options is an integral part of a rehabilitation specialist's role.

The attorney, on the other hand, is interested in acquiring a financial settlement for the client, which is usually based on a documented loss of function and an inability to provide for one's family. The attorney must be able to document and demonstrate those activities that the client can no longer perform so that the client receives the largest cash settlement possible for the injury. Therefore, some attorneys consider the rehabilitation process to be a deterrent to the ultimate financial settlement made on behalf of the injured worker. In an attempt to protect their client, these attorneys object to the rehabilitation specialist's involvement.

An attorney's involvement can increase the burden on the medical providers. In an effort to document "disability," some attorneys advise their clients to continue with medical treatment and therapies, even after they may no longer be warranted. Physicians are then put into the uncomfortable position of hearing patients say that their attorneys have advised them *not* to return to work, even when there are no medical contraindications to this activity.

The workers' compensation boards in many states are no longer receptive to settlement agreements made without the injured party having a concrete vocational goal. They recognize that the lump sum settlement obtained by the injured worker may not be sufficient to pay ongoing expenses and that, without a viable employment plan, these cash settlements are not, by themselves, solutions for the disabled individual. With regulations from state departments administering industrial accident claims, attorneys are increasingly allowing their clients to avail themselves of rehabilitation services. It is in the client's best interest for rehabilitation specialists and attorneys to communicate openly about client goals. If attorneys understand how rehabilitation can be effective in offering their clients realistic, viable, and practical options for future consideration, usually they will allow the use of rehabilitation services.

If the attorney requests it, the rehabilitation specialist will conduct the initial client meeting in his/her office. The rehabilitation goal remains to evaluate current functioning and future planning. However, the joint meeting also provides each party the opportunity to explain his/her point of view, and agreements can be reached about specific legal and rehabilitation goals. Meeting together with the attorney can decrease clients' apprehension about receiving conflicting advice from two different professionals involved in their overall care.

In summary, regardless of eventual claims issues that must be settled between the insurance company and the attorney on behalf of the injured worker, everyone should be in agreement that ultimately it is in the client's best interest to resume a productive, active lifestyle. It is toward this end that the rehabilitation specialist strives.

INITIAL EVALUATION

Initially, the rehabilitation specialist meets separately with the client, employer, and physician to obtain a comprehensive understanding of the particular injured worker's situation and to identify any obstacles that might impede the client's ultimate recovery and ability to return to work. The initial goal of the rehabilitation evaluation process is to assess (1) the client's current level of functioning, (2) how it has changed as a result of the accident, (3) what medical treatment is being given, and (4) how the injury affects the client's ability to perform the job.

During the first client interview the rehabilitation specialist begins to create an atmosphere of trust by listening carefully to the injured worker's concerns, making note of any perceived problems, and discussing how the injury has affected the client's overall functioning and lifestyle. Regardless of the clinical factors, it is the client's understanding and feelings about the injury that become the key to the development of a successful rehabilitation program. The rehabilitation specialist *must start where the client is* and use the relationship to help the client develop a new self-concept before he or she can begin to think about successful vocational planning, as in the following case example.

> Mr. F is a 44-year-old laborer. He worked vigorously and steadily, except for layoffs in the winter when inclement weather prohibited working outside. One day, while digging in a trench, another laborer's shovel severed the fifth digit on Mr. F's left hand. Subsequently Mr. F had surgery in which the tip of his finger was removed. At 8 months postinjury, rehabilitation services were requested. By that time Mr. F perceived himself as totally disabled and unable to resume work. He complained of intense pain, said he had gone to several doctors, and claimed nothing could be done. He felt very limited in what he could do and where he could go. He thought his finger was "in his way" and that it prevented him from using his entire hand.

He spent most of his time at home watching television.

Mr. F's self-perception was that his pain made him totally disabled and unable to resume a productive lifestyle. This self-concept greatly limited his activities of daily living. Despite a physician's reassurance that he could work and his employer's willingness to re-employ him, Mr. F *felt* disabled. The challenge for the rehabilitation specialist was to listen to Mr. F such that he felt sufficiently heard to be able to trust and then move on with his life. The rehabilitation specialist took Mr. F to a physician, who in fact discovered a neuroma and surgically repaired it. Even after the pain decreased, Mr. F, whose cultural background taught him that any imperfection meant he was "useless," was not receptive to returning to work. Mr. F needed the opportunity not only to be heard but to have his point of view validated. Slowly, with rehabilitation counseling, he began to recognize that even though he had lost the tip of one finger, he had remaining abilities that could be used constructively.

Once the rehabilitation specialist has an opportunity to hear the client's point of view, it is critical to discuss the client's situation with the employer and the physician. Initially a job analysis is performed of the job that the client did at the time of injury. It includes information about special training and tools used on the job and an evaluation of the exact physical demands of the job, such as how much climbing, stooping, pushing, pulling, bending, walking, standing, and lifting are required and the frequency of each activity. During the visit to the employer, the rehabilitation specialist also learns about other, less physically demanding jobs that might be available and about the possibility of modifying the client's current job.

The last step in the initial evaluation process is the meeting with the physician, in which the rehabilitation specialist has an opportunity to discuss treatment modalities, prognosis, and most importantly, the client's physical capacities. Obtaining the results of a physical (functional) capacities evaluation is critically important to the development of a viable vocational plan for the client. The face-to-face meeting enables the rehabilitation specialist to establish a rapport with the physician and to obtain the doctor's recommendations regarding a return to work based on a job analysis of the specific physical demands of the position.

At this point the rehabilitation specialist has already had contact with all the key players in the client's life pertaining to the industrial accident. The foundation for the subsequent work of coordinating programs and being a liaison among all involved parties is thus laid.

HINDERING FACTORS

The rehabilitation specialist is particularly skilled in identifying hindering factors, deterrents preventing a client from resuming a productive lifestyle. Most of these factors are secondary to the injury. Some examples of deterrents are described in the cases below.

1. Because of his injury, Mr. C. cannot look forward to earning what he formerly earned and therefore becomes resistant to engaging in any kind of work. The rehabilitation specialist works sensitively with him to assist him in recognizing his *current* level of functioning so that he can utilize his existing abilities. Entering any new field requires starting at or near the bottom, and once the client recognizes that there is potential for growth, this barrier is often resolved. Furthermore, in many states, workers' compensation benefits provide a wage incentive; that is, they supple-

ment an income that is lower than the preinjury wage so long as the lower wage is due to the residual disability. Once an injured person understands this fact, he may become more receptive to starting work at a lower salary.

2. Mr. R's self-image is at risk. He was raised to feel that his manliness is directly related to his ability to perform strenuous physical responsibilities at work. Since he can no longer perform these physical requirements, his very core feels threatened. The rehabilitation specialist explores other ways in which Mr. R can maintain his sense of self while accepting both a new self-image and a less physically stressful job.

3. Mr. T's wife took a job to supplement the now lower family income while her husband has been receiving workers' compensation benefits. As a result, the injured worker has become the primary caregiver for the T's two preschool-aged children. He cannot return to work unless adequate child care is arranged. The rehabilitation specialist works with existing community resources to find appropriate child care so that Mr. T can return to work.

4. There is no objective evidence for persistent pain and disability, yet Mrs. Y complains of constant, debilitating pain. Physicians have stopped listening to her because of her relentless whining and her apparent inability to hear that there is nothing more than can be done medically to improve her situation. She is frustrated and angry at the entire system. The rehabilitation specialist, who is a skilled listener, provides Mrs. Y with the opportunity to vent and be understood fully. The specialist also identifies whatever activities Mrs. Y is already doing so that they can be increased at regular intervals, thereby preparing her for increased productivity. A home activity chart is developed that notes increased demands on a daily or weekly basis, thereby allowing Mrs. Y to begin to recognize what she *can* do in preparation for a more structured lifestyle that will ultimately include work. The criti-

cal issue with individuals such as Mrs. Y is to acknowledge their personal frustration regarding their functional losses while concurrently reinforcing their strengths.

5. Mr. N's attorney advised him not to return to work until he has obtained a financial settlement from the insurance company. Yet, Mr. N has been meeting with his rehabilitation specialist regularly to develop a future vocational plan. Consequently, Mr. N becomes confused about whether he should continue to remain as involved with his rehabilitation specialist.

Rehabilitation efforts focus on working with the physician to identify Mr. N's capabilities and develop viable future vocational options. Claims issues are left for the attorney and the insurance company to resolve. The rehabilitation specialist explains to Mr. N and his attorney that, no matter what the lump sum settlement may eventually be, Mr. N is entitled to develop a safe plan for his ultimate return to work with a rehabilitation professional who takes into consideration his physical capabilities, physician recommendations, employer's attitude, and a variety of other aspects that will contribute to his ultimate success.

6. Mr. A is worried that there are no longer jobs that he can perform. His employer insists that no light duty jobs are available and that job modification is not a viable option. The rehabilitation specialist works closely with Mr. A's employer, conducting job analyses of various jobs in the plant and showing the employer the physical capacities evaluation (provided by the physician) so that together they can determine if there are, in fact, any realistic opportunities for Mr. A. If no possibilities exist with the former employer, the rehabilitation specialist will then explore alternate fields based on transferable skills and the information from the physical capacities evaluation. If it is ultimately determined that Mr. A has no existing marketable transferable skills, then appro-

priate, short-term retraining is considered. *What initially seemed hopeless to Mr. A becomes an organized, step-by-step progression to appropriate employment.*

The critical tasks of the rehabilitation specialist are the identification and, subsequently, the resolution of each hindering factor as it arises. Every client has a particular set of needs and in an attempt to meet these needs can, without even being aware of it, create hindering factors that seem appropriate for dealing with the situation. These seemingly immobile hindering factors cause considerable frustration for physicians who are treating injured workers. When physicians collaborate with rehabilitation specialists, they can reduce their sense of helplessness with these difficult patients. The rehabilitation specialist identifies barriers that inhibit progress and works with the client, other involved parties, and community resources to resolve them, thereby freeing the physician to deal more directly with medical issues, as in the following case example:

Mr. G worked in a tool manufacturing company. While demonstrating a machine to some new employees he badly damaged his dominant, right hand. All fingers were partially amputated, and his hand function was impaired severely. At their first encounter, he greeted the rehabilitation specialist at the door by saying, "I work to earn money; I live to play clarinet." The rehabilitation specialist, listening carefully to what Mr. G was saying, appreciated that, regardless of the medical outcome and his potential to return to work, his personal need to play his clarinet was going to become a dominant factor in his overall recovery. His self-image as a musician and his desire and need to continue to pursue his music, even though it did not provide him with a livelihood, were critical to his entire healing process. Therefore, while Mr. G continued receiving medical care, the rehabilitation specialist and he worked together to determine ways he could resume his music. Initially Mr. G thought he could have his hand reconstructed, but with time he became aware, with the assistance of rehabilitation counseling, that a reconstructed hand would not provide the function necessary to play his instrument. Having accepted this reality, the rehabilitation specialist and Mr. G then worked together to have his clarinet rebuilt so that the keys would fit the remaining stubs on his hand. Engaging Mr. G in this process gave him the hope he needed to cooperate fully with all aspects of his medical care. In fact, he worked diligently with physicians and therapists and did not burden them with his preoccupying concern about his clarinet playing. While meeting with his rehabilitation specialist, he clearly had the feeling that what was *really* important in his life was being addressed. Indeed, the day Mr. G picked up his reconstructed clarinet, he returned to a modified job at work. Mr. G was thus involved in the entire rehabilitation process, and, most importantly, attention was given to his entire self-image, which, in the last analysis, is what assists human beings in overcoming the crises they face in life.

The rehabilitation process addresses more than just the physical recovery of clients. As in the case of Mr. G above, sometimes clients' self-image is challenged. Sometimes, their fears take over, making it difficult for them to go on with their lives. Sometimes, clients develop a chronic disability syndrome that increases their dependence on the workers' compensation system. Unique to the workers' compensation system is that recipient receive both a wage reimbursement and medical care as part of their benefit package. Therefore, it is the injury itself that provides their livelihood while they are receiving benefits. *Reaching maximum medical improvement without having a clear idea of a vocational direction can be terrifying.* The injured worker becomes afraid of being cut off from insurance benefits while lacking skills for gainful employment.

For example, a young man needs his hands to operate a tool manufacturing machine. As the result of an accident, three of his fingers have been amputated, making it impossible for him to manipulate the levers on the machine. He has never done any other work, is not a high school graduate, and has few transferable skills. In his mind, he *must* stay disabled in order to receive his wage reimbursement. Unless vocational counseling is provided concurrent with his medical treatment, he unconsciously resists improving. His fear of reaching a medical maximum improvement and having no job overwhelm him, and consequently he becomes dependent on the system. The same person, however, can move on with his life if he has early rehabilitation intervention. The rehabilitation specialist has the ability to evaluate his transferable skills and recommend job areas that are appropriate given his potential limitations, so that this person does not feel hopeless about his vocational future. Individuals who have the benefit of these services seem to be able to move on with their lives more smoothly.

The overall goal is to enable clients to assume primary responsibility for their own recovery and to gain a personal desire to resume an active lifestyle. It is the rehabilitation specialist's task to create incentives to encourage clients to achieve these goals.

TEAM APPROACH

The rehabilitation specialist is committed to developing relationships not only with the client but also with the attorney, employer, physician, and all other interested parties so that the client can be ensured the best possible services available and so that each party can participate in the eventual success of the injured worker's recovery process.

Physician Cooperation

Injured individuals, by the very nature of being injured, develop a dependent relationship with their treating physician. They rely on the doctor to advise them on all aspects of their recovery and to treat them responsibly so that they can resume a normal lifestyle once they are healed.

Physicians, by the very nature of their training, are best suited to resolve the medical issues at hand. Their busy schedules do not always allow them the luxury of listening to all the other nonmedical factors that affect the client's progress.

Rehabilitation specialists, by their training, are required to look at a variety of life issues that affect individuals and that ultimately become the basis for their decisions. These issues often interfere with the client's overall progress. Therefore, an injured individual can have a surgical success and remain unable to resume a productive lifestyle.

As soon as the client is seen by a rehabilitation specialist, the specialist initiates contact with the physician. It is the partnership between the physician and rehabilitation specialist that holds the greatest promise for a successful outcome. The rehabilitation specialist, in the unique position of being in regular communication with all parties involved with the injured worker's recovery, has a broad perspective on the client's overall coping mechanisms, the attorney's input, the employer's willingness to modify a job, the outlook in the labor market for alternative employment, and many other factors that

could impinge on the client's potential for full recovery and return to productivity. Therefore, it is critical that the physician and the rehabilitation specialist work closely together so that the latter has a clear understanding of a patient's current and/or potential functional capacities. The success of a rehabilitation program is increased with clear knowledge of the client's functional capacities.

The physician has everything to gain from a cooperative relationship with the rehabilitation specialist. Together they can direct the case, developing trust with the client/patient. When rehabilitation specialists attend meetings between the doctor and patient, they can work together to prepare and encourage the injured individual for the current course of treatment and vocational plan. The rehabilitation specialist can continue to counsel the client after they leave the physician's office, thereby facilitating compliance with recommendations and enhancing patient/doctor trust. In short, the rehabilitation specialist actually extends the impact the physician has on his patient by reinforcing medical recommendations and encouraging timely follow-up.

Some physicians do not readily collaborate with the rehabilitation specialist. This lack of cooperation could be a result of their not understanding the role of the rehabilitation specialist, a lack of confidence to share control of the case, or a lack of interest in confronting the psychosocial forces that must be resolved. When these obstacles cannot be overcome, it might be in everyone's best interest to refer the patient to a physician who is prepared to deal with the psychosocial, legal, and economic issues and who is willing to work with the other professionals who are necessary to manage these problem clients.

Collaboration with Physicians and Therapists

The rehabilitation specialist works collaboratively with physicians, physical therapists, and occupational therapists in a variety of ways. Most importantly, the rehabilitation specialist obtains a physical capacities evaluation from the physician and/or therapist so that any vocational plan is well within the client's physical capabilities. The rehabilitation specialist can be helpful in ensuring that a patient complies with the instructions given by the physician and/or therapist. Often exercises must be done on a daily basis at home, and during the visits to the client's home, the rehabilitation specialist can evaluate compliance with the exercise regimen. A thorough job analysis presented to the physician and/or therapist enables them to have a more informed opinion about the prognosis for a return to that job or to render an opinion regarding what modifications are needed to ensure a safe return to work. Physicians and therapists can obtain a clearer understanding of the work demands and environment of a particular patient, making it easier to understand just what level of recovery must be attained before a patient can be released to work. Often, the physician, physical and/or occupational therapist, and the rehabilitation specialist work together to assist their patients in understanding their physical capacities so that they can feel more confident about a return to work.

Because the philosophical goals of the therapist and the rehabilitation specialist are similar—to provide injured workers with tools to maximize their potential—the collaboration of these two professionals is usually comfortable and supportive. The occupational/physical therapist is often the professional who meets most frequently with the individual who has an upper extremity injury. In casual discussion while developing and demonstrating appropriate exercises, the therapist often learns about other aspects of the individual's life and coping mechanisms. Close communication between the therapist and the rehabilitation specialist can lead to shared planning for resumed activity within a realistic time frame.

Employer Contact

Rehabilitation specialists have frequent interaction with employers. They conduct on-site visits with employers who have injured employees. They convey the client's progress based on physician input. They contact employers to explore viable options for injured workers who are seeking alternate employment. They discuss ways to modify jobs to suit the particular needs of a disabled individual based on medical input. This daily dialogue with the world of work provides the rehabilitation specialist with a unique perspective regarding job availability and opportunities in a specific geographical area. Employers usually welcome the rehabilitation specialist's input because they are committed to having a safe work place where the number of injuries is kept low and losses are reduced. Their collaboration with the rehabilitation specialist is part of a broader risk management program.

VOCATIONAL PLACEMENT

In addition to restoring good health, rehabilitation services are designed to restore the ability to work. Therefore, concurrent with medical management, rehabilitation services include vocational assessment and job placement. Early in the rehabilitation process a transferable skills analysis is conducted to determine abilities that an individual has acquired through training, education, and experience. These transferable skills are then matched with the client's physical capacities to determine actual job areas in which the client can work.

Return to Work

Same Job/Same Employer

The primary goal is to return a client to the same job and employer. Therefore, once an injured worker's physical capacities and transferable skills are well understood, the rehabilitation specialist meets with the employer to ascertain how the injured worker can be reintegrated into the work place. Understanding both the client's physical abilities and the physical demands of various jobs puts the rehabilitation specialist in a unique position of being able to match the injured worker with an appropriate job that will most likely ensure success at work. Only if the employer absolutely cannot accommodate the former employee is consideration given to outside employment.

Alternative Employment

Looking for a new job can be a discouraging task, even for someone who has the skills to do it. For injured workers who have lost some confidence in their ability to be gainfully employed and who must now, because of a disability, enter a new field, this task is even more formidable. The intervention of a rehabilitation specialist makes the task much more palatable. It is critical to assess carefully what a client's capabilities really are so that the injured worker does not develop unrealistic aspirations.

Sometimes the injured worker is resistant to any exploration of alternative employment. Despite the severity of the injury, a client may state that he *only* wants to resume his former occupation. "My fa-ther and grandfather were carpenters. I am, too. It is all I know and it is all I want to do for the rest of my life." When a rehabilitation specialist hears this statement from a man who has had a partial amputation of four digits on his dominant hand and may no longer be able to hold tools to do his work, the professional must think creatively of ways to assist him to maintain his dignity and optimism, and still have the tools to move ahead with his life. It would be counterproductive to eliminate the injured person's hope.

This vocational counseling process is reminiscent of the process that high school seniors go through when applying to college. A student might say, "I will only go to an Ivy League school." If he only applies to Ivy League schools he runs the risk of being rejected and having no school to attend when the fall approaches. College counselors wisely recommend that a student apply to whatever Ivy League schools he likes and, in addition, to a range of other schools, including "safety schools." Again, it would be counterproductive to eliminate hope.

Establishing job goals with a client follows much the same principle. The rehabilitation specialist can maintain the client's goal of returning to his carpenter's job. During the medical recovery period, other job areas are developed, some of which demand much less fine motor coordination. Then, once the injured worker reaches maximum medical improvement, he will have a choice of vocational options and can select the one(s) that is most appropriate to his physical capabilities. If he has sufficient dexterity to assume the carpenter's tasks, then he can return to his former employment. If, however, his physical capabilities are more limited, he will have appropriate options from which he can choose. This approach does not, then, unequivocally eliminate any possibilities, but it also does not leave to chance end point physical capabilities that might be highly unrealistic and might make the client feel even more discouraged and more defeated with the end result. The key is to maintain the client's interest and to continue an ongoing discussion of vocational issues and vocational goals throughout the recovery period so that the concept of alternate jobs or modified employment is not a novel one at the time a medical end result is achieved.

When considering alternate job areas, a labor market survey is conducted. Employers in the identified field are contacted to determine whether jobs are available, what they pay, and what they require in skills and physical demands. Careful records are kept of every contact, and the client is encouraged to participate in the process.

While the job exploration is in progress, the rehabilitation specialist assists the client in preparing a resume and a cover letter to accompany it. They work together on interviewing skills, how to explain the injury to prospective employers, and any other issues that contribute to the client's ability to gain employment.

After being out of work for any extended period of time, a person can become quite insecure about re-entering the labor market. Many clients harbor the impression that losing work because of a disability is a stigma that can be used against them. Therefore, the rehabilitation specialist gives whatever assistance is necessary to smooth this job seeking process, ultimately facilitating a successful job placement.

Once appropriate job areas are identified, a job search begins. During this phase, both the rehabilitation specialist and the client arrange actual job interviews. Frequently the rehabilitation specialist contacts prospective employers after the job interview. Talking with them about how the client has done gives the rehabilitation specialist the opportunity to assist the client to improve interview-

ing skills for subsequent interviews. The goal is to use each interviewing experience as a learning and growth experience for the client.

After a specific job is offered, a job analysis can be conducted and submitted to the attending physician. This analysis serves to verify that the intended job is within the limitations specified by the doctor. It also reassures the employer that the client can indeed perform the duties of the job. Additionally, it provides injured workers with the confidence that they are considering a job for which they are highly qualified.

Once a client begins to work, the rehabilitation specialist stays in close contact with both the client and the employer to ensure there are no major problems and to resolve immediately any concerns that might arise. The length of this involvement varies from 30 to 60 days depending on the issues in the case or specific state laws. These postplacement services are an integral part of the rehabilitation process because they provide support to both the new employer and employee as they adjust to each other. Misunderstandings can be resolved before they become major obstacles to successful continued employment.

Thus far, two approaches for placing a client in the job market have been presented. One is to explore the possibility for return to the former place of employment. The other is to do extensive job development in an effort to find a job using a client's transferable skills. There are times when neither of these lead to a job goal, and then retraining is considered.

VOCATIONAL TRAINING

There are two major types of vocational training: on-the-job training (OJT) and formal (school) training. The former is a commitment by an employer to teach an employee a skill as an apprentice. Typically the rehabilitation specialist creates an arrangement with the insurer whereby the client/employee receives partial payment from the new employer and partial payment through workers' compensation benefits while learning the new skills necessary for the job. Upon completion of an OJT, the client is trained specifically for the demands of that particular job. The benefit is that the employee/client feels confident about his/her skills, the employer has a new employee who already knows the requirements of the job and can be productive immediately, and the insurer is assured that in a specified time period this injured individual will be fully employed and therefore no longer receiving compensation benefits.

If more formal training is required, the rehabilitation specialist thoroughly investigates its appropriateness to ensure the client's marketability upon graduation. As with the exploration of job areas, a labor market survey is conducted to explore employment possibilities within a specific field given a certain amount of training and to establish the marketability of an individual who graduates from a specific training program. Only with documentation that a client would be highly marketable after a formal training program is a recommendation for such a program made. As the client nears the end of a training program, the rehabilitation specialist becomes increasingly involved with the injured worker to ensure prompt job placement after graduation. The job search efforts that ensue are quite like those described when conducting a job search using transferable skills without formal retraining.

CONCLUSION

Rehabilitation services are a necessary component in the overall successful recovery of an injured worker. Collaborat-

ing with insurance carriers, attorneys, physicians, occupational and physical therapists, employers, and other significant people in the injured worker's life, the rehabilitation specialist creates a team approach that allows each player to contribute his or her expertise fully while the client benefits in a systematic way. The ability of the rehabilitation specialist to take a complicated system that gives a myriad of advice to injured workers and to ensure that they obtain consistent, nonfragmented care that will ultimately allow them to progress gives cohesiveness to an otherwise overwhelming and confusing system. Rehabilitation intervention can free the physician to focus on medical issues. The collaborative efforts of the rehabilitation specialist and the physician contribute to a coordinated effort for the injured worker, increase trust, and ensure continuity of care outside the doctor's office.

In most cases, the injured worker initially only wants to heal and return to the lifestyle held before his injury. With the passage of time, disappointment, increased disillusionment, loss of function, and fear of the future ensue and the client's ultimate recovery becomes more doubtful. Therefore, early intervention by a rehabilitation specialist creates the environment in which injured individuals have the opportunity to maximize their potential by obtaining both timely and appropriate medical care and concrete, viable vocational options.

REFERENCES

1. Stein J, ed: Random House Dictionary of the English Language. Random House, New York, 1967
2. Kubler-Ross E: On Death and Dying. Macmillan Co, New York, 1969

SUGGESTED READINGS

Benner CL, Schilling AD, Klein L: Coordinated teamwork in California industrial rehabilitation. J Hand Surg 12A:936, 1987

Brena SF, Chapman SL: Pain and litigation, p. 832. In Wall PD, Melzak R (eds): Textbook of Pain, Churchill Livingstone, Edinburgh, 1984

Hadler NM: Illness in the workplace: the challenge of musculoskeletal symptoms. J Hand Surg 10A:451, 1985

Melzack R, Katz J, Jeans ME: The role of compensation in chronic pain: analysis using a new method of scoring the McGill Pain Questionnaire. Pain 23:101, 1985

Talso S, Hendler N, Brodie J: Effects of active and completed litigation on treatment results: workers' compensation patients compared with other litigation patients. J Occup Med 31:265, 1989

Welch EM: Workers' Compensation: Strategies for Lowering Costs and Reducing Workers' Suffering. LRP Publications, Fort Washington, PA, 1989

20

Impairment and Disability Evaluation

William H. Bowers, M.S., M.D.

As a physician, one might think that impairment rating should come easily—a natural consequence of the many evaluations and decisions that occur in the course of medical management. I have not found this to be true. At the end of care, many factors come to the fore that tend to cloud one's judgment. Contradictions, which are not often voiced, make this process difficult. For instance, the better a physician's result is judged, the smaller the impairment award to the injured. A skilled worker whose wages are good recovers nicely from a severe arm and wrist injury and is rated at a 20 percent permanent partial impairment only to find, to his dismay, that he cannot perform his previous work either to his or his employer's satisfaction. "If you can't do it at 100%, don't come back until you can" is often heard from employers who have "always treated me right before." The physician says, "But you're doing well; you're ready to go—I can't get you any better—here's your rating. They will settle with you."

Emotions run high in this process. Anger, frustration, and displaced guilt are focused on this event where the final cards are played and the cords of compensation are cut.

Physicians who rate impairment must consider the environment in which they function, the forces at play, the consequences of the event, and the misunderstandings that are possible. It is not uncommon for workers to begin to view compensation awards unrealistically—perhaps planning to buy a new car or house or to finance a new career—only to find the laws providing them with what they consider to be a token amount. Physicians have even been physically or legally threatened as a consequence of misunderstandings generated in the ratings process.

Following the process described below is helpful when preparing a permanent partial impairment rating. It begins after the injury has been treated and evaluated and the rehabilitation process completed.

1. Well in advance of the expected time of maximum medical benefit (MMB), arrange a meeting of the patient, therapist, rehabilitation counselor, employer representative, and family members to assess progress and to plan the work re-entry process.
2. Enlist vocational counselors, psychologists, and supporting individuals, to help with problems uncovered in the meeting.

3. Counsel patients about the laws and process of rating in the state in which you are providing the rating.
4. Evaluate and test the patient's physical capabilities and compare them with those of the previous job. Assess realistically return-to-work possibilities and discuss with the patient. Set goals.
5. Help select alternative job opportunities with rehabilitation and vocational specialists if return to the previous work is not possible. Review and approve new or different job placements. Do on-site visits as required.
6. Support the patient during the return to work. See frequently and assess the patient's progress.
7. Perform permanent partial impairment rating *only* when successful job re-entry is accomplished *or* the level of impairment is well understood and patient has participated in the other options available.
8. Explain again the laws governing the rating process and their purpose, as well as your part of the event.
9. Do the permanent partial impairment rating and discuss the results with the patient.

An impairment rating generated in this manner is the conclusion to a process in which the informed patient has participated actively. When such a process is followed, problems are less likely to occur.

WHEN AND WHY DO WE RATE IMPAIRMENT?

Individuals who have an injury that produces a derangement or loss of a body part, function, or system eventually reach a point in their care when the end result of the event can be assessed. The physician, the patient, a compensation car-rier, or others may then request that the degree of loss be assessed. The end point (or a prolonged plateau) may be fairly assumed by all to represent "permanency" and the degree of loss to be the individual's "impairment." As noted above, the assessment of permanent impairment is of extreme importance. It generally signifies the official end of medical care for the condition. The compensation carrier can begin to wind up its financial responsibility, which generally includes some form of a lump sum payment to the patient for the loss of health. For patients, T.S. Eliot's phrase, "to make an end is to make a beginning," was never more true. They must truly begin to live and work with the loss and consequences. To define the end point accurately and to render an accurate assessment of impairment often means as much to the parties involved as does the care itself.

DISTINCTION BETWEEN IMPAIRMENT (IMPAIRMENT RATINGS) AND DISABILITY (DISABILITY RATINGS)

Impairment is an alteration in an individual's health status. It usually is a loss of body parts, functions, or systems. An impairment rating can be considered an inventory of equipment missing and remaining after damage to the human machine. The assessment is made after optimum medical care has been rendered. It is a *patient-oriented* analysis of the anatomic, functional, and cosmetic effect of the loss and is the domain of the medical community.[1]

Disability implies that one is not able or has decreased ability to meet personal, social, or occupational demands or statutory or regulatory requirements. A disability rating is an estimation of the gap between what an individual can do and what he or she needs, wants, or is required to do. The rating of disability includes information on impairment, but is a nonmedical, administrative, *task-oriented* assessment of what an individual can or cannot do with the physical equipment remaining after impairment.

The term *handicapped* is defined under the provisions of "federal law" as an impairment that substantially limits one or more life activities, including work.

HISTORY OF IMPAIRMENT RATINGS

Impairment ratings, for compensation purposes, is a centuries-old process, perhaps dating to 2050 B.C. The law of Ur-Nammau, King of Ur in Sumaria, delineated compensation for fractures of the hand, foot, and nose.[2] Early laws of the Greeks, Romans, Arabs, and Chinese provided similar recompense for loss. For example, under early Arab law, a joint of the thumb or great toe was worth half the value of a finger. Calculation for the loss of a penis was based on its length and an ear upon its surface area. In 1924 a standard permanent disability schedule was published by the U.S. Department of Labor. In 1936 Earl McBride[3] published his text, *Disability Evaluation and Treatment*, that established much of the basis for our current system. During World War II, Sterling Bunnel, emphasized the importance of separate anatomic and functional disabilities. In 1946 Donald Slocum presented his rating system based on the hands' functional components of hook, pinch, and grasp. The American Academy of Orthopaedic Surgery first presented an instructional course on Impairment Evaluation in 1949, and many

have been presented since. The American Medical Association (AMA) created a committee on medical rating of impairment and published the first AMA guide in 1958. This guide has been republished in 1971, 1984, 1988, and the upper extremity revision of the 1988 guide, upon which this chapter's recommendations are based, was published in early 1991.[1] In 1963, a committee of the American Society for Surgery of the Hand (ASSH), including Daniel Riorden, John Adams, and Alfred Swanson, presented a report to ASSH in a pamphlet that became the most valuable guide for use by hand professionals. Swanson's efforts to improve and standardize rating methods continued and resulted in acceptance of a system by the International Federation of Societies for Surgery of the Hand (IFFSH) in 1980. The Clinical Assessment Committee of the American Society for Surgery of the Hand began a review of methods for rating impairment in 1985. Their work has eventually collated with that of the IFSSH and AMA during the late 1980s.[4] The combined efforts of the IFSSH, ASSH and AMA are reflected in the revised upper extremity section of the AMA guide published in 1991.[1]

The effort for consensus has been commendable. The rewards will be forthcoming in improved care of the injured and impaired patient. I strongly recommend that these standards and methods come to be well understood, widely accepted, and applied.

WHO SHOULD RATE IMPAIRMENT OF THE UPPER EXTREMITY?

Physicians interested and experienced in treating impairments of the upper extremity should accept the responsibility for rating impairment for at least two good reasons. First, a knowledge of the natural history of the impairing event with or without intervention is essential to an accurate assessment of the reasonable end point of care (permanency). Second, although a rating is ideally objective and impartial, the end result is an arbitrary estimate representing the examining physician's own personal opinion. The best guide for this estimation has been constructed by a consensus of those experienced in hand and upper extremity disorders. It follows that these guides are likely to be best understood and applied by those who use the process daily in evaluating their own treatment. The guides provide a basis for uniformity of estimation, and experience provides the basis for accuracy. Significant aberrations in the final result can best be avoided if those requesting a permanent impairment rating insist the rating be done by hand professionals.

EQUIPMENT AND PERSONNEL REQUIRED FOR AN ACCURATE ASSESSMENT OF IMPAIRMENT

Physician Requirements

- a sound knowledge of normal functional anatomy
- a specialized knowledge of anatomic, cosmetic, and functional loss as it relates to the hand and upper extremity and its use in activities of daily living and work
- an ability to consider and analyze reports regarding the patient's psychological, sociologic, environmental, and economic status
- an ability to record and narrate data in a clear and understandable way

Data Records, Standard References, and Equipment

- *AMA Guides to the Evaluation of Permanent Impairment.* 3rd Ed. Rev., 1991
- a chart or record for the accumulation of data, such as that in the *Guides*
- references for evaluating norms of strength, sensation, etc.
- camera for recording the cosmetic effect and other hard-to-describe factors of impairment
- a small and large goniometer
- a device for testing two-point discrimination
- a dynamometer for recording grip
- a pinch meter
- a ruler
- familiar objects for tactile identification
- a computer and software for entering and collating data

Other Personnel

Because impairment evaluations are often data and labor intensive, a team approach is useful. Occupational or physical therapists who have acquired skills in hand therapy are both adept and concerned with the accuracy and professionalism required by an impairment rating. Psychologists and social workers are helpful in extensive evaluations. Although these nonphysician personnel are desirable, they should be under the direct supervision and in direct contact with the physician evaluator whose final opinion and presentation will go on record.

RATING OF IMPAIRMENT BY FUNCTIONAL TESTING—THE FUTURE

The best guides available are based on relative values, which are of historical legislative design. The award for amputation of an arm is greater than for a leg; a thumb is greater than for a finger. These are arbitrary values that serve to expedite legal requirements for lump sum settlements. They have no known scientific basis. Nevertheless, these relative values have become ingrained in and have even shaped our thinking to such an extent that they may appear reasonable, especially when modified in as sophisticated a fashion as the current AMA *Guides*. They provide us, at best, with an anatomic impairment index that may have only coincidental relationship to the effect of the impairment on the individual. An individual with an amputation of an arm is permanently impaired at a 60 percent level of the "whole man." There is no argument, however, that for bimanual tasks the impairment approaches 100 percent, whereas for certain tasks the impairment may be minimal.

Functional testing is a global assessment concept that ignores, to a larger degree, the specific loss. In theory, it provides an assessment of the individual's ability to function with the loss. This "ability index," in order to be meaningful, must be standardized, and the testing methods must be of sufficient variety as to represent the motor performance required in most vocational settings.

Ergonomic engineers have been evaluating motor performance in industrial settings for a number of years. Most tasks can be divided into performance characteristics that can eventually be tested and normed, including motion, timed motion, strength, endurance, reach, positioning, pinch versus power grip, applying pressure, etc.

Given time and effort, a battery of functional tests should be developed that would allow an impaired individual to be compared to performance norms. The ability index would then provide a true measure of the effect of the impairment on an individual. An obvious spin-off would be to provide a scientific basis for job alteration or modification that could maximize the usefulness of the impaired individual.

This is not a dream. The concept is in place in some hand practices today. For general acceptance and usage, the concept will require further research into methods and applications. The development of an ability index is a practical and attainable goal for physician scientists and may provide the desired interface with legal and industrial interests that has been so elusive.

RECOMMENDED METHODS OF EVALUATION

The most useful method for evaluating upper extremity impairment is detailed in the AMA *Guides*, specifically, the revision of Chapter 3 published in January, 1991.[1] The evaluation is based on a detailed examination of the patient to determine the anatomic aspects of impairment. Cosmetic evaluation assesses the reaction by the patient and society to the impairment and results of surgical treatment. It is, by definition, a subjective evaluation that may be included at the examiner's discretion. A method for cosmetic evaluation is found in another chapter of the *Guides*. Functional evaluation, although acknowledged as valuable, has not been sufficiently developed for current testing and is generally excluded, except for a highly restricted usage of strength testing. Pain is acknowledged in the derivation of ratings for amputation, sensory loss, deficits in range of motion, and peripheral nervous and vascular disorders and is not evaluated as a separate parameter.

Before the evaluation, the examiner should review Chapter 3 of the *Guides*[1] and be familiar with the elements of examination and methods of recording and calculation. The charts and tables are useful and may be reproduced without permission. The examiner should accumulate and evaluate historical records, laboratory tests, x-rays, and other data. A detailed history sheet should include vital statistics, details of the impairing event, subsequent therapy, and general historical facts that might bear on the event. Records of previous psychological testing should be noted, and a judgment made for the inclusion of additional testing coincident with the impairment evaluation. Photographic and roentgen evaluation should be included as well.

This chapter does not repeat the information provided in the AMA *Guides*. The *Guides* are comprehensive, complete, and as fair as a system based on the ancient system of relative values can be. They do, however, require close attention to detail and experience. The remainder of this chapter may be considered a guide to the *Guides*.

For any type of upper extremity loss, the basis for comparison is the effect of loss by amputation. The relative values for loss by amputation can be determined by consulting the AMA *Guides*; the loss at any level can be converted to a higher level by using tables in the *Guides*. For instance, the loss of a digit can be converted to its effect on the hand or, in turn, to the upper extremity and the whole man. At the whole man level, the impairment may be combined with other losses. These basic figures and tables are the benchmark of any impairment evaluation and should be reviewed until one is at ease with their principles.

Elements of loss that are included in the *Guides* and are rated by comparison to amputation loss values are

- sensation
- motion and ankylosis
- peripheral nervous system disorders

(considering pain, sensory and/or motor loss)
- entrapment neuropathy
- peripheral vascular disorders
- other disorders to include joint crepitation, swelling, digital lateral deviation, rotational deformity, joint subluxation, instability, and both implant and resection arthroplasty
- strength of grip and pinch

The examiner should accumulate the data for each category in which the patient's impairment could be considered.

Amputation

One should record the record level of amputation in each digit, hand, or arm, being as specific as the various charts allow.

Sensation

For each impaired digit or portion of the hand, one should record the sensory loss that is believed to contribute to the impairment. Such loss should be unequivocal and permanent. The sensory loss is evaluated by the two-point discrimination method and judged either total (greater than 15 mm), partial (7 to 15 mm), or normal (6 mm or less). The distribution of loss is characterized as transverse (both digital nerves) or longitudinal (one digital nerve). It is also estimated according to level as a percent of the digit. The ratings now give consideration for the relative importance of various sensory locales, i.e., outer borders of the digits are rated more highly.

Motion/Ankylosis

Motion is evaluated for each joint using the full range of active motion possible. If a joint cannot be moved by the patient or examiner, the position of ankylosis is recorded. The ranges are measured using the principle that neutral is the zero degree position. The charts in the *Guides* give weight to all normal motions, and the specific techniques of measurement are well described.

Evaluation of Peripheral Nervous System Disorders (Including Entrapment Neuropathy)

The peripheral nerve disorders may be rated only when static or well stabilized after management and rehabilitation. These disorders, in order to be rated using this section of the *Guides*, must be associated with a specific peripheral spinal root, trunk, or nerve. Evaluation assesses the loss of function due to sensory deficits or pain and motor deficits as evidenced by loss of power. The examination should thus include a specific sensory dermatomal distribution for the sensory deficit or pain and a manual muscle examination of all muscle groups supplied by the root, plexus, trunk, or nerve. It is important to note that loss of motion, ankylosis, or sensory disturbances attributed to the peripheral nerve disorder are weighted in the values for this section. These impairments should not be rated additionally using other portions of the *Guides*. Specifically, the examiner should not double rate the sensory loss using this and the sensory evaluation section. Entrapment neuropathies may be rated if they are irreversible and do not respond to treatment; a special table is used that excludes other methods of rating.

Impairment Due To Vascular Disorders

In these disorders, claudication, edema, loss of pulses, subcutaneous tissue disturbances, arterial calcifications, Raynaud's phenomenon, and ulcers are quantified according to frequency, degree, and control by medication and other physical measures. The values are classified according to severity and given proportional impairment values, which are then combined with amputation impairment values using the combined values chart.

Other Disorders

This section of the *Guides* gives examiners a way to rate specific impairments that in their opinion have not been rated adequately by the basic section of the *Guides*. It is the examiner's responsibility to avoid duplication of impairment values when these sections are used. For example, a physician might use this section to rate an individual who has normal range of motion but whose joints crepitate, are swollen, and demonstrate lateral deviation or malrotation or whose x-rays show evidence of carpal instability. This section also recognizes impairment due to resection or implant arthroplasty of each upper extremity joint. The principle employed is that any joint resected (40 percent impairment) or replaced (50 percent impairment) loses normal functioning attributes and should be considered impaired even though the surgical result might be considered good. The values derived from the arthroplasty table and the joint evaluation table are then combined with range of motion and other equivalent losses to derive an impairment value.

Strength

In general, strength deficits have been considered an integral part of the derivation of values for amputation, sensory loss, neural and vascular disorders, joint

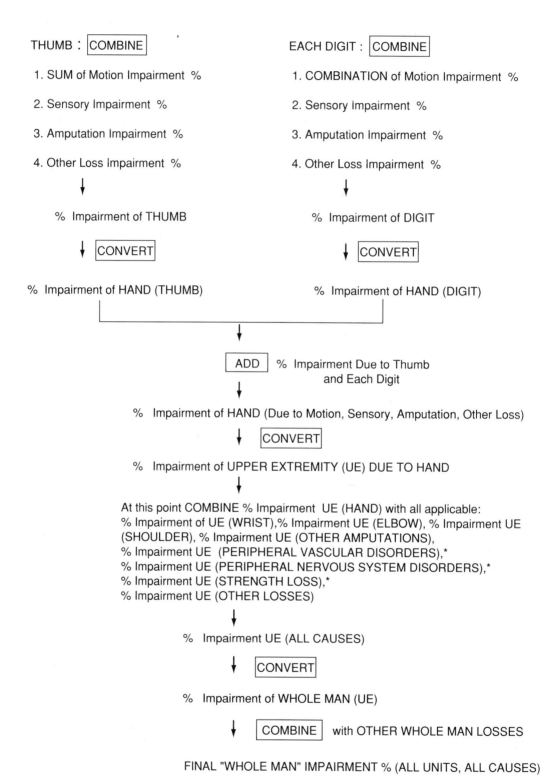

Fig. 20-1. Steps in the computation of impairment. Particular attention should be given to the use of addition, combination, and conversion. Combination and conversion tables are provided in the *Guides*.[1] Asterisks mean that special instructions are provided for integration of these values in the scheme.

dysfunction, etc. This last section provides a way to consider loss of strength if the examiner feels that it represents an additional factor that has not been not rated satisfactorily. The testing is recognized as a functional testing method and is affected by many factors, including patient cooperation. It therefore should be repeated at intervals. More than 20 percent variation is considered to represent less than full effort. The testing provides a value that is subtracted from the normal values given in the *Guides*. Division of this number by the normal gives a percentage strength index, which is then converted to the percentage impairment of the upper extremity.

COMPUTATION OF IMPAIRMENT

Three methods are used in computation: addition, combination, and conversion (Fig. 20-1).

Combination is used to derive a rating when multiple impairments act on a particular level. All impairment factors must be combined for each subunit before that subunit value is converted to a percentage of the unit as a whole. For example, a digit impaired by partial amputation, decreased range of motion, sensory impairment, and/or other disorder (e.g., joint replacement) has a value for each impairment that can be combined using a combined values table. The combined value is expressed as a percentage of 100 for that digit and is then converted to its value as a part of the next higher subunit (the hand) using the conversion tables. Multiple digital impairments converted to hand percentages are then added to give the total percentage of impairment

of the hand. The hand percentage impairment derived by addition of digital impairments is then converted to upper extremity percentages. At this level it may be combined with other losses as rated individually: loss of strength, other amputations; elbow, shoulder, and wrist range of motion deficits; peripheral neurologic or vascular disorders; other stand-alone disorders; and perhaps entrapment neuropathies. The combined upper extremity rating is then converted to a percentage of the whole man and at this level may be combined with deficits of other extremities or the trunk to give a final rating. See Figure 20-1 for the process of computing upper extremity impairment.

The rating should include adequate documentation. The entire record need not be submitted as a part of the rating, but it should remain in the patient's chart and be available if required. The appropriate rating may be then submitted to the workers' compensation or medical board and substantiated by physician testimony as required.

REFERENCES

1. Committee on Medical Rating of Physical Impairment: the extremities, spine and pelvis. In *Guides to the Evaluation of Permanent Impairment*. 3rd Ed. Rev. American Medical Association, Chicago, 1988
2. Kramer SN: History Begins at Sumer. Thames and Hudson, London, 1958
3. McBride ED: Disability Evaluation: Principles of. Treatment of Compensible Injuries. JB Lippincott, Philadelphia, 1963
4. Swanson AB, deGroot Swanson G, Blair SJ: Evaluation of impairment of hand and upper extremity function, p. 73. In Barr JS (ed): Instructional Course Lectures 38. American Academy of Orthopaedic Surgeons, Park Ridge, IL, 1989

Index

Page numbers followed by f *indicate figures; those followed by* t *indicate tables.*